Evidence Based Handbook on Diagnosis and Staging in Oncology

Satyajit Pradhan • Ashutosh Mukherji
Prashanth Giridhar
Editors

Evidence Based Handbook on Diagnosis and Staging in Oncology

Springer

Editors
Satyajit Pradhan
Department of Radiation Oncology
MPMMCC & HBCH, Varanasi, Units of
Tata Memorial Centre and affliated with
Homi Bhabha National Institute
Mumbai, India

Ashutosh Mukherji
Department of Radiation Oncology
MPMMCC & HBCH, Varanasi, Units of
Tata Memorial Centre and affliated with
Homi Bhabha National Institute
Mumbai, India

Prashanth Giridhar
Department of Radiation Oncology
MPMMCC & HBCH, Varanasi, Units of
Tata Memorial Centre and affliated with
Homi Bhabha National Institute
Mumbai, India

ISBN 978-981-95-9700-0 ISBN 978-981-95-9701-7 (eBook)
https://doi.org/10.1007/978-981-95-9701-7

This Springer imprint is published by the registered company Springer Nature Singapore Pte Ltd.
The registered company address is: 152 Beach Road, #21-01/04 Gateway East, Singapore 189721, Singapore

Foreword

The editors of *Evidence Based Handbook on Diagnosis and Staging in Oncology* need to be commended for compiling a succinct and informative book. The text integrates the radiological, pathological, and clinical aspects of evaluation of all malignancies. There is often doubt in the minds of clinicians both in tertiary oncology setting and primary healthcare setting regarding the right investigations to evaluate a suspected malignancy. This book effectively provides evidence-based information regarding various evaluation modalities to arrive at a diagnosis and also stage a tumor appropriately. I am confident that this book will help all clinicians immensely. The information in this book is presented in a logical and straightforward manner, thus offering an enjoyable learning experiencc. It is a privilege for me to write a foreword for this book. I am confident that many clinicians would significantly benefit from the information provided by the authors.

The field of oncology has witnessed remarkable advances in imaging, molecular diagnostics, and pathological techniques, substantially enhancing our ability to diagnose and manage cancer. At the same time, the expanding array of available investigations has made clinical decision-making increasingly complex. In the absence of clear guidance, this may result in inappropriate selection of tests, leading to over- or under-investigation, increased costs, and delays in initiating definitive treatment. There is therefore a pressing need for evidence-based resources that provide clarity and standardization in diagnostic and staging practices across cancer sites.

This book addresses this important gap by offering a systematic, site-wise and histology-wise approach to the investigations required for diagnosis, staging, prognostication, treatment planning, and follow-up of cancer patients. The recommendations are firmly grounded in evidence, with due emphasis on test performance parameters such as sensitivity, specificity, and predictive values, ensuring their relevance to everyday clinical practice. Designed for oncology residents as well as practicing faculty in surgical, medical, and radiation oncology, this work will serve as a valuable reference to support multidisciplinary decision-making and promote rational, timely, and patient-centered cancer care.

Director, Tata Memorial Centre, Mumbai, India Sudeep Gupta

Preface

With the advent of multiple new imaging modalities, molecular markers of cancer and onco-pathological testing, clinicians are often unsure of the ideal tests to be utilized to adequately diagnose and stage malignancies. Certain specific investigations are also necessary to prepare patients for treatment. Absence of clarity sometimes leads to under- or over-investigating and delays in starting treatment.

This book covers subsite-wise (histology-wise in some sections) ideal investigations to diagnose, stage, prognosticate, and predict outcome of treatments. The recommendations are evidence-based (based on sensitivity, specificity, negative predictive value, etc.) and provide healthcare providers concise information to share with colleagues and patients. Each chapter also includes a section dedicated to investigations necessary during follow-up of cancer patients after various forms of treatment.

The book is especially meant for Oncology residents (Surgical, Medical, and Radiation Oncology) and junior and senior faculty members to update their knowledge and apply it in the clinic.

Varanasi, Uttar Pradesh, India — Satyajit Pradhan
Varanasi, Uttar Pradesh, India — Ashutosh Mukherji
Varanasi, Uttar Pradesh, India — Prashanth Giridhar

Contents

Chapter 1
Presentation and Evaluation of Pediatric CNS Tumors

Ninad Patil, Zarmina Alam, and Shreya Shukla

1.1 Introduction and Epidemiology

Each year, over 4000 CNS (intracranial and spinal cord) tumors are diagnosed in children, with 5% occurring in the 0–14-year age group [1, 2]. Gliomas and embryonal tumors constitute most of the malignant pediatric CNS tumors [3] (Fig. 1.1).

N. Patil (✉) · Z. Alam
Department of Radiation Oncology, MPMMCC/HBCH Varanasi, Units of Tata Memorial Centre, and Homi Bhabha National Institute, Mumbai, India

S. Shukla
Department of Radio-diagnosis, MPMMCC/HBCH Varanasi, Units of Tata Memorial Centre, and Homi Bhabha National Institute, Mumbai, India

S. Pradhan et al. (eds.), *Evidence Based Handbook on Diagnosis and Staging in Oncology*, https://doi.org/10.1007/978-981-95-9701-7_1

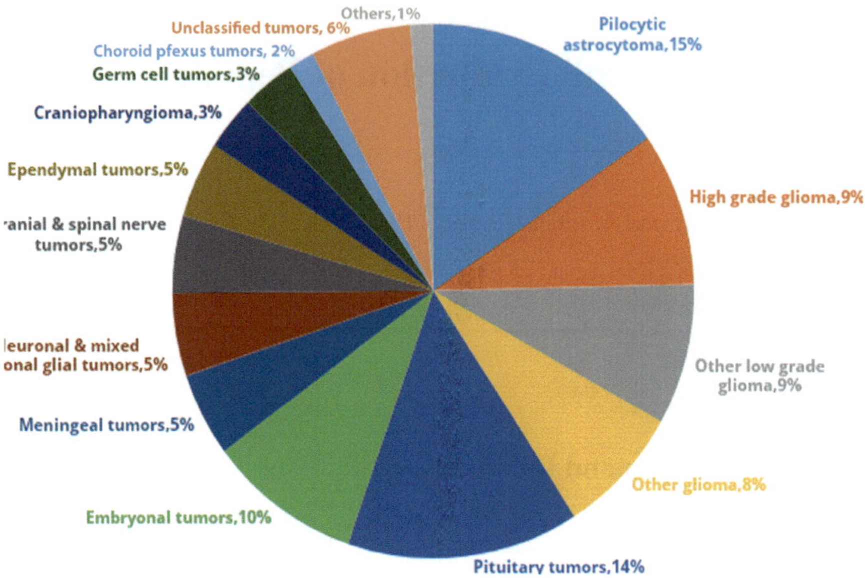

Fig. 1.1 Distribution of all primary CNS tumors in children and adolescents aged 0–19 years [3]

1.2 Risk Factors

The exact cause of most pediatric CNS tumors remains unknown, but certain genetic and environmental factors are associated with increased risk. Well-established risk factors include inherited cancer predisposition syndromes and exposure to ionizing radiation. Particularly, exposure to ionizing radiation has been most commonly linked to tumors like meningioma, glioma, and nerve sheath tumors, with the risk being notably higher in younger children [4]. Less than 5% of CNS tumors in the pediatric population are associated with a known genetic predisposition, and for most cases, no predisposing factors can be identified (Table 1.1) [5].

1.3 WHO 2021 Classification

In the WHO Classification of CNS tumors, the fifth edition (2021), the histologic and molecular features are integrated to distinguish between "pediatric-type" and "adult-type" tumor categories [16].

Pediatric-type diffuse low-grade gliomas have been sub-classified into

1. Diffuse astrocytoma, *MYB*- or *MYBL1*-altered
2. Angiocentric glioma
3. Polymorphous low-grade Neuro-epithelial tumor of the young
4. Diffuse low-grade glioma, MAPK pathway-altered

Table 1.1 Inherited syndromes associated with pediatric CNS tumors

Syndrome	Gene(s)	CNS tumor type(s)	Non-CNS tumors
Cowden syndrome [6]	PTEN	Dysplastic gangliocytoma of the cerebellum, meningiomas	Thyroid cancer, breast cancer, endometrial cancer
Hereditary retinoblastoma [7]	Rb	Pineoblastoma, glioma, meningioma	Retinoblastoma, osteosarcoma, malignant melanoma
Li-Fraumeni syndrome [8]	TP53	Gliomas, meningiomas, medulloblastomas, choroid plexus carcinoma	Sarcoma, adrenocortical tumor, acute leukemia, premenopausal breast cancer, broncho-alveolar cancer
Neurofibromatosis type 1 [9]	NF-1	Neurofibroma, optic nerve glioma, brainstem glioma	
Neurofibromatosis type 2 [9]	NF-2	Cranial and peripheral nerve schwannoma, meningioma, spinal ependymoma	
Gorlin's syndrome [10]	PTCH	Medulloblastoma, meningiomas	Basal cell carcinoma
Turcot syndrome [11, 12]	APC, hMLH1	Medulloblastoma, glioblastoma	Colorectal adenomas, colorectal adenocarcinoma
Tuberous sclerosis [13]	TSC1, TSC2	Sub-ependymal giant-cell astrocytoma	
von Hippel-Lindau syndrome [14]	VHL	Hemangioblastoma	
Rubenstein-Taybi syndrome [15]	CBP	Medulloblastoma, oligodendroglioma, meningioma	

Pediatric-type diffuse high-grade gliomas have been sub-classified into

1. Diffuse midline glioma H3 K27-altered
2. Diffuse hemispheric glioma, H3 G34-mutant
3. Diffuse pediatric-type high-grade glioma, H3-wild type and IDH-wild type
4. Infant-type hemispheric glioma

1.3.1 Embryonal Tumors

Medulloblastoma, a type of embryonal tumor, is the most common malignant brain tumor found in children [17]. In the recent WHO classification, medulloblastoma is sub-classified into four principal molecular groups (Table 1.2):

1. Medulloblastoma, molecularly defined
    - Medulloblastoma, WNT-activated
    - Medulloblastoma, SHH-activated and TP53-wildtype
    - Medulloblastoma, SHH-activated and TP53-mutant
    - Medulloblastoma, non-WNT/non-SHH

Table 1.2 Common types of pediatric CNS tumors based on location of tumor [29]

Supratentorial (25–40%)	Infra-tentorial (45–60%)
Low-grade glioma (10–20%)	*Medulloblastoma (20–30%)*
High-grade glioma (5–10%)	*Low-grade glioma (10–20%)*
Ependymoma (2–5%)	*Diffuse intrinsic pontine glioma (diffuse midline glioma) (5%)*
Ganglioglioma (1–5%)	*Ependymoma (5%)*
Oligodendroglioma (1–5%)	Others (5%)
Germ cell tumor (1%)	
Choroid plexus tumors (1%)	
Meningioma (1%)	
Others (5%)	

1.4 Clinical Presentation

The clinical presentation of pediatric CNS malignancies differs depending on tumor location, the patient's age at diagnosis, and sometimes the tumor type.

Common signs and symptoms include the following.

(a) Raised intracranial pressure:

Manifests as worsening headaches, early morning vomiting, a change in personality, cranial nerve VI palsy, papilledema, and macrocephaly in neonates. It may occur due to a tumor, brain edema, or obstructed cerebrospinal fluid (CSF) flow.

(b) Seizures

(c) Weakness in one side of the body (hemiparesis) or a single limb (mono-paresis)

(d) Cranial nerve deficits

(e) Ataxia

(f) Sensory loss

(g) Speech difficulties (dysphasia or aphasia)

(h) Memory problems

(i) Increasing head circumference (seen in neonates in whom fontanels are open)

(j) Loss of developmental milestones

(k) Personality changes and declining school performance

The signs and symptoms listed above also vary depending on the growth rate, with high-grade tumors typically causing more symptoms than lower-grade ones.

Features such as Diencephalic syndrome, macrocephaly, short stature, and disordered pubertal development are specific to pediatric CNS tumors and are not observed in adults (Tables 1.3 and 1.4).

Table 1.3 Signs and symptoms as per tumor location [29]

Cause/location	Symptoms
Cerebellar tumor	Unsteady gait, intention tremor, scanning speech, dysdiadochokinesis, nystagmus, ataxia
Brain stem tumor	Long tract signs, spastic palsies, horizontal ophthalmoplegia, cranial nerve palsies
Cerebellopontine tumor	Torticollis, facial paralysis, and hearing loss
Cerebral hemispheric tumor	Cerebral seizures, paresis/paralyses, sensory impairments
Suprasellar tumor/chiasma/ hypothalamus tumors	Vision loss, narrowing of the visual field, nystagmus
Tumor of the hypophyseal and hypothalamic region	Disordered pubertal development, eating disorders, short stature, diabetes insipidus
Diencephalic tumors	Diencephalic syndrome: Cachexia observed in infants who sometimes appear euphoric, normal intake
Pineal/midbrain tumor	Parinaud syndrome: Convergence retraction, upward gaze palsy, light-near dissociation, and bilateral lid retraction

Table 1.4 Differential diagnosis of the common presenting symptoms

1. Seizures	*Metabolic causes*: Inborn errors of metabolism, dyselectrolytemia, hypoglycemia *Infections*: Meningitis, encephalitis *Vascular*: Intracranial thrombosis, hemorrhage *SOLs*: Inflammatory granulomas (tuberculoma, neurocysticercosis) *Miscellaneous*: Febrile seizures, drug poisoning, epilepsy syndrome
2. Raised ICT	*Vascular*: Intracranial or intraventricular hemorrhage *Infections*: Brain abscess, encephalitis *Congenital*: Aqueduct stenosis, Dandy Walker syndrome [18], Arnold Chiari syndrome [19] *Miscellaneous*: Pseudotumor cerebri
3. Focal neurological deficit	*Vascular*: Intracranial hemorrhage (etiologies: Head trauma, AV malformation, aneurysm), thrombosis, or embolism (coagulopathy) *Infections*: Cerebral abscess, meningitis, encephalitis *Miscellaneous*: Moya Moya disease [20], transient cerebral arteriopathy
4. Developmental delays	*Chromosomal disorders*: Trisomy 21, 18 *Inborn errors of metabolism*: Tay Sachs disease, mucopolysaccharidosis *Infections*: Toxoplasmosis, CMV, meningitis *Miscellaneous*: Iodine deficiency

50% and more of all CNS tumors in children occur in the posterior cranial fossa or in the brainstem. A tumor in this region may obstruct CSF drainage, thereby increasing intracranial pressure.

In neonates and young infants, traditional signs of increased intracranial pressure might be missing. Instead, they could present with macrocephaly and failure to thrive.

1.5 Evaluation for a Pediatric CNS Tumor

1.5.1 Neuroimaging

Imaging plays a crucial role in evaluating patients with suspected or confirmed brain tumors, with magnetic resonance imaging (MRI) being the preferred method. Conventional MRI of the brain and/or spine, performed with and without gadolinium contrast, remains the gold standard for tumor diagnosis due to its superior soft tissue contrast and lack of ionizing radiation. Essential MRI sequences include pre- and post-contrast T1-weighted images, T2-weighted images, Fluid-Attenuated Inversion Recovery (FLAIR), and ideally a 3D sequence. Additional techniques such as diffusion-weighted imaging (DWI), MR perfusion, and MR spectroscopy can complement standard MRI to enhance diagnostic precision. MRI axial slices should typically have a thickness of 3–4 mm.

Identifying whether a lesion is intra-axial or extra-axial is essential for diagnosis. An extra-axial lesion typically exhibits these characteristics (Table 1.5):

- Displaced and expanded subarachnoid space
- Displaced sub-arachnoid vessels
- CSF cleft sign
- Bony reaction
- Cortical gray matter between mass and white matter
- Dural tail

1.6 Magnetic Resonance Spectroscopy (MRS)

Magnetic resonance spectroscopy (MRS) is a non-invasive method that measures metabolites in brain tissue. In glial tumors, MRS usually shows increased choline, decreased or nearly absent N-acetyl aspartate (NAA), and lower total creatine levels [21]. It can be a valuable tool for tumor grading and the selection of biopsy sites (Fig. 1.2).

1.7 Diffusion-Weighted Imaging (DWI)

MR diffusion imaging tracks the movement of water molecules, known as Brownian motion, within the brain. From these images, an apparent diffusion coefficient (ADC) map is derived. Malignant lesions restrict water molecule movement, resulting in low intensity on the ADC map. This imaging technique effectively characterizes tissue, evaluates tumor cellularity, grades tumors, and differentiates between various tissue types [22–24].

Table 1.5 Imaging features of pediatric CNS tumors

Supratentorial (25–40%)	
1. Low-grade glioma (e.g., oligodendroglioma grade 2) T1: hypointense T2: hyperintense Contrast: minimal enhancement No necrosis No intra-tumoral bleed	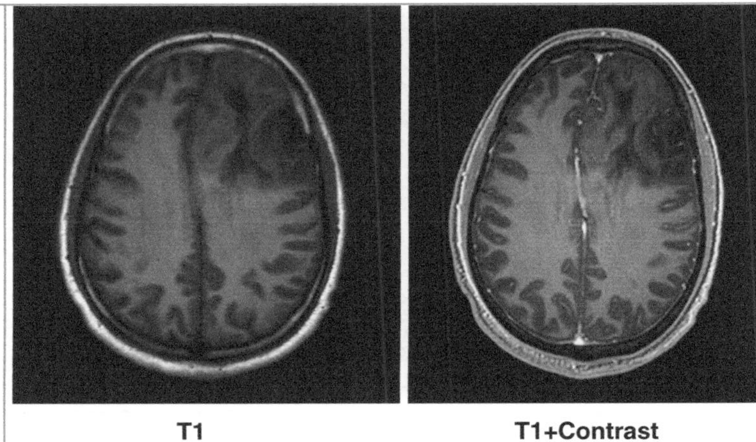

(continued)

Table 1.5 (continued)

2. *High-grade glioma* Intra-axial mass in subcortical white matter T1: isointense T2: heterogeneously hyperintense showing a few hemorrhagic signals Contrast: patchy peripheral enhancement Mass effect in the form of midline shift	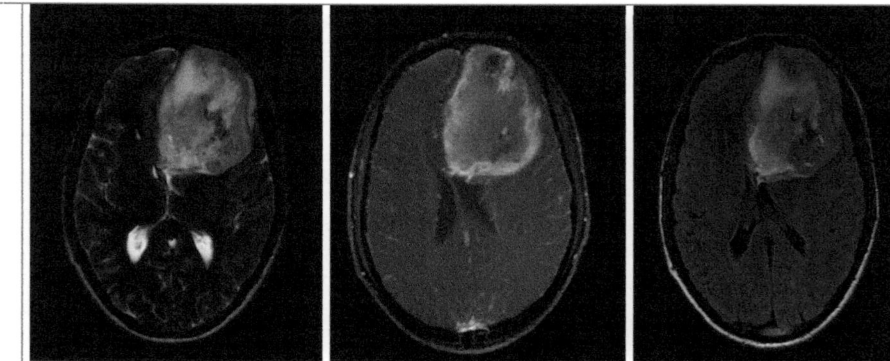
3. *Ependymoma* Intraventricular mass T1: heterogeneously isointense T2: hyperintense Contrast: intense heterogeneous enhancement Calcific focus Cystic spaces	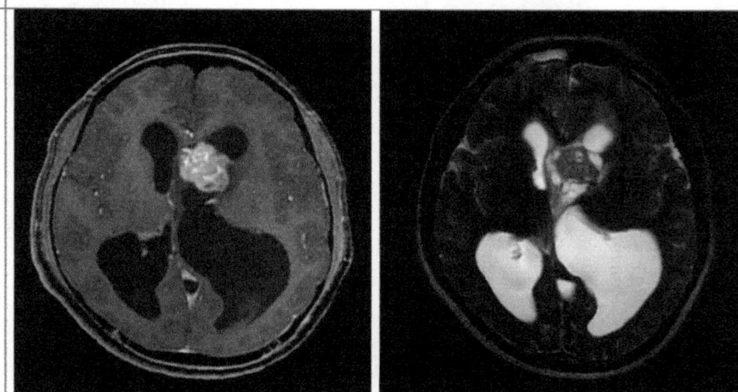

4. Ganglioglioma Location: in the supratentorial temporal lobe Circumscribed cyst with mural nodule T1: contrast enhancement is variable T2: hyperintense solid component	
5. Oligodendroglioma Location: in the supratentorial; frontal lobe T1: variable enhancement T2: typically hyperintense Calcification is seen as an area of blooming	
6. Germ cell tumor T1: homogenous contrast uptake in the pineal or hypophysis region Do not show T2 hyperintensity in the posterior lobe of the hypophysis	
7. Meningioma Extra-axial, intracranial lesion Dural based T1: Isointense T2: Intermediate Contrast: homogeneous enhancement	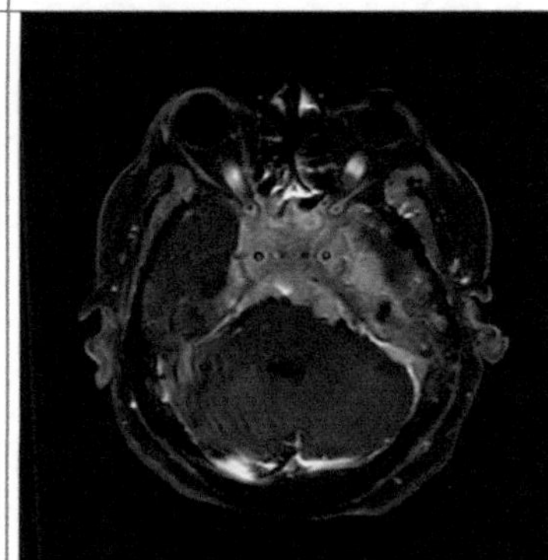 T1+Contrast

(continued)

Table 1.5 (continued)

Infra-tentorial (45–60%)	
A. Medulloblastoma Posterior cranial fossa lesion in the region of the fourth ventricle T1: hypointense T2: hyperintense Contrast: mild heterogeneous enhancement Cystic areas Necrosis	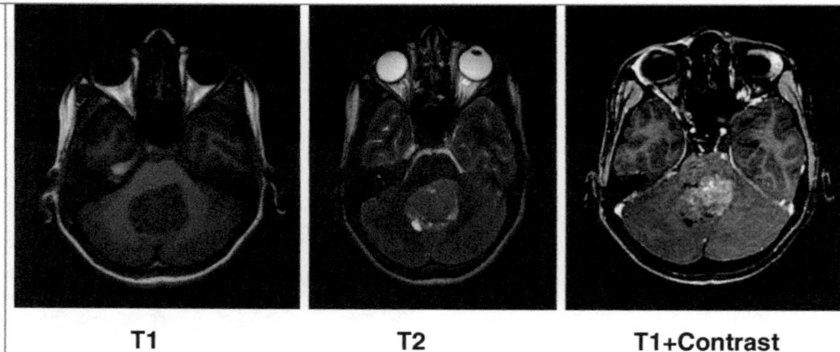
B. Low-grade glioma	
C. Diffuse intrinsic pontine glioma (diffuse midline glioma) Expansile lesion involving the brainstem, extending into the right cerebral peduncle T2: intermediate with multiple interspersed hyperintense areas Contrast: patchy peripheral enhancement Obstructive hydrocephalus	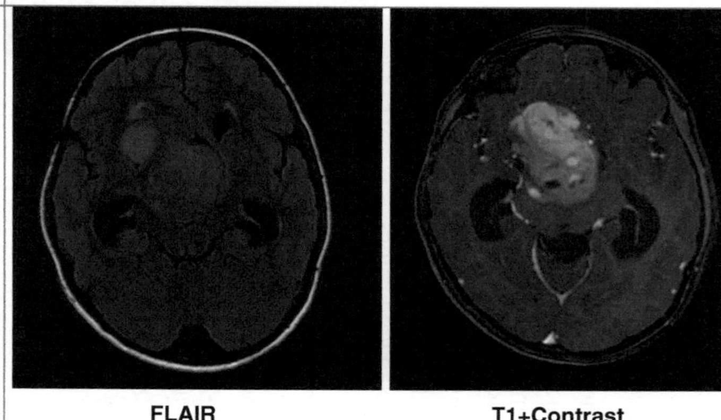

D. Ependymoma Irregular, lobulated mass arising from the fourth ventricle Internal cystic/necrotic component Obstructive hydrocephalus T1: isointense T2: hyperintense Contrast: heterogeneous enhancement	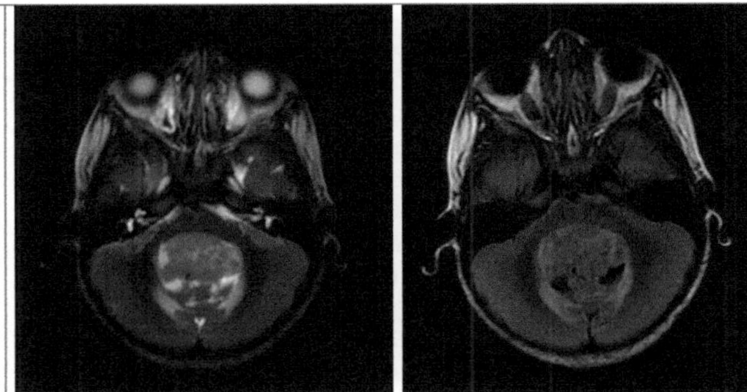 T2 FLAIR

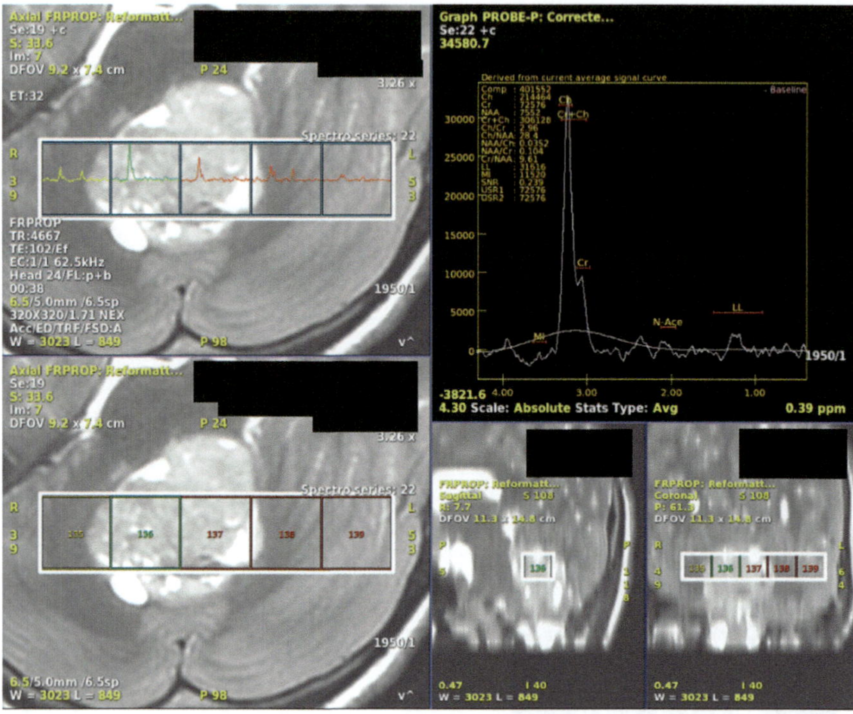

Fig. 1.2 MRS showing Cho peak with fall in NAA, with Cho:Cr ratio of 2.96 in a case of medulloblastoma

1.8 Magnetic Resonance Perfusion Imaging

Perfusion imaging evaluates cerebral perfusion dynamics by analyzing relative cerebral blood volume (rCBV), relative cerebral blood flow, and mean transit time. Research shows a positive correlation between rCBV and tumor grade [25]. This technique is valuable for targeting lesions for biopsy, grading tumors, evaluating response, and identifying malignant degeneration and pseudoprogression (Fig. 1.3).

1.8.1 CT Scan (With or Without Contrast)

A head CT scan is often the first imaging choice. It helps identify acute intracranial hemorrhage, ventriculomegaly, calcifications, and shunt complications. However, for suspected space-occupying lesions in the brain, MRI is generally preferred, except when MRI is not an option.

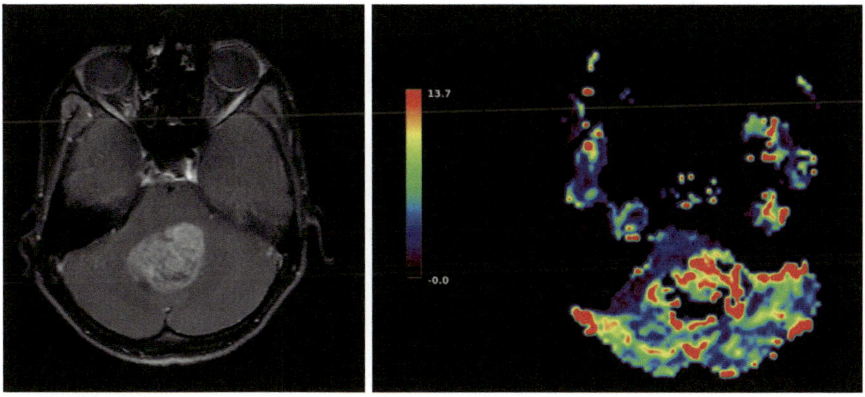

Fig. 1.3 MR perfusion showing mild diffuse hyperperfusion with rCBV ratio of 1.72 in a case of medulloblastoma

Benefits of a CT scan include shorter acquisition time and suitability for acutely emergent or immediate post-operative settings. However, CT scans have limited soft tissue contrast, and metal causes streak artefacts that limit evaluation.

1.9 Positron Emission Tomography (PET)

Positron emission tomography (PET) can act as an imaging biomarker for assessing tissue metabolic activity. The most common radiotracer used is fluorodeoxyglucose (FDG), although healthy brain tissue also shows high metabolic activity. New radiotracers being developed for brain tumor evaluation include fluorothymidine, fluoro-DOPA, fluoromisonidazole, and carbon-11 methionine [26]. PET may also serve the purpose of grading tumors and identifying biopsy targets. Limitations of PET include its lower spatial resolution compared to brain CT and MRI, inconsistent availability of radioisotopes, and increased radiation exposure.

1.10 CSF Study

CSF cytology is crucial for staging tumors prone to CSF spread, such as medulloblastoma, germ cell tumors, ependymoma, and CNS lymphoma. Tumor spread in the CSF can manifest as abnormal biochemical and cellular findings: raised CSF pressure, elevated protein levels, reduced glucose levels, and the presence of tumor cells on cytologic examination. Additionally, tumor markers in the CSF can assist in making the diagnosis [27]. The ideal time to perform CSF sampling is either before surgery or more than 3 weeks afterward to avoid false-positive results.

1.11 Pathology

Diagnosing a pediatric CNS tumor involves a comprehensive approach utilizing histologic, immunohistochemical, and molecular data.

1.11.1 Commonly Used IHC and Molecular Markers for Pediatric CNS Tumors [28]

Astrocytic Tumors

- Pilocytic astrocytoma—Grade I; locations: cerebellar, optic pathway, brainstem, cerebral, diencephalic; KIAA1549–BRAF fusion, BRAF mutation, 7q34 gain.
- Pleomorphic xanthoastrocytoma—Grade II; BRAF mutation, 9p loss.
- Diffuse astrocytoma (pediatric)—Grade II; BRAF mutation.
- Glioblastoma (pediatric/DIPG)—Grade IV; H3F3A, ATRX, DAXX mutations; ADAM3A homozygous deletion; PDGFRA amplification/mutation; IHC: ATRX, DAXX.

Neuronal Tumor

- Ganglioglioma—Grade I; BRAF mutation, trisomy 7.

Ependymal Tumor

- Ependymoma—Posterior fossa A (Grade II–III): 1q gain.
- Ependymoma—Posterior fossa B (Grade II): 6q loss, 22q loss, 9q gain, 15q gain, 18q gain; IHC: LAMA2, NELL2.

Embryonal Tumors

- Medulloblastoma—WNT subgroup (Grade IV): CTNNB1, MLL2/MLL3, SMARCA4, DDX3X mutations; monosomy 6; IHC: CTNNB1, DKK1.
- Medulloblastoma—SHH subgroup (Grade IV): PTCH1, SUFU mutations; GLI and MYCN amplification; 9q deletion; TP53 germline mutation; IHC: SFRP1, GLI1, GAB1.
- Medulloblastoma—Group 3 (Grade IV): MYC amplification, SMARCA4 mutation; 10q loss, 1q gain, 5q loss, i17q; IHC: NPR3.
- Medulloblastoma—Group 4 (Grade IV): KDM6A mutation; i17q; IHC: KCNA1.
- PNET—Grade IV; IDH1 mutation, CDKN2A homozygous deletion, PDGFRA amplification; 1q gain, 19p gain.
- ATRT—Grade IV; SMARCB1 and SMARCA4 mutations; 22q loss; IHC: SMARCB1 loss.

Germ Cell Tumor

- Germinoma—KIT mutation; Trisomy X, i12p; IHC: KIT.

DIPG—diffuse intrinsic pontine glioma; PNET—primitive neuroectodermal tumor; ATRT—atypical teratoid/rhabdoid tumor.

References

1. American Cancer Society. Key statistics for brain and spinal cord tumors in children. 2022.
2. American Cancer Society. Cancer facts and figures. 2022.
3. Ostrom QT, Patil N, Cioffi G, Waite K, Kruchko C, Barnholtz-Sloan JS. CBTRUS statistical report: primary brain and other central nervous system Tumors diagnosed in the United States in 2013–2017. Neuro-Oncology. 2020;22(Supplement_1):iv1–iv96.
4. Ron E, Modan B, Boice JD, Alfandary E, Stovall M, Chetrit A, et al. Tumors of the brain and nervous system after radiotherapy in childhood. N Engl J Med. 1988;319(16):1033–9.
5. Baldwin RT, Preston-Martin S. Epidemiology of brain tumors in childhood—a review. Toxicol Appl Pharmacol. 2004;199(2):118–31.
6. Garofola C, Jamal Z, Gross GP. Cowden disease. In: StatPearls [Internet]. Treasure Island: StatPearls Publishing; 2023.
7. Lohmann DR, Gallie BL. Retinoblastoma. In: Adam MP, Feldman J, Mirzaa GM, et al., editors. GeneReviews® [Internet]. Seattle: University of Washington, Seattle; 2000. Available from: https://www.ncbi.nlm.nih.gov/books/NBK1452/.
8. Mai PL, Best AF, Peters JA, DeCastro RM, Khincha PP, Loud JT, et al. Risks of first and subsequent cancers among TP53 mutation carriers in the National Cancer Institute li-Fraumeni syndrome cohort. Cancer. 2016;122(23):3673–81.
9. Campian J, Gutmann DH. CNS tumors in neurofibromatosis. J Clin Oncol Off J Am Soc Clin Oncol. 2017;35(21):2378–85.
10. Lo Muzio L. Nevoid basal cell carcinoma syndrome (Gorlin syndrome). Orphanet J Rare Dis. 2008;3:32.
11. Hamilton SR, Liu B, Parsons RE, Papadopoulos N, Jen J, Powell SM, et al. The molecular basis of Turcot's syndrome. N Engl J Med. 1995;332(13):839–47.
12. Kim H, Lim KY, Park JW, Kang J, Won JK, Lee K, et al. Sporadic and lynch syndrome-associated mismatch repair-deficient brain tumors. Lab Investig J Tech Methods Pathol. 2022;102(2):160–71.
13. Grajkowska W, Kotulska K, Jurkiewicz E, Matyja E. Brain lesions in tuberous sclerosis complex. Review. Folia Neuropathol. 2010;48(3):139–49.
14. Maher ER, Neumann HP, Richard S. von Hippel–Lindau disease: a clinical and scientific review. Eur J Hum Genet. 2011;19(6):617–23.
15. Boot MV, van Belzen MJ, Overbeek LI, Hijmering N, Mendeville M, Waisfisz Q, et al. Benign and malignant tumors in Rubinstein-Taybi syndrome. Am J Med Genet A. 2018;176(3):597–608.
16. Louis DN, Perry A, Wesseling P, Brat DJ, Cree IA, Figarella-Branger D, et al. The 2021 WHO classification of Tumors of the central nervous system: a summary. Neuro-Oncology. 2021;23(8):1231–51.
17. Rossi A, Caracciolo V, Russo G, Reiss K, Giordano A. Medulloblastoma: from molecular pathology to therapy. Clin Cancer Res. 2008;14(4):971–6.
18. I Kh Almadhoun MK, Hattab AW, Alazzeh NN, Aladwan ST, Ta'amneh O. Diagnosis and treatment of Dandy-Walker syndrome with two types of ventriculoperitoneal (VP) shunts: a case report. Cureus. 2023;15(10):e46564.
19. Rodríguez-Blanque R, Almazán-Soto C, Piqueras-Sola B, Sánchez-García JC, Reinoso-Cobo A, Menor-Rodríguez MJ, et al. Chiari syndrome: advances in epidemiology and pathogenesis: a systematic review. J Clin Med. 2023;12(20):6694.
20. Scott RM, Smith ER. Moyamoya disease and Moyamoya syndrome. N Engl J Med. 2009;360(12):1226–37.
21. Zarifi M, Tzika AA. Proton MRS imaging in pediatric brain tumors. Pediatr Radiol. 2016;46(7):952–62.
22. Pierce T, Kranz PG, Roth C, Leong D, Wei P, Provenzale JM. Use of apparent diffusion coefficient values for diagnosis of pediatric posterior fossa tumors. Neuroradiol J. 2014;27:233–44.
23. Kitis O, Altay H, Calli C, Yunten N, Akalin T, Yurtseven T. Minimum apparent diffusion coefficients in the evaluation of brain tumors. Eur J Radiol. 2005;55:393–400.

24. Bulakbasi N, Guvenc I, Onguru O, Erdogan E, Tayfun C, Ucoz T. The added value of the apperent diffusion coefficient calculation to magnetic resonance imaging in the differentiation and grading of malignant brain tumors. J Comput Assist Tomogr. 2004;28:735–46.
25. Aronen HJ, Gazit IE, Louis DN, Buchbinder BR, Pardo FS, Weisskoff RM, et al. Cerebral blood volume maps of gliomas: comparison with tumor grade and histologic findings. Radiology. 1994;191(1):41–51.
26. Chung JK, Kim Y, Kim S, Lee Y, Paek S, Yeo J, et al. Usefulness of 11C-methionine PET in the evaluation of brain lesions that are hypo- or isometabolic on 18F-FDG PET. Eur J Nucl Med Mol Imaging. 2002;29(2):176–82.
27. Bruschi M, Petretto A, Cama A, et al. Potential biomarkers of childhood brain tumor identified by proteomics of cerebrospinal fluid from extraventricular drainage (EVD). Sci Rep. 2021;11:1818.
28. Ichimura K, Nishikawa R, Matsutani M. Molecular markers in pediatric neuro-oncology. Neuro-Oncology. 2012;14(Suppl 4):iv90–9.
29. Louis DN, Perry A, Wesseling P, et al. The 2021 WHO classification of tumors of the central nervous system: a summary. Acta Neuropathol. 2021;141(3):341–62.

Chapter 2
Presentation and Evaluation of Adult CNS Tumors

Supriya Mallick, Adrija Ghosh, and Abhilash Dagar

2.1 Introduction

The clinical presentation of brain tumors can be diverse. It requires a trained brain to recognize the myriad ways in which a brain tumor can present to the clinic. Even in this era of modern, sophisticated imaging, clinical symptomatology plays an important role as an adjunct in the diagnosis of brain tumors.

2.2 General Background [1, 2]

- Clinical presentation is not specifically linked to the specific tumor type.
- Symptoms depend upon the location of the tumor.
- Patients can present with focal or generalized symptoms.
- Direct infiltration by tumor into neural tissue causes focal symptoms.
- Initially, especially in low-grade tumors, symptoms are focal, depending on tumor location.
- As tumor size increases, it manifests more generalized symptoms, including headache, nausea, and vomiting, hinting at increased intracranial pressure.
- Vasogenic edema caused by disruption of the blood-brain barrier leads to most of the symptoms.
- Mechanisms of presenting symptomatology may depend on tumor factors or peri-tumoral factors.

S. Mallick (✉)
Department of Radiation Oncology, National Cancer Institute, AIIMS, New Delhi, India

A. Ghosh · A. Dagar
Department of Radiation Oncology, All India Institute of Medical Sciences, New Delhi, India

S. Pradhan et al. (eds.), *Evidence Based Handbook on Diagnosis and Staging in Oncology*, https://doi.org/10.1007/978-981-95-9701-7_2

- Tumor factors include histology, grade, and location.
- Low-grade gliomas cause neuronal denervation hypersensitivity and a more epileptogenic microenvironment. Hence, more commonly associated with seizures.
- Certain locations correlate with certain histologies:

  Glioneuronal tumors and astrocytomas appear to favor the temporal lobe. Oligodendrogliomas prefer the frontal lobe.

- Peritumoral factors, including regional hypoxia blood–brain barrier breakdown, may predispose to seizure and localized neuronal dysfunction.

2.3 Generalized Clinical Features

2.3.1 Headache [3–7]

- Headache is an almost ubiquitous finding in brain tumor patients (64%), although it is rarely the only symptom (8%).
- The location of the headaches is not always characteristic and often misleading. It is probably due to a stretching of the dura incident to a local or generalized increase in pressure.
- Frequently associated with frontal, brainstem, cerebellar, and suprasellar tumors.
- The "classic" presentation of tumor headache is of dull, constant character and of severe intensity, immediately after awakening, and associated with nausea and vomiting.
- The **American Academy of Neurology** published guidelines for red flags of headache, which merit further evaluation: Abnormal neurologic examination, headache worsened by Valsalva maneuver, headache causing awakening from sleep, new onset headache in the older population, progressively worsening headache, or headache not fulfilling the strict definition of migraine.

2.3.2 Nausea and Vomiting [4, 8]

- Tumors trigger the CTZ (Chemoreceptor trigger zone) in the area postrema at the floor of the fourth ventricle.
- Vomiting usually indicates raised intracranial pressure.
- In brainstem tumors, it can be due to direct compression of the CTZ by the tumor.
- Occurs usually at the peak of the accompanying headache.
- Projectile vomiting, seen usually in posterior fossa tumors in children, is uncommon in adults.
- Recurrent vomiting associated with headache, having no relation to meals or unaccompanied by abdominal distress, warrants an investigation of the central nervous system.

- Ictus emeticus or vomiting as an ictal phenomenon can, rarely, be a manifestation of tumors involving the insula and mesial temporal lobe.

2.3.3 *Altered Mental Status [4, 9, 10]*

- Neuropsychiatric manifestations associated with intracranial tumors are not limited to lesions of the frontal lobe and may arise from involvement of adjacent or deep brain regions. Focal neurocognitive deficits such as aphasia, agnosia, abulia, alexia, and apraxia possess important localizing significance; however, are frequently misinterpreted as features of generalized cognitive decline.
- In contrast, nonspecific alterations in mental status are more subtle and occur more commonly. Early manifestations may include irritability, emotional lability, impaired memory, reduced initiative, and psychomotor slowing, which can gradually progress to apathy and lethargy. Such symptom patterns may indicate tumors affecting deep cerebral structures, including thalamocortical pathways, the corpus callosum, the reticular activating system, and occasionally the frontal lobes.
- Behavioral withdrawal and diminished motivation are often mistakenly attributed to depressive disorders. Lesions involving the amygdala may present with aggressive or impulsive behavior, while auditory hallucinations—frequently regarded as hallmarks of primary psychotic illness—can be an early manifestation of tumors arising in the temporal lobe.
- When psychiatric or cognitive symptoms occur in conjunction with features suggestive of raised intracranial pressure, such as persistent headache or recurrent vomiting, an underlying organic intracranial pathology should be strongly considered and appropriately investigated.

2.3.4 *Optic Symptoms*

- Pituitary tumors show early diminution of vision (segmental/quadrantal/bitemporal hemianopsia).
- Occipital or temporal lobe tumors can potentially compress and destroy the optic pathway, causing homonymous hemianopsia.
- Visual hallucinations may accompany temporal or frontal lobe tumors.
- Papilledema may be present as an indicator of increased intracranial pressure, more commonly in children.
- Papilledema due to raised intracranial pressure is usually bilateral, although it may not be symmetric.

2.3.5 Seizure [11–15]

- Brain tumors may cause seizures by direct mass effect, vascular modifications, recruitment of microglia, or by disturbing the balance of GABA-glutamate neurotransmitters, which are also growth factors for tumor cells.
- Peritumoral factors like blood-brain barrier disruption, pH imbalance, and metabolic changes due to vascular disturbance, cytokine and glutamate concentrations, localized immunologic interactions, and hypoxia also trigger seizures.
- Slow-growing tumors are the most epileptogenic.
- New-onset seizures garner early attention and act as a good predictive factor.
- Recurrence or worsening of seizures during the disease course implies tumor progression.
- Levetiracetam is the drug of choice for brain tumor-related epilepsy (BTE).
- One-third of BTEs show pharmacoresistance. Polytherapy is synergistic in managing these.
- The antitumor effects of valproic acid as a histone deacetylase inhibitor (HDACi) in glioblastoma (GBM) have gained attention.

2.4 Clinical Features of CSF Obstruction [16–19]

- Monro-Kellie doctrine and its later elaborations postulated that the brain, blood, and CSF are incompressible and contained within a rigid skull. Hence, all space-occupying lesions lead to raised CSF pressure once the capacity for "compensation" is exhausted.
- Severe subarachnoid obstruction of CSF flow, leading to impaired CSF absorption at the superior sagittal sinus, is the main cause of raised CSF pressure with supratentorial tumors.
- Identification is essential as they warrant urgent medical attention.
- Symptoms and signs that should trigger warning bells include generalized intermittent headache, blurred vision, papilledema, urinary incontinence, memory deficits, seizure, coma, hemiparesis, and normal-pressure hydrocephalus.
- Third and fourth ventricle tumors (ependymomas, choroid plexus carcinomas, or papillomas, and meningiomas) can obstruct the outflow of CSF and cause hydrocephalus.
- Leptomeningeal tumors can lead to communicating hydrocephalus.
- Hydrocephalus and raised intracranial pressure may occur as a delayed complication of hemispheric tumors such as glioblastoma and metastases.

2.5 Brain Herniation Symptoms [20]

- Herniation syndrome is a rare presentation in undiagnosed brain tumors.
- Usually seen late in the course of the disease, when it has progressed despite treatment.
- Subfalcine herniation: Cingulate gyrus displacement under the falx cerebri compresses the anterior frontal lobes, causing cognitive issues.
- Uncal herniation: Due to a mass lesion, the uncus of the temporal lobe protrudes through the tentorium cerebelli.
- The key clinical sign is **ipsilateral oculomotor nerve palsy** with a fixed and dilated pupil due to compression by the medial temporal lobe.
- Ipsilateral hemiparesis is a false localizing sign due to compression of the contralateral cerebral peduncle against the tentorium (Kernohan notch).
- Central herniation: pressure from a mass on the diencephalon may lead to coma.
- Tonsillar herniation: cerebellar tonsils herniate through the foramen magnum, blocking the outflow of the fourth ventricle and compressing the medulla, causing sudden death.
- Upward brainstem herniation is seen in patients with posterior fossa tumors.

2.6 Localizing Symptoms and Signs of Intracranial Neoplasms

The ability to localize brain tumors to a particular location helps in narrowing down the diagnosis to a few probable differentials, even before histopathological confirmation. This is based on a certain inherent affinity of specific tumors to specific locations.

2.6.1 Frontal Lobe Tumors [21–24]

- Subtle and non-specific symptoms.
- Progressive symptoms or association with features of raised intracranial pressure/seizure should prompt investigation.
- Higher mental functions are affected in deeper lesions.
- Personality change and flattening of affect are typical features that may progress to apathy.
- Disinhibition sometimes leads to striking social lapses.
- Often only relatable retrospectively.

- Severe urgency, frequency, and incontinence can also occur in the absence of dementia, indifference, or lack of social concern.
- Gait apraxia is associated with the involvement of frontal eye fields, where patients have difficulty in initiating gait.
- Speech disturbances occur when the dominant hemisphere is affected.
- Lesions in the posterior inferior frontal gyrus relate to the classical Broca's aphasia (expressive difficulty and repetition deficits).
- Lesions in the posterior aspect of the frontal lobe may result in motor weakness.
- If limited in size, it affects the lower extremity if superior and medial, or the upper extremity and face if more lateral (Motor Homunculus).

2.6.2 *Temporal Lobe Tumors [25–29]*

- Seizures (temporal lobe epilepsy): most common with temporal lobe lesions.
- Partial complex seizures are the most common.
- Half of temporal lobe tumor patients have seizures.
- Visual field defects: due to disruption of the optic radiation.
- Meyer's loop is associated with homonymous upper quadrant defects.
- Dysphasia.
- Cognitive and memory dysfunction.
- Non-dominant temporal lobe tumors may not show symptoms until they become very large.
- Tumors on the dominant side can cause more significant cognitive problems in both verbal and non-verbal functions.
- Cognitive disturbances and mental impairment features are indistinguishable from the frontal lobe tumors.
- Occasionally, patients present with schizophrenia-like features, including hallucinations, which may cause diagnostic confusion.
- Epileptic auras can cause abnormal subjective experiences such as déjà vu, overwhelming fears, and sudden emotional changes, making diagnosis difficult.

2.6.3 *Parietal Lobe Tumors [5, 30–32]*

- Seizures are most commonly seen with motor cortex lesions.
- Focal seizures are characteristic of parietal-lobe masses, in particular those in the region of the motor cortex.
- Sensory abnormalities:

- Dominant-hemisphere lesions are typically associated with agraphesthesia, left-right confusion, and finger agnosia.
- Non-dominant hemisphere lesions are classically associated with unilateral neglect phenomena.
- Visual disturbances: lesions affecting the optic radiations.
- Inferior quadrant defects.
- Dyspraxia: Body and spatial disturbances of voluntary motor function.
- Dysphasia: Receptive speech disorders.
- More complex associative features than classical Wernicke's aphasia.
- Less likely to cause psychological changes.
- Communication difficulties may hinder the ability to gain the patient's attention and cooperation.

2.6.4 Occipital Lobe Tumors [5]

- Visual defects are synonymous with occipital mass lesions.
- Homonymous hemianopsia is typical.
- Macular sparing is characteristic but not universal.
- Nystagmus is often associated.
- Seizures less likely.
- Increased risk of raised intracranial pressure causing a disturbance of consciousness.

2.6.5 Diencephalic Tumors [5, 33, 34]

- Mass effect on the third ventricle.
- CSF obstruction can cause raised intracranial pressure and hydrocephalus.
- Memory impairment, often with confabulation, hypersomnia, and akinetic mutism, is characteristic.
- Hyperphagia, somnolence, and hypersomnia are seen when the hypothalamus is affected.
- Hypersomnolence to be differentiated from impaired consciousness of raised intracranial hypertension.
- Other hypothalamic disorders include amenorrhea, diabetes insipidus, or disturbances of thermoregulation.
- Pineal region lesions can lead to delayed or precocious puberty or, by pressure on the tectum of the midbrain and along with oculomotor dysfunction, cause the classic Parinaud's syndrome of vertical-gaze paresis.
- Thalamic tumors: Cause early and severe dementia.

2.6.6 Pituitary Region Tumors [33]

- Raised intracranial pressure symptoms
- Pituitary disturbances
- Visual field defects (close relation to optic chiasma)

2.6.7 Cerebellar Tumors [33–35]

- Hydrocephalus is caused by the proximity of the cerebellum to the fourth ventricle and is most common with midline cerebellar lesions. Larger lateral cerebellar lesions may also do the same.
- Lateral cerebellar lesions: Limb ataxia, disturbed motor coordination, nystagmus.
- Midline lesions are likely to present with CSF obstruction and more midline ataxia.
- Significant cognitive and behavioral sequelae of hydrocephalus: cerebellar cognitive affective syndrome.

2.6.8 Brainstem Tumors [36–38]

- Contralateral motor dysfunction: proximity to cranial nerves and corticospinal tract ipsilateral VI nerve palsy and contralateral hemiparesis.
- Cranial neuropathies:

  Pontine lesions: VI, VII, V (sensory)
  Medullary lesions: lower cranial nerves (IX, X, XI, XII)

- Medullary lesions are associated with quadriplegic deficits.
- Diffuse brainstem gliomas have been associated with ataxia, cerebellar signs, and long-tract signs.
- Subtle changes in scholastic performance.
- Swallowing disturbances causing micro-aspiration can lead to recurrent URTIs.

2.6.9 Cerebellopontine Angle Tumors [33, 34]

- Cranial nerve: involvement, especially VIII.
- Mass effect on the adjacent cerebellum.

- Facial nerve involvement is also often seen, given the immediately adjacent location of the extra-axial part of the facial nerve to the acoustic neuroma.
- Vestibular schwannoma/acoustic neuroma is the classic tumor seen at this location, presenting with vertigo, tinnitus, or hearing loss as the presenting symptom.

2.7 Investigating a Brain Tumor [33, 39–46]

- When clinical symptoms raise suspicion of a brain tumor, it becomes imperative to conduct investigations to reach a diagnosis.
- After a detailed history, a full medical examination, including a neurological examination, becomes mandatory.
- This is to be augmented by visual field testing by perimetry, especially if the tumor is suspected to be in the vicinity of the pituitary.
- Audiometry becomes important when suspecting a cerebellopontine angle tumor.
- Almost all Schwannomas are associated with sensorineural hearing loss.
- Hematological and biochemical investigations, a part of the basic diagnostic armamentarium of any disease, confer information about the general well-being of the patient.
- Endocrinological examination to assess the functioning of the hypothalamo-pituitary axis in patients suspected of having a tumor in this location.
- Neuroimaging by an MRI is the most important tool to diagnose brain tumors.
- EEG can be done in patients who present with seizures.
- Cytology of CSF is unreplaceable in the postoperative staging of tumors prone to have a leptomeningeal spread.

2.7.1 MRI Neuroimaging

- Gold standard for diagnosing brain tumors.
- Excellent tissue contrast and resolution help detect small lesions.
- No artefact by overlying bone.
- Gadolinium enhancement helps delineate tumor margins from surrounding edema.
- Various MRI sequences (T1, T2, FLAIR) and their variants, including perfusion, diffusion, spectroscopy, and angiography in combination, help diagnose brain tumors by defining tumor volumes, characteristics, and evaluation of blood flow and metabolites.
- Indicators of an aggressive, high-grade glioma (HGG) include contrast enhancement and certain morphologic features like mass effect, necrosis, and hemorrhage.

- Contrast enhancement in particular is strongly correlated to malignancy, but is non-specific.
- There are no conventional MRI features that reliably differentiate between the different glioma subtypes, such as grade II astrocytoma and oligodendroglioma.
- Pilocytic astrocytoma (WHO grade I): Cerebellar location is most common, hypo-isointense on T1w, and hyperintense on T2w with intense homogenous enhancement.
- Astrocytomas:

  WHO grade II are well-defined, homogenous masses; they are hypointense on T1w, hyperintense on T2w, and have calcification in 50%.
  WHO grade III have less well-defined borders, heterogeneous mass; they have more mass effect, vasogenic edema, and heterogeneous enhancement.

- GBMs are poorly defined, have a mass effect, massive vasogenic edema, and common intra-tumoral hemorrhage. They are heterogeneous on both T1w and T2w, have satellite tumor location, spread along white matter tracts, and have infiltrative borders.
- Oligodendroglioma: Heterogeneous signal intensity, isointense on T1w, hyperintense on T2w, and frequent calcification (blooming effect on susceptibility sequences).
- Medulloblastoma: Posterior fossa tumors with risk of spinal drop metastasis, heterogeneous signal intensity, frequent calcification, cyst formation may be present, isointense with grey matter on T1w, and hyperintense on T2w.
- Ependymoma: Posterior fossa tumor in children, spinal cord tumor in adults, risk of CSF dissemination, hypo to isointense on T1, hyperintense on T2w, and supratentorial ependymoma indistinguishable on MRI from astrocytoma
- Meningioma: Extra-axial tumor with dural tail sign, hypo to isointense on T1w, isointense on T2w, and has homogeneous enhancement
- Craniopharyngioma: Sellar to suprasellar location, calcification, cystic component, hyperintense on T1w, and mixed signal on T2w. The solid portion shows enhancement with contrast
- Primary central nervous system lymphoma:

  Immunocompetent: single lesion, peripheral location
  Immunosuppressed: multiple lesions with deeper location (basal ganglia)
  Hypo to isointense on T1w and T2w with intense contrast enhancement.

2.7.2 *Functional Imaging in Brain Tumors*

- Positron emission tomography (PET) and single-photon emission computed tomography (SPECT) allow the detection of tumors as a result of their neurochemical and physiological responses, such as increased blood flow to the tumor, protein production, or glucose consumption.

- Radiation necrosis is often difficult to distinguish from a tumor with CT or MRI.
- The radiolabeled amino acids commonly used in clinical studies are methyl-11CL-methionine (MET), 3,4-dihydroxy-6-[18F]-fluoro-L-phenylalanine (FDOPA), and 18F-fluoroethyltyrosine (FET).
- [11C]-MET-PET is superior to [18F]-FDG-PET for defining tumor extent.
- MRI and FET-PET in combination can result in 93–94% sensitivity and specificity.
- PET-FET is a superior indicator of post-surgery residual tumor volume which has a strong prognostic impact.
- FDOPA-PET helps distinguish between true and pseudo-progression.

References

1. Chang SM, Parney IF, Huang W, et al. Patterns of care for adults with newly diagnosed malignant glioma. JAMA. 2005;293(5):557–64. https://doi.org/10.1001/jama.293.5.557.
2. Jaeckle KA. Signs of focal lesions and of increased intracranial pressure in brain tumors. Handb Clin Neurol Neuro-Oncol Part. 1998;1:139–65.
3. Vázquez-Barquero A, Ibáñez F, Herrera S, Izquierdo J, Berciano J, Pascual J. Isolated headache as the presenting clinical manifestation of intracranial tumors: a prospective study. Cephalalgia. 1994;14(4):270–1. https://doi.org/10.1046/j.1468-2982.1994.1404270.
4. Courville CB. Brain tumor: its presenting symptoms. Calif West Med. 1929;31(2):100.
5. Alther B, Mylius V, Weller M, Gantenbein A. From first symptoms to diagnosis: initial clinical presentation of primary brain tumors. Clin Trans Neurosci. 2020;4(2):17. https://doi.org/10.1177/2514183X20968368.
6. Forsyth PA, Posner JB. Headaches in patients with brain tumors: a study of 111 patients. Neurology. 1993;43(9):1678–83.
7. Schaefer PW, Miller JC, Singhal AB, Thrall JH, Lee SI. Headache: when is neurologic imaging indicated? J Am Coll Radiol. 2007;4(8):566–9.
8. Chen C, Yen DJ, Yiu CH, Shih YH, Yu HY, Su MS. Ictal vomiting in partial seizures of temporal lobe origin. Eur Neurol. 1999;42(4):235–9.
9. Weitzner MA. Psychosocial and neuropsychiatric aspects of patients with primary brain Tumors. Cancer Investig. 1999;17(4):285–91. https://doi.org/10.3109/07357909909040599.
10. Malamud N. Psychiatric disorder with intracranial tumors of limbic system. Arch Neurol. 1967;17(2):113–23. https://doi.org/10.1001/archneur.1967.00470260003001.
11. van Breemen MS, Wilms EB, Vecht CJ. Epilepsy in patients with brain tumours: epidemiology, mechanisms, and management. Lancet Neurol. 2007;6(5):421–30.
12. Vecht CJ, Kerkhof M, Duran-Pena A. Seizure prognosis in brain tumors: new insights and evidence-based management. Oncologist. 2014;19(7):751–9.
13. Pallud J, Capelle L, Huberfeld G. Tumoral epileptogenicity: how does it happen? Epilepsia. 2013;54:30–4.
14. Krauze AV, Myrehaug SD, Chang MG, Holdford DJ, Smith S, Shih J, Tofilon PJ, Fine HA, Camphausen K. A phase 2 study of concurrent radiation therapy, temozolomide, and the histone deacetylase inhibitor valproic acid for patients with glioblastoma. Int J Radiat Oncol Biol Phys. 2015;92(5):986–92.
15. Beaumont A, Whittle IR. The pathogenesis of tumour associated epilepsy. Acta Neurochir. 2000;142:1–5.
16. Langfitt TW. Increased intracranial pressure: chapter XXI. Neurosurgery. 1969;16:436–71.
17. Van Crevel H. Papilloedema, CSF pressure, and CSF flow in cerebral tumours. J Neurol Neurosurg Psychiatry. 1979;42(6):493–500.

18. Dandy WE. Diagnosis, localization and removal of tumors of the third ventricle. Bull Johns Hopkins Hosp. 1922;33:188–9.
19. Desai KI, Nadkarni TD, Muzumdar DP, Goel AH. Surgical management of colloid cyst of the third ventricle—a study of 105 cases. Surg Neurol. 2002;57(5):295–302.
20. Posner JB. Plum and Posner's diagnosis of stupor and coma. USA: Oxford University Press; 2007.
21. Jefferson G. Tumours of the frontal lobe. Postgrad Med J. 1950;26(293):133.
22. Sachs E. Meningiomas with dementia as the first and presenting feature. J Ment Sci. 1950;96(405):998–1007.
23. Avery TL. Seven cases of frontal tumour with psychiatric presentation. Br J Psychiatry. 1971;119(548):19–23.
24. Keschner M, Bender MB, Strauss I. Mental symptoms associated with brain tumor: a study of 530 verified cases. JAMA J Am Med Assoc. 1938;110(10):714–8.
25. Gabr M, Lüders H, Dinner D, Morris H, Wyllie E. Speech manifestations in lateralization of temporal lobe seizures. Ann Neurol. 1989;25(1):82–7.
26. Arseni C, Petrovici IN. Epilepsy in temporal lobe tumours. Eur Neurol. 1971;5(4):201–14.
27. Serafetinides EA, Falconer MA. Speech disturbances in temporal lobe seizures: a study in 100 epileptic patients submitted to anterior temporal lobectomy. Brain. 1963;86(2):333–46.
28. Cole M, Zangwill OL. Deja vu in temporal lobe epilepsy. J Neurol Neurosurg Psychiatry. 1963;26(1):37.
29. Bingley T. Mental symptoms in temporal lobe epilepsy and temporal lobe gliomas with special reference to laterality of lesion and the relationship between handedness and brainedness; a study of 90 cases of temporal lobe epilepsy and 253 cases of temporal lobe glioma. Acta Psychiatr Neurol Scand Suppl. 1958;120:1–51.
30. Salanova V, Andermann F, Rasmussen T, Olivier A, Quesney LF. Tumoural parietal lobe epilepsy clinical manifestations and outcome in 34 patients treated between 1934 and 1988. Brain. 1995;118(5):1289–304.
31. Liouta E, Stranjalis G, Kalyvas AV, Koutsarnakis C, Pantinaki S, Liakos F, Komaitis S, Stavrinou LC. Parietal association deficits in patients harboring parietal lobe gliomas: a prospective study. J Neurosurg. 2018;130(3):773–9.
32. Critchley M, Russell WR, Zangwill OL. Discussion on parietal lobe syndromes. Proc R Soc Med. 1951;44(4):337–46.
33. David D, Fleminger S, Kopelman M, Lovestone S, Mellers J. Lishman's organic psychiatry: a textbook of neuropsychiatry. Wiley-Blackwell; 2012.
34. Alentorn A, Hoang-Xuan K, Mikkelsen T. Presenting signs and symptoms in brain tumors. Handb Clin Neurol. 2016;134:19–26.
35. Schmahmann JD, Sherman JC. The cerebellar cognitive affective syndrome. Brain. 1998;121(4):561–79.
36. Jallo GI, Biser-Rohrbaugh A, Freed D. Brainstem gliomas. Childs Nerv Syst. 2004;20:143–53.
37. Recinos PF, Sciubba DM, Jallo GI. Brainstem tumors: where are we today? Pediatr Neurosurg. 2007;43(3):192–201.
38. Sun T, Wan W, Wu Z, Zhang J, Zhang L. Clinical outcomes and natural history of pediatric brainstem tumors: with 33 cases follow-ups. Neurosurg Rev. 2013;36:311–20.
39. Rees J. Advances in magnetic resonance imaging of brain tumours. Curr Opin Neurol. 2003;16(6):643–50.
40. Abd-Ellah MK, Awad AI, Khalaf AA, Hamed HF. A review on brain tumor diagnosis from MRI images: practical implications, key achievements, and lessons learned. Magn Reson Imaging. 2019;61:300–18.
41. Rehman L, Rehman UL, Azmat SK, Hashim AS. Magnetic resonance spectroscopy: novel non-invasive technique for diagnosing brain tumors. J Coll Physicians Surg Pak. 2015;25(12):863–6.

42. Leung D, Han X, Mikkelsen T, Nabors LB. Role of MRI in primary brain tumor evaluation. J Natl Compr Cancer Netw. 2014;12(11):1561–8.
43. Chen W. Clinical applications of PET in brain tumors. J Nucl Med. 2007;48(9):1468–81.
44. Herholz K, Langen KJ, Schiepers C, Mountz JM. Brain tumors. In: Seminars in nuclear medicine, vol. 42, no 6. WB Saunders; 2012. p. 356–70.
45. Pierallini A, Bonamini M, Bozzao A, Pantano P, Stefano DD, Ferone E, Raguso M, Bosman C, Bozzao L. Supratentorial diffuse astrocytic tumours: proposal of an MRI classification. Eur Radiol. 1997;7:395–9.
46. Taphoorn MJ, Bromberg JE. Neurological effects of therapeutic irradiation. Continuum. 2005;11(5):93–115.

Chapter 3
Presentation and Evaluation of Spinal Tumors

Kanika Sood Sharma and Aditi Tanwar

3.1 Introduction

Tumors originating in or around the spinal cord can be either primary or metastatic. Primary spinal cord tumors arise from cells within or adjacent to the spinal cord. Metastatic tumors are deposits in the cord from primary tumors anywhere else in the body. Primary spinal cord tumors constitute 2–4% of all central nervous system tumors. The scarcity of information regarding the frequency of spinal tumors can be attributed to their infrequent manifestation.

3.2 Classification

Spinal cord tumors, based on their site of origin, are classified into three categories: epidural tumors, intradural extramedullary tumors, and intramedullary tumors.

Further stratification can be done based on whether these tumors are benign or malignant in nature.

K. S. Sharma (✉) · A. Tanwar
Dharamshila Narayana Superspeciality Hospital, New Delhi, India

S. Pradhan et al. (eds.), *Evidence Based Handbook on Diagnosis and Staging in Oncology*, https://doi.org/10.1007/978-981-95-9701-7_3

3.3 Clinical Presentation

3.3.1 *Pain*

The majority of the patients present with pain in the back as the primary symptom. This pain can either be an isolated regional pain or a radiating pain, depending on the extent of the lesion and location in the spine. Regional pain or local pain is the result of periosteal stretching by intraosseous tumor and neoplastic inflammatory mediators. The patient experiences a dull aching pain usually in the night and is usually responsive to anti-inflammatory medications and palliative radiation.

The pain can also be mechanical, resulting from loss of integrity of the spinal column, thereby limiting the ability of the spine to provide structural stability. This type of pain gets worsened with weight bearing and/or ambulation. It typically improves in the recumbent position but rarely responds to analgesics or palliative radiation.

Often, patients present with radicular pain radiating along the involved dermatome. It occurs due to nerve root compression by either direct tumor extension or collapse of the vertebral body.

3.3.2 *Neurological Dysfunction*

Neurological dysfunction can be seen as a severe complication of spinal metastasis. The symptoms are a result of direct contiguous expansion of spinal bony tumors into the spinal canal or encasing neural foramina, causing compressive symptoms pertaining to the nerve root or spinal cord. Pathological fractures of the vertebral bone can also lead to compression of neural elements. According to the degree of involvement, neurologic symptoms range from radiculopathy to myelopathy. Radiculopathy refers to motor weakness or sensory loss corresponding to the involved nerve roots.

3.3.3 *Myelopathy*

Myelopathy is due to spinal cord compression. The patient experiences a specific sensory level of impairment, which may or may not be accompanied by extremity weakness. Myelopathy can begin with difficulty in motor activities and can further progress to bladder or bowel dysfunction, saddle anesthesia, and erectile dysfunction.

3.3.4 *Pathological Fractures*

Direct extension of the tumor into the vertebral body can lead to collapse and pathological fracture. It usually manifests with pain on weight bearing and can progress to neurological compromise.

3.3.5 *Spinal Deformities*

A large or destructive tumor may cause anatomical deformities in the spine, like scoliosis.

3.4 Differential Diagnosis

1. Potts spine
2. Trauma
3. Disc herniation
4. Spinal cord abscess
5. Spinal arteriovenous malformation
6. Multiple myeloma
7. Syringomyelia
8. Spondylolisthesis
9. Aneurysmal bone cyst
10. Spinal stenosis
11. Other conditions mimicking spinal tumors—cauda equina and conus medullaris syndromes, epidural hematoma, and intervertebral disc disorders.

3.5 Clinical Evaluation

A detailed history of the presenting symptom, which is usually pain in case of spinal tumors, forms the basis of clinical evaluation. Assessment includes the site of pain, weakness, or numbness, the nature of pain (local or radiating), and associated symptoms. A thorough neurological evaluation of sensory and motor functions is mandatory. Assessing exacerbating and alleviating elements, comprehensive prior medical records, potential history of trauma, chronic ailments, or surgical procedures, among other factors, aids healthcare providers in reaching an accurate diagnosis. The nature of radicular pain can help in identifying the involved dermatome, and hence, the level of the spinal cord being affected can be localized. Efficient clinical evaluations play a crucial role in making well-considered decisions regarding the necessity of additional radiological investigations.

3.6 Radiological Evaluation

3.6.1 X-Ray

An X-ray of the spine is the first investigation in a low-resource country and is a valuable tool for detecting many vertebral tumors. Its diagnostic effectiveness stems from its relatively high sensitivity and spatial resolution in capturing images of bone. This imaging technique can provide clear visualization of bone size, structure, and any bone-related abnormalities in the skeletal system. It can also reveal bone destruction and periosteal reactions, which result from changes in bone mineral density caused by variations in calcium concentration within the spine. Although X-rays are not effective in localizing the spinal cord tumors, they may be used in assessing pathological fractures or any bony deformities in the spine that may be caused by the tumor. Additionally, its utility is limited when it comes to examining and analyzing cartilage lesions due to inherent constraints. Furthermore, tumors located adjacent to or beneath structures such as the adnexa can be easily overlooked. Despite its limitations, plain X-ray film remains the fundamental method for tumor diagnosis.

3.6.2 CT Scan (Computed Tomography)

CT scan offers notable advantages, characterized by its swift scan speed and production of high-resolution images. Multi-row CT scans have notably truncated scan durations and minimized motion-related artifacts. Notably, this technology has elevated the Z-axis resolution, facilitating the clear visualization of minute lesions. This has been particularly instrumental in the early detection of primary spinal osseous tumors, effectively circumventing the limitations of conventional plain X-ray films.

CT scan of the vertebral column aids in giving information about the integrity of the bony anatomy of the spinal column and provides initial information on the presence and location of spinal tumors. Any paravertebral mass or tumor in the cord itself is suggested by widening of the spinal canal. Although CT scans are effective in visualizing the bones, they have limitations in imaging the soft tissues and neural structures. Hence, its utility is limited in diagnosing spinal tumors, and a CT scan is not the best modality for providing detailed information about a spinal cord tumor.

3.6.3 MRI (Magnetic Resonance Imaging)

An MRI is the most reliable investigation in diagnosing a spinal tumor, allowing notable benefits like exceptional spatial resolution as well as the ability to capture images from various angles and sequences. It also exhibits high sensitivity in the determination of the extent of the lesion and can diagnose a tumor even in its early stages. It is very effective in localizing the site of the tumor, assessing its relation with the surrounding structures, level and extent of nerve root compression, spinal cord compression, etc. Contrast-enhanced images can localize the blood vessels in and around the spinal cord and are useful in assessing the treatment response. Diffusion weighted images can represent tumor necrosis both pre and post treatment. Magnetic resonance is useful to study associated soft tissue extension, marrow infiltration, and intraspinal extension and can differentiate between intradural-extramedullary, intramedullary, and extradural tumors. Additionally, the employment of T2-weighted imaging (T2WI) sequences in MRI enables the visualization of the lesion's relationship with nearby blood vessels, nerves, and muscles within the adjacent vertebral segments. This aspect greatly aids in assessing the extent of the lesion's impact on the surrounding soft tissues, allowing for effective determination of tissue violations. MRI provides most of the information needed by the surgeons and radiation oncologists for treatment purposes. It is necessary to acquire an MRI scan for patients planned for SBRT of the spine for precise delineation of the spinal cord and cauda equina in relation to the spinal canal.

3.6.4 Spinal Angiography

Spinal angiography is an elaborate evaluation of the vascular supply and venous outflow of the spinal cord, vertebrae, and surrounding soft tissue. It can be done for investigating patients with suspected primary vascular lesions of the spinal cord. Neurosurgeons operating on patients with spinal cord compression utilize a spinal angiogram for the identification of the native spinal artery supply for the surgical approach.

3.6.5 CSF Analysis

In patients with a suspicion of spread of tumor along the meninges (drop mets from primary) or infection along with tumor, a lumbar puncture may be done to assess the CSF for the presence of tumor cells or infections, etc.

3.6.6 Neurological Testing

Nerve conduction velocity studies and electromyography can help in the functional assessment of nerves and muscles affected by the tumor itself or due to compression of neural foramina.

Table 3.1 Sensitivity, specificity, and positive predictive value of PET CT for spinal tumors

	Sensitivity (%)	Specificity (%)	PPV (%)
Intradural extramedullary	93.2	92	93.6
Intramedullary	93.3	97	88.5
Extradural	88.5	97.7	90.2

3.6.7 PET CT Scan (Positron Emission Tomography)

It is not uncommon for spinal tumors to be a part of metastasis and not a primary tumor. In such cases, a detailed clinical history may suggest the need for assessing the primary tumor somewhere else in the body. A PET CT is highly useful in detecting the primary tumor and also gives a good anatomical and metabolic detail about the spinal metastasis, its location, paravertebral soft tissue component, cord compression, etc.

The sensitivity of PET/CT for the diagnosis of spinal metastases is 92.19%, and the specificity is 78.95% [1].

The sensitivity of MRI in the diagnosis of spinal metastases is 78.13%, and the specificity is 56.25%.

The sensitivity of MRI for primary spinal tumors varies according to the site of the disease (Table 3.1) [1].

3.7 Pathological Evaluation

Although MRI is highly effective in diagnosing a spinal tumor, particularly primary, it cannot substitute for a histopathological evaluation. Like any other neoplastic etiology, a spinal tumor (primary or metastatic) needs a tissue diagnosis. Biopsy can be performed as fine needle aspiration, core biopsy, or incisional or excisional biopsy. Fine needle biopsy and Tru-Cut biopsy are feasible if the tumor can be approached percutaneously. Biopsy in spinal tumors carries a risk of contamination of the tract by tumor cells and, hence, is performed away from the neurovascular structures by small incisions, which could then be removed with the tumor mass in a definitive surgical procedure.

Lumbar puncture is sometimes indicated if meningeal spread of disease is suspected. Presence of tumor cells or infectious cells in the CSF further demands a battery of tests to rule out an ascending infection or spread of disease.

Apart from histopathological proof, certain laboratory investigations are also mandatory in diagnosing and treating spinal tumors. Complete blood count, erythrocyte sedimentation rate (ESR), or C-reactive protein (CRP) help distinguish between neoplastic and infectious processes. A comment on alkaline phosphatase, serum calcium can also point towards a neoplastic etiology. Serum electrophoresis or urine electrophoresis is performed when multiple myeloma or plasmacytoma is suspected.

3.8 Take-Home Message

Spinal tumors, while constituting a minority of central nervous system tumors, present intricate features that pose clinical challenges. The most common presenting symptoms are pain and neurological deficit. These tumors may emerge as either primary growths within the spine or as a manifestation of systemic metastasis, often stemming from common sources like lung or breast carcinoma. In the primary setting, MRI is the modality of choice for diagnosis, and it helps in accurately identifying the location of the tumor, its relation with the adjacent structures, including blood vessels and nerve roots. MRI is of great help in guiding neurosurgeons and radiation oncologists in planning and executing treatment. PET CT has been found to be helpful when the spinal tumor presents as part of metastasis from a primary elsewhere in the body. While a multitude of imaging technologies are at our disposal, none can replace the value of sound clinical judgment. A comprehensive patient history and a thorough physical examination remain pivotal not only in reaching an accurate diagnosis but also in shaping the course of subsequent investigations. It is imperative that no invasive treatment should start without a histopathological proof, sparing some rare scenarios where conservative treatment will not suffice, and immediate intervention is required. After an adequate diagnosis, the management part involves a collaborative effort across diverse medical specialties. The goal is to intervene promptly before irreversible damage takes hold.

Reference

1. Luo ZH, Lu PX, Qi WL, Jin AF, Liu Q, Zeng QY, et al. The sensitivity and specificity of ^{18}F-FDG PET/CT in spinal leptomeningeal metastases: the synergistic effect of the ^{18}F-FDG PET-CT to gadolinium-enhanced MRI. Quant Imaging Med Surg. 2023;13(10):6863–75.

Chapter 4
Genetic Syndromes Associated with CNS Tumors

Ashutosh Mukherji and Tanvee Singla

4.1 Introduction

- Central nervous system (CNS) tumors are a rare group of malignancies associated with significant morbidity and mortality across all age groups. The highest incidence of CNS malignancies occurs in children aged 0–14 years [1].
- They account for 20–25% of all pediatric malignancies [2].
- Brain tumors may be classified as malignant or benign, with malignant tumors comprising the majority and having an incidence of 3.55 per 100,000 population. In comparison, non-malignant CNS tumors are less frequent, with an incidence of 2.6 per 100,000 population [1]. Survival varies according to histology as well as age at diagnosis in brain tumors [3].
- The most common histology seen in pediatric CNS tumors is pilocytic astrocytoma, followed by low-grade glioma, malignant glioma, and medulloblastoma.
- Among non-malignant tumors, pituitary malignancies are most common.

A. Mukherji (✉) · T. Singla
Department of Radiation Oncology, MPMMCC & HBCH, Varanasi, Units of Tata Memorial Centre and affiliated with Homi Bhabha National Institute, Mumbai, India

S. Pradhan et al. (eds.), *Evidence Based Handbook on Diagnosis and Staging in Oncology*, https://doi.org/10.1007/978-981-95-9701-7_4

Distribution of CNS Tumors

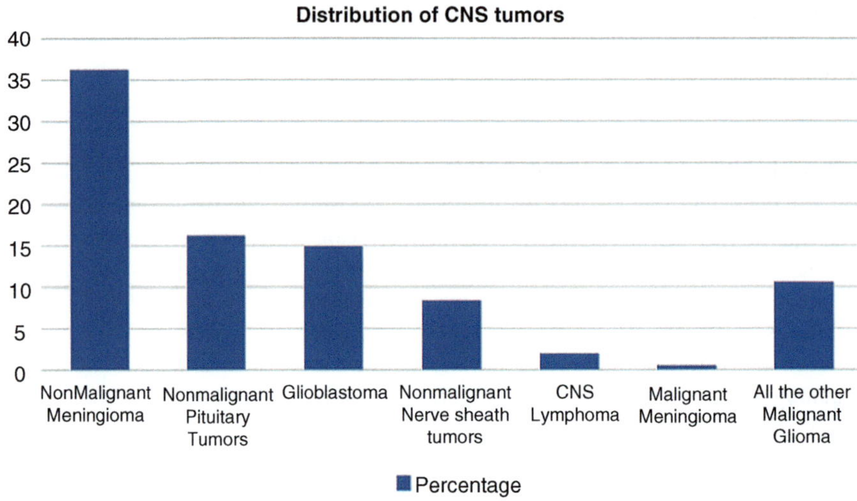

Risk Factors

- The principal etiological factors implicated in the development of CNS tumors include inherited genetic syndromes and exposure to ionizing radiation.
- The association between ionizing radiation and CNS tumors is more frequently observed in the pediatric population and demonstrates a dose-dependent relationship. For meningiomas, the excess relative risk (ERR) per gray (Gy) of ionizing radiation exposure is 4.63, whereas for gliomas, the ERR is 1.98 [4].
- Other risk factors include birth weight and non-chromosomal structural birth defects [5].
- *Various syndromes associated with CNS tumors are listed below:*

Genetic Syndromes

Syndrome	Gene involved (chromosome locus)	CNS tumors	Clinical findings and other associated features
Li-Fraumeni syndrome	TP53 (17p13)	Astrocytoma; cPNET; Medulloblastoma, choroid plexus tumor	Osteosarcoma, acute leukemia Breast cancer and adrenal cortical tumors
Cowden syndrome	PTEN (10q23)	Dysplastic cerebellar gangliocytoma	Melanoma Breast cancer Endometrial cancer Rectal cancer Trichilemmoma Thyroid disorders Gastrointestinal polyps Macrocephaly

Syndrome	Gene involved (chromosome locus)	CNS tumors	Clinical findings and other associated features
Von Hippel-Lindau syndrome	VHL (3p25)	Hemangioblastoma	Neuroendocrine tumor Paraganglioma Retinal tumor Clear cell RCC Pheochromocytoma Pancreatic neuroendocrine tumor
Neurofibromatosis-1	NF1 (17q11)	Optic pathway glioma and other astrocytoma	RMS Neuroblastoma Café au lait spots Neurofibroma Scoliosis Behavioral issues
Neurofibromatosis-2	NF2 (22q12)	Bilateral vestibular schwannomas, peripheral schwannomas, meningioma, astrocytoma, spinal ependymoma	Café au lait spots Neurofibroma
Goltz-Gorlin syndrome (basal cell nevus syndrome)	PTCH (9q31)	Medulloblastoma	Odontogenic keratocyst Palmar and/or plantar pits Ectopic calcifications of the falx cerebri
Tuberous sclerosis	TSC1 (9q34) TSC2 (16p13)	Sub-ependymal giant cell astrocytoma (SEGA)	Neurodevelopmental defects Renal angiomyolipoma Cardiac rhabdomyoma Ash-leaf spots Shagreen patches

4.2 Syndromes and Diagnostic Criteria

1. *Classic Li-Fraumeni Syndrome*—It is diagnosed when the person has all the following criteria
   (a) A sarcoma diagnosed before age 45.
   (b) A first-degree relative, parent, sibling, or child with any cancer before age 45.
   (c) Any cancer before age 45 or a sarcoma at any age in a first-degree or second-degree relative or grandchild.
2. *Familial Adenomatous Polyposis Syndrome*

   Evaluation of Familial Adenomatous Polyposis (FAP) Following Diagnosis by Colonoscopy

Assessment for extra-colonic manifestations of FAP is essential and should include the following:

- Upper gastrointestinal endoscopy to evaluate the stomach and duodenum, initiated between 20 and 25 years of age.
- Yearly abdominal examination to screen for the presence of desmoid tumors.
- In patients who have undergone colectomy and have a family history of desmoid tumors, postoperative abdominal imaging with computed tomography (CT) or magnetic resonance imaging (MRI) may be considered.
- Annual clinical thyroid examination along with thyroid ultrasonography for surveillance of thyroid malignancy.

No screening for CNS tumors

3. *Cowden Syndrome* [6]

Major criteria	Minor criteria
Patient must fulfill two major criteria to be diagnosed with Cowden syndrome:	Patients with one major and three of the following minor criteria or four minor criteria may be diagnosed with Cowden disease
(*One of the two must be either Lhermitte-Duclos disease or macrocephaly.)	Genitourinary tumors or malformations
Lhermitte-Duclos disease*	Lipoma
Thyroid carcinoma	Fibroma
Macrocephaly*	Mental retardation
Breast cancer	Fibrocystic disease of the breast
	Gastrointestinal hamartomas Other thyroid lesions, such as goiter Muco-cutaneous lesions or palmoplantar keratosis can meet the criteria alone if six or more are present

4. *VHL Syndrome*

   VHL can be classified as

Type 1 (without pheochromocytoma)
Type 2 (with Pheochromocytoma).
Type 2 is further classified as
Type 2A: Pheochromocytoma with CNS hemangioblastomas but no RCC.
Type 2B: Pheochromocytoma with both CNS hemangioblastomas and RCC.
Type 2C: Pheochromocytoma without hemangioblastomas or RCC

Evaluation: Clinical criteria for diagnosis

More than one CNS hemangioblastoma
OR
One CNS hemangioblastoma and a visceral manifestation of VHL
OR
Any manifestation with a family history of VHL

5. *Neurofibromatosis 1*
   Diagnostic Criteria

   A. *A Patient with no family history should have two or more of the following*:
      - Six or more café-au-lait macules over 5 mm (before puberty) and over 15 mm (after puberty)
      - Freckling in the axillary or inguinal region
      - Two or more neurofibromas of any type or one plexiform neurofibroma
      - Optic pathway glioma
      - Two or more iris Lisch nodules, choroidal abnormalities
      - A distinctive osseous lesion such as sphenoid dysplasia, bowing of the tibia, or pseudarthrosis of a long bone
      - A pathogenic *NF1* variant

   B. *A child with a positive family history can have only one or more criteria in A*

6. *Neurofibromatosis 2*
   The clinical diagnosis of NF2 is based on
   Presence of any one of the following criteria:

   - Bilateral vestibular schwannomas less than 70 years of age
   - Unilateral vestibular schwannoma before age 70 years and a first-degree relative with NF2

   Any two of the following:

   - Meningioma, schwannoma (non-vestibular), neurofibroma, glioma, cerebral calcification, cataract, and a first-degree relative to NF2 *OR* unilateral vestibular schwannoma and negative LZTR1 testing
   - Multiple meningiomas and unilateral vestibular schwannoma or any two of the following: schwannoma (non-vestibular), neurofibroma, glioma, cerebral calcification, and cataract
   - Constitutional or mosaic pathogenic *NF2* gene mutation from the blood or by the identification of an identical mutation from two separate tumors in the same individual

7. *Goltz-Gorlin Syndrome or Basal Cell Naevus Syndrome (BCNS)*
   Diagnosis of BCNS requires the presence of two major or one major and two minor clinical criteria [7].

   Major criteria: Multiple (>2) BCCs or 1 BCC by ≤20 years of age, odontogenic keratocysts of the jaw proven by histology, palmar or plantar pitting, bilamellar calcification of the falx cerebri, bifid/fused/splayed ribs, and a first-degree relative with BCNS.

   Minor criteria: Medulloblastoma, increased circumference of the head, congenital malformations (frontal bossing, coarse facies, cleft lip/palate, moderate or severe hypertelorism), other skeletal abnormalities (Sprengel deformity, marked pectus deformity, marked syndactyly of the digits), radiologic abnormalities (bridging of the sella turcica, hemivertebrae, fusion or elongation of the vertebral bodies, modeling defects of the hands and feet, or flame-shaped lucencies of the hands or feet), and ovarian and cardiac fibromas.

8. *Tuberous Sclerosis* [8]

   Diagnostic criteria for tuberous sclerosis include the following major and minor features:

   Major features

   - Hypomelanotic macules (>2, at least 5 mm in diameter)
   - Angiofibromas (>2) or a fibrous cephalic plaque
   - Ungual fibromas (>1)
   - Shagreen patch
   - Multiple retinal hamartomas
   - Cortical dysplasias
   - Subependymal nodules
   - Subependymal giant cell astrocytoma
   - Cardiac rhabdomyoma
   - Lymphangioleiomyomatosis
   - Angiomyolipomas (>1)

   Minor features

   - Confetti skin lesions
   - Dental enamel pits (>3)
   - Intraoral fibromas (>1)
   - Retinal achromic patch
   - Multiple renal cysts
   - Nonrenal hamartomas

A confirmed diagnosis is made when a patient demonstrates either two major criteria or one major criterion accompanied by at least two minor criteria. A diagnosis is considered "possible" when a patient presents with one major criterion or with two or more minor criteria.

References

1. Ostrom QT, Patil N, Cioffi G, Waite K, Kruchko C, Barnholtz-Sloan JS. CBTRUS statistical report: primary brain and other central nervous system tumors diagnosed in the United States in 2013–2017. Neuro-Oncology. 2020;22(12 Suppl 2):iv1–iv96. https://doi.org/10.1093/neuonc/noaa200.
2. Gittleman HR, Ostrom QT, Rouse CD, et al. Trends in central nervous system tumor incidence relative to other common cancers in adults, adolescents, and children in the United States, 2000 to 2010. Cancer. 2015;121:102–12.
3. Surawicz TS, Davis F, Freels S, Laws ER Jr, Menck HR. Brain tumor survival: results from the National Cancer Data Base. J Neuro-Oncol. 1998;40(2):151–60. https://doi.org/10.1023/a:1006091608586.
4. Ostrom QT, Adel Fahmideh M, Cote DJ, et al. Risk factors for childhood and adult primary brain tumors. Neuro-Oncology. 2019;21:1357–75.

5. Georgakis MK, Kalogirou EI, Liaskas A, et al. Anthropometrics at birth and risk of a primary central nervous system tumour: a systematic review and meta-analysis. Eur J Cancer. 2017;75:117–31.
6. Eng C. Will the real Cowden syndrome please stand up: revised diagnostic criteria. J Med Genet. 2000;37(11):828–30. https://doi.org/10.1136/jmg.37.11.828. PMID: 11073535; PMCID: PMC1734465.
7. Kimonis VE, Goldstein AM, Pastakia B, Yang ML, Kase R, DiGiovanna JJ, et al. Clinical manifestations in 105 persons with nevoid basal cell carcinoma syndrome. Am J Med Genet. 1997;69(3):299–308.
8. Northrup H, Krueger DA; International Tuberous Sclerosis Complex Consensus Group. Tuberous sclerosis complex diagnostic criteria update: recommendations of the 2012 International Tuberous Sclerosis Complex Consensus Conference. Pediatr Neurol. 2013;49(4):243–54.

Chapter 5
Evaluation of Patients in Follow-Up After Treatment of CNS Tumors

Supriya Mallick, Aashita, and Abhilash Dagar

The aim of evaluation in patients with brain tumors who have completed treatment is to monitor disease recurrence, manage late treatment-related side effects, and improve quality of life.

The tools for such evaluation would be:

1. History and physical examination
2. Neuro-imaging
3. Blood tests
4. Rehabilitation exercises, physiotherapy, yoga, speech therapy, etc.
5. Management of chronic medicines

When and how to follow up varies with the tumor type.

5.1 Follow-Up

The first follow-up should be scheduled after 4–6 weeks of completion of radiation. On this day, the patient should be evaluated clinically for symptoms suggesting residual disease or radiation-associated toxicities.

Frequency of neuroimaging is suggested based on the grade of the primary tumor, with a shorter follow-up interval for high-grade tumors or if symptoms recur.

Assessment of hypothalamic-pituitary axis (HPA)-associated hormones should be evaluated and monitored if the radiation dose delivered to the HPA was higher than 30 Gy, with worsening of levels over time.

S. Mallick (✉) · Aashita · A. Dagar
Department of Radiation Oncology, AIIMS, New Delhi, India

Department of Radiation Oncology, National Cancer Institute, AIIMS, New Delhi, India

S. Pradhan et al. (eds.), *Evidence Based Handbook on Diagnosis and Staging in Oncology*, https://doi.org/10.1007/978-981-95-9701-7_5

5.2 Symptoms of Recurrence

Symptoms can mimic those of the primary diagnosis or be of higher intensity, including headaches, seizures, feeling of being sick, drowsiness, loss of consciousness, diplopia or blurring of vision, and changes in speech and mood.

5.3 Symptoms of Radiation-Associated Toxicities

Anatomic location	Time	Injury
Brain	Acute injury (days to weeks after RT)	Fatigue, headache, anorexia, nausea, and vomiting Worsening of pre-existing neurologic symptoms Acute encephalopathy
	Early delayed injury (1–6 months after RT)	Fatigue, headache, anorexia, nausea, and vomiting Worsening of pre-existing neurologic symptoms Acute encephalopathy Somnolence syndrome Pseudo-progression Brainstem syndrome—ataxia, dysarthria, diplopia, nystagmus, and hearing loss
	Late delayed injury (>6 months after RT)	Delayed cognitive impairment that varies from mild memory loss to severe dementia Leukoencephalopathy Radiation necrosis (symptoms depend on the location of the lesion and can include focal neurologic deficits or more generalized signs and symptoms of increased intracranial pressure) Cerebrovascular complications Arteritis Intracranial aneurysm Cavernous malformation (hemorrhagic vasculopathy) Stroke-like migraine attacks after RT (SMART syndrome) Mineralizing micro-angiopathy—dystrophic calcification Chronic expanding encapsulated hematoma Cranial nerve impairment Endocrine complications Radiation-induced secondary normal pressure hydrocephalus—(progressive memory loss, reduced attention, gait difficulties, urinary incontinence, and fatigue) Secondary neoplasms

Anatomic location	Time	Injury
Spine	Early delayed injury (1–6 months after RT)	Lhermitte sign
	Late delayed injury (>6 months after RT)	Osteoradionecrosis Spinal cord myelopathy Secondary neoplasms

5.4 Neurological Examination

1. Performance status
2. Alertness, consciousness, and orientation
3. Higher mental function—memory, mathematical calculation, and attention
4. Sensory and motor function examination of limbs
5. Gait
6. Cranial nerve examination
7. Ophthalmological and PTA examination
8. Reflexes—superficial and deep reflexes
9. Signs of meningeal irritation
10. Growth monitoring with growth charts in case of pediatric patients
11. Signs of attaining puberty in case of pediatric patients
12. Neuropsychological assessment with MMSE

5.5 Neurological Imaging

	Characteristics	T1W + contrast	T2W	DWI/ADC	MRS	MRP	PET-CT	SPECT-CT
Progression	Can occur any time after treatment	Heterogeneous contrast enhancement seen in the tumor, Ring-like enhancement seen	Hyperintense core, surrounding edema	Hypointense signal surrounding Hyperintense core, decreased diffusion around the ring Low ADC value (~1.7)	Increased choline (3.2 ppm), choline/creatine ratio—1.17, and choline/NAA ratio >1.11 Lactate/lipid can increase in GBM Myo-inositol (3.5 ppm) can increase in low-grade glioma and decrease in high-grade glioma	Increased blood volume Elevated rCBV, k-trans	Higher local radiotracer uptake is proportional to local perfusion, with higher sensitivity and better resolution	Higher local radiotracer uptake is proportional to local perfusion
Pseudo progression	Seen more in MGMT methylated tumors who received radiation with concurrent temozolamide	Ring-like enhancement	Hyperintense around the ring	Increased diffusion around the ring	Elevated lipid signals Low Cho/NAA ratio	Lower rCBV compared with regions of viable tumor	Will have reduced uptake	Will have reduced radio-tracer uptake

	Characteristics	T1W + contrast	T2W	DWI/ADC	MRS	MRP	PET-CT	SPECT-CT
Radiation necrosis	Months–years after RT	Central hypodensity, ring enhancement, high edema to enhancing tumor ratio Swiss cheese pattern Seen in the region of high radiation dose	"Cut pepper" or "soap bubble–like" or "Swiss cheese–like" appearance	Higher ADC (~2.3)	Increased lipid/lactate peak; decreased NAA, choline, and creatine peaks Low cho/NAA <1.11 and cho/creat <1.17	rCBV <0.6, higher fractional anisotropy value—0.89 ± 0.15	Low uptake	Low uptake
Contrast agents used		Gadolinium is used					11C-methionine (MET), PSMA, F18-DOPA, and F18-FET/FLT, DOTA-PET	99mTc-GHA is used

5.6 SPECT-CT Images (Fig. 5.1)

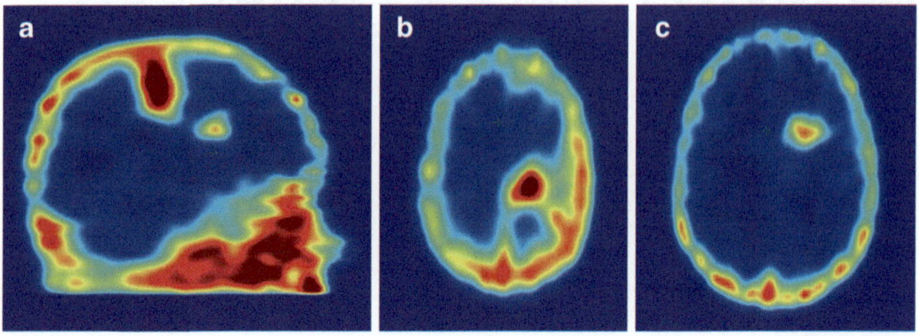

Fig. 5.1 (**a**) A 45-year-old male with anaplastic oligodendroglioma CNS WHO Grade 3 who had undergone maximal safe resection followed by adjuvant radiation with concurrent Temozolomide. Follow-up MRI was indistinguishable between radiation necrosis and tumor recurrence. GHA-SPECT was advised, which was suggestive of multifocal viable recurrent tumor with GHA index 5.5 (**b**) and 3.8 (**c**), respectively

5.7 PSMA-PET Brain (Fig. 5.2)

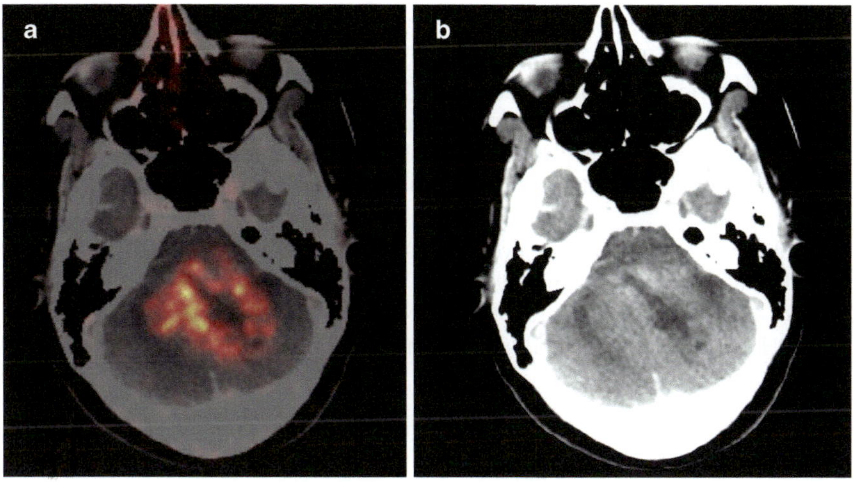

Fig. 5.2 (**a**) PSMA PET and (**b**) corresponding CT images showing disease recurrence in a case of a 25-year-old follow-up case of Medulloblastoma CNS WHO Grade 4 post maximal safe resection and adjuvant radiation and adjuvant chemotherapy. Was on regular follow-up with an interim MRI brain showed only post-treatment changes, however the patient was symptomatic hence a PSMA PET-CT was done

5.8 Blood Investigations

Disease or the treatment (surgery or radiation) can alter the hypothalamic-pituitary axis (HPA) and result in deficiencies or excesses of hormones, and that depends on the radiation dose received by the HPA.

Hormone deficiency	Observed at the radiation dose (Gy)
Growth hormone	>18
FSH/LH	>30
TSH	>30
ACTH	>30
Prolactin increase	>50

The incidence of radiation-induced hypopituitarism correlates with the time elapsed since radiation, with hormonal deficiency progressing throughout the follow-up period and largely in the first 5 years.

It has been observed that GH deficiency occurs the earliest (mean 2.6 years), with gonadotropin deficiency and hyperprolactinemia at 3.8 years, ACTH deficiency at 6 years, and TSH deficiency at 11 years. Multiple pituitary hormone deficiencies have been seen in 30–60% of patients after a follow-up period of 10 years.

5.9 Testing for Dysfunction

1. Thyroid—clinical examination, TSH, FT3, FT4 (Normal values: TSH: 0.5–4.5 mU/l; FT4: 9–24 pmol/l)
2. Growth hormone—growth assessment, IGF-1 (GH levels: normal: >6 μg/l; partial deficiency: 3–6 μg/l; severe deficiency: ≤3 μg/l)
3. LH/FSH panel—puberty assessment, LH/FSH/testosterone/estradiol (LH levels at 1–3 h > 5 IU/l; estradiol at 24 h > 50 pg/ml; testosterone in males—less than 300 ng/ml)
4. Prolactin—serum prolactin levels (Normal prolactin—<450 mU/l)
5. Adrenal—clinical examination, ACTH, and cortisol (Serum cortisol—>540 nmol/l; hypocortisolism is excluded; hypocortisolism: <100 nmol/l)
6. ADH deficiency (Serum sodium >145 meq/l; urine osmolarity <300 mosm/kg)

5.10 RANO Criteria [1]

Response Assessment in Neuro-Oncology (RANO) criteria is used as an objective tool to assess treatment response in high-grade gliomas. Response is classified based on new lesions, need for steroids, clinical status, T1 contrast, and T2/FLAIR findings on MRI brain.

Criteria [1]	Complete response	Partial response	Stable disease	Progressive disease
New lesion	Absent	Absent	Absent	Present
Steroid use	Nil or physiologic replacement	Stable or lower	Stable or decreasing	Required
Clinical status	Stable/improving	Stable/improving	Stable/improving	Worsening
T1 contrast-enhanced disease	None	≥50% decrease	<50% decrease <25% increase	>25% increase
T2/FLAIR	Improved non-enhancing	Improved non-enhancing	Stable non-enhancing	Increasing
	All features to be present	All features to be present	All features to be present	If anyone is present

5.11 Timing for Evaluation After Radiation Therapy According to RANO

The interval between completion of radiotherapy and subsequent imaging is a critical factor in the interpretation of post-treatment scans. According to the *Response Assessment in Neuro-Oncology (RANO)* criteria, the first 12 weeks following the completion of chemoradiation represent a period with a high likelihood of treatment-related imaging changes. During this time frame, radiological progression should be diagnosed only if new contrast enhancement is identified outside the irradiated volume, specifically beyond the high-dose region or the 80% isodose line.

When a new or increasing enhancement is confined within the radiation field, a diagnosis of progressive disease cannot be made on imaging alone; in such cases, definitive confirmation of viable tumor requires histopathological evidence obtained through tissue sampling.

5.12 Specific Recommendations

1. Craniospinal irradiation for medulloblastoma/embryonal tumors/choroid plexus tumors/pineal tumors

   CEMRI brain + spine every 3–4 months for 2 years, then every 6 months up to 5 years, and annually thereafter
2. Benign diseases and low-grade glioma

   CEMRI every 6 months for 2 years, then annually
3. High-grade glioma

   Every 3–4 months for 2 years, then every 6 months up to 5 years, and annually thereafter
4. Sellar tumors

   CEMRI every 6 months for 2 years, then annually

5.13 Surveillance Guidelines for Genetic Syndromes Associated with CNS Tumors [2, 3]

Syndrome	CNS tumors	Associated tumors	Surveillance
Ataxia telangiectasia	Meningioma, glioblastoma, pilocytic astrocytoma, medulloblastoma	Leukemia, lymphoma, breast, and gastric carcinomas	Annual physical examination, complete blood count, and metabolic profile

Syndrome	CNS tumors	Associated tumors	Surveillance
Cowden syndrome	Dysplastic cerebellar gangliocytoma, glial tumors	Follicular thyroid, breast, and endometrial carcinomas	1. Annual MRI breast or 2-yearly mammography 2. USG thyroid and abdomen 3. Baseline colonoscopy and skin examination
Familial adenomatous polyposis	Medulloblastoma, astrocytoma, ependymoma	Colorectal carcinoma	1. Colonoscopy at 1–2 year intervals from 10 to 12 years in suspected FAP and 18–20 years in suspected AFAP 2. Thyroid palpation and ultrasound 2–5 yearly
Hereditary non-polyposis colorectal cancer	Glioblastoma, other glial tumors	Colorectal carcinoma	1. Colonoscopy every 1–2 years from 20 to 25 years 2. TVUS, CA-125, and endometrial sampling annually from 30 to 35 years
Gorlin syndrome	Desmoplastic medulloblastoma, meningioma, oligodendroglioma, craniopharyngioma	Basal cell carcinoma, cardiac/ ovarian fibromas	1. Annual skin and dental examination 2. Pelvic USG every 3 years 3. Brain MRI every 3–5 years
Li-Fraumeni syndrome	Astrocytoma, choroid plexus carcinoma, medulloblastoma, primitive neuroectodermal tumor	Breast cancer, bone/ soft-tissue sarcomas, adrenocortical carcinoma, melanoma	1. Clinical examination every 6 months 2. Annual whole body MRI 3. Upper GI endoscopy and colonoscopy every 2–5 years 4. Annual dermatologic examination

Syndrome	CNS tumors	Associated tumors	Surveillance
Multiple endocrine neoplasia 1	Pituitary microadenoma and macroadenoma	Parathyroid adenoma, pancreatic, and duodenal neuroendocrine tumors	1. Annual calcium and PTH, gastrin, glucagon, vasointestinal polypeptide, pancreatic polypeptide, chromogranin A, insulin, fasting glucose level, prolactin, and IGF-I 2. Abdomen CT or MRI and brain MRI every 3 years
Neurofibromatosis type 1	Optic/chiasmatic gliomas, plexiform neurofibromas, pilocytic astrocytoma, glioblastoma	Leukemia, pheochromocytoma, rhabdomyosarcoma	1. Clinical examination 2. Visual screening 3. Annual MRI breast or mammography
Neurofibromatosis type 2	Vestibular schwannoma, meningioma, ependymoma	None	Annual brain and spine MRI
Tuberous sclerosis	Subependymal giant cell astrocytoma	Cardiac rhabdomyoma, renal angiomyolipoma	CEMRI of the CNS and abdomen every 1–3 years
von-Hippel Lindau	Hemangioblastoma, endolymphatic sac tumor	Clear cell RCC, renal angioma, pancreatic serous cystadenoma, pheochromocytoma	1. Annual retinal, hearing, and neurological inspection 2. CEMRI of the CNS (brain and neuroaxis), including the inner ear and abdomen 3. Annual plasma metanephrine and plasma normetanephrine 4. Annual pediatric examination

5.14 Management of Chronic Medicines

5.14.1 *Steroids*

- Prophylactic use of steroids peri-operatively or during radiation with brain tumors is not recommended.
- Patients with clinical symptoms should be treated as long as clinical benefit is observed at the minimum dose that provides sufficient symptom control with minimum side effects. They should be closely monitored with regular clinical examinations to decide whether tapering can be considered to minimize side effects. Three days may be an adequate trial for many situations (e.g., headache), with tapering soon after initiation. Steroids should be discontinued if not found to benefit within a week.
- For long-term steroid users, a dose reduction over 2–4 weeks will be appropriate, but patients with long-term steroid use may require an even longer period until complete tapering.
- Appropriate pneumocystis jiroveci prophylaxis, e.g., with trimethoprim-sulfamethoxazole, should be considered in patients requiring steroid treatment of >4 weeks, in those undergoing radiotherapy or chemotherapy, or with a lymphocyte count <1000/ml.

5.14.2 *Antiepileptics*

Prophylactic antiepileptics are not recommended in brain tumor patients. If the patient remains seizure-free for a period of 2 years after initiation of antiepileptics, they can be tapered and stopped.

5.14.3 *Class of Antiepileptic Drugs and Side Effects [3, 4]*

Drugs	Mechanism of action	Side effects
Carbamazepine	Voltage-gated Na^+ channel blockade	Sedation, drowsiness, cognitive dysfunction, ataxia, blurred vision, hypersensitivity reactions, bone density loss, dilutional hyponatremia (increased ADH secretion), hepatotoxicity, leukopenia, hematological toxicity (aplastic anemia, agranulocytosis, potent inducer of metabolizing enzyme)
Clobazam	Prolongs GABA-A Cl– opening	Sedation, lethargy, tolerance, dependence
Clonazepam	Prolongs GABA-A Cl– opening	Sedation, lethargy, tolerance, dependence

Drugs	Mechanism of action	Side effects
Ethosuximide	T-type (low-voltage-activated) Ca^{2+} channel blockade	Nausea, anorexia, mood changes, headaches, lethargy
Gabapentin	Binds α2-δ subunit of L-type voltage-regulated Ca^{2+} channels (high-voltage activated class)	Sedation, dizziness, ataxia, nystagmus
Levetiracetam	SV2A synaptic vesicle protein 2A inhibitor	Sedation, dizziness, weakness, irritability, hallucinations
Phenytoin	Voltage-gated Na^{+} channel blockade	Ataxia, vertigo, diplopia, nystagmus, tissue overgrowth (gingival hirsutism), megaloblastic anemia, altered vitamin D metabolism, altered folate metabolism, a weak inducer of drugs metabolism, fetal malformation
Pregabalin	Binds the α2-δ subunit of L-type voltage-gated Ca^{2+} channels	Sedation, dizziness, ataxia, nystagmus
Valproic acid	Increased GABA-ergic transmission. Reduced release and/or effects of excitatory amino acids (NMDA?) voltage-gated Na^{+} channel blockade. Modulation of dopaminergic and serotonergic transmission	Vomiting, nausea, alopecia, curling of hairs, hepatotoxicity, pancreatitis, rashes, obesity, increased ammonia, teratogenic (causes neural tube defects), thrombocytopenia, enzyme inhibitor, weight gain, drowsiness, tremor

5.15 Management of Radiation-Induced Endocrinopathy [5]

Deranged hormone profile as a result of radiation to the hypothalamo-pituitary axis (HPA) needs evaluation and management as follows:

Hormone deficiency	Management	Contra-indications
Growth hormone	Dose—Initially 150–300 μg/day; gradually increased if required Maximum—1 mg/day Used at the minimum effective dose Required dose may decrease with age	Active malignancy, intracranial hypertension
FSH/LH/testosterone	Females: Pre-menopausal—Combined estrogen and progesterone Post-menopausal—Estrogen alone Males—Testosterone replacement	Females—VTE Males—Breast cancer in men, prostate cancer, history of primary liver tumors, hypercalcemia, and nephrotic syndrome
ACTH	15–25 mg hydrocortisone/day in two to three divided doses	–

Hormone deficiency	Management	Contra-indications
Thyroid	Levothyroxine replacement (FT4 level in the upper quartile of the normal range)	In panhypopituitarism or adrenal insufficiency, corticosteroid therapy is initiated before starting thyroxine
Prolactin	Dopamine agonist (cabergoline) Dose—Started at 0.25 mg twice a week Dose is increased in increments of 0.25 mg twice a week, no more frequently than every 4 weeks, depending on the patient's prolactin level Maximum dose—1 mg twice a week	–

5.16 Neurocognition

Neurocognitive assessment should be done at baseline and on follow-up after radiation to monitor the decline in various cognitive domains.

1. Due to surgery

   Depends on the site of the tumor.

   Cognitive alterations are observed in 15–50% of patients.

   Attention and information processing speed are the most frequently declined cognitive domains.
2. Due to radiation

   Depends on the total dose of radiation, dose per fraction, use of concurrent chemotherapy, time since treatment, use of concurrent antiepileptics, and steroids.

   Cognitive alterations are observed in 50–90% of patients.

   Domains affected by radiation are verbal and non-verbal memory, executive function, attention, and information processing speed.

5.17 Workup of Cognitive Decline

Symptoms of cognitive decline need to be evaluated, and the affected domain should be identified.

1. CE MRI with perfusion with spectroscopy Brain (to rule out residual/recurrence)
2. Change antiepileptics (side effects of antiepileptics include drowsiness and cognitive decline. Use of newer antiepileptics can help reduce those side effects, e.g., levetiracetam)

3. Reduce the dose of steroids if possible, as it has been observed that long-term use of steroids leads to memory loss (Mechanism—Prolonged exposure to glucocorticoids inhibits glucose utilization, which increases the concentration of glutamate and leads to excitotoxic neuronal death. It also reduces synaptic plasticity in hippocampal neurons)
4. Check hormonal profile—Serum TSH, cortisol, testosterone
5. Check nutritional deficiency—Serum folate/B12

5.18 Management of Cognitive Decline

1. Fatigue—Patient encouraged for regular physical exercise and sleep hygiene. Armodafinil, a CNS stimulant, can be used at 150 mg OD 1 h before work.
2. Memory loss—Memantine 5 mg OD or Donepezil 5 mg OD can be used. The patient would need help from family and social support.
3. Attention deficit—Psychological counselling and behavioral therapy are helpful. Methylphenidate 20 mg OD can be used.

References

1. Leao DJ, Craig PG, Godoy LF, Leite CC, Policeni B. Response assessment in neuro-oncology criteria for gliomas: practical approach using conventional and advanced techniques. Am J Neuroradiol. 2019;41(1):10–20. https://doi.org/10.3174/ajnr.a6358.
2. Vijapura C, Saad Aldin E, Capizzano AA, Policeni B, Sato Y, Moritani T. Genetic syndromes associated with central nervous system tumors. Radiographics. 2017;37(1):258–80. https://doi.org/10.1148/rg.2017160057.
3. Mallick S, Giridhar P, Rath GK. Evidence based practice in neuro-oncology. 1st ed. Springer; 2021. https://doi.org/10.1007/978-981-16-2659-3.
4. Chong DJ, Lerman AM. Practice update: review of anticonvulsant therapy. Curr Neurol Neurosci Rep. 2016;16(4):39. https://doi.org/10.1007/s11910-016-0640-y.
5. Sathyapalan T, Dixit S. Radiotherapy-induced hypopituitarism: a review. Expert Rev Anticancer Ther. 2012;12(5):669–83. https://doi.org/10.1586/era.12.27.

Chapter 6
Evaluation and Staging in Nasopharyngeal Cancer

Sambit Swarup Nanda and Samapika Bhaumik

6.1 Introduction and Epidemiology

Nasopharyngeal carcinoma (NPC) is a rare malignancy globally, with age-standardized rates generally below 1 per 100,000 person-years. It is most commonly observed in the Cantonese population of southern China, and intermediate rates are found in indigenous populations in Southeast Asia, the Arctic region, North Africa, and the Middle East [1]. As per GLOBOCAN 2020, the incidence of NPC worldwide was 1,33,354 and an estimated 80,008 deaths occurred from it, making it the 22nd most common cancer and 21st most common cause of cancer death worldwide [2]. NPC is most commonly found in Asia, specifically eastern and southern China (including Hong Kong), Singapore, Vietnam, and the Philippines.

6.2 Risk Factors for Nasopharyngeal Cancers

There are a variety of risk factors contributing to nasopharyngeal carcinoma, some modifiable and some non-modifiable. Non-modifiable factors include male gender (2–3 times more than females), age, family history, and ethnicity. Modifiable risk factors can be diet, smoking, alcohol consumption, and some viral infections like EBV and HPV. Diets rich in salt-cured fish and meats increase the risk of NPC, while diets rich in fruits, vegetables, nuts, and low dairy products confer some protection from NPC, as per some studies [3]. Nitrosamine in salted foods is considered a probable carcinogen. Infection by certain strains of EBV and HPV and consumption of tobacco and alcohol have also been linked to NPC [3].

S. S. Nanda (✉) · S. Bhaumik
Department of Radiation Oncology, MPMMCC/HBCH Varanasi, Units of Tata Memorial Centre; Also affliated with Homi Bhabha National Institute, Mumbai, India

S. Pradhan et al. (eds.), *Evidence Based Handbook on Diagnosis and Staging in Oncology*, https://doi.org/10.1007/978-981-95-9701-7_6

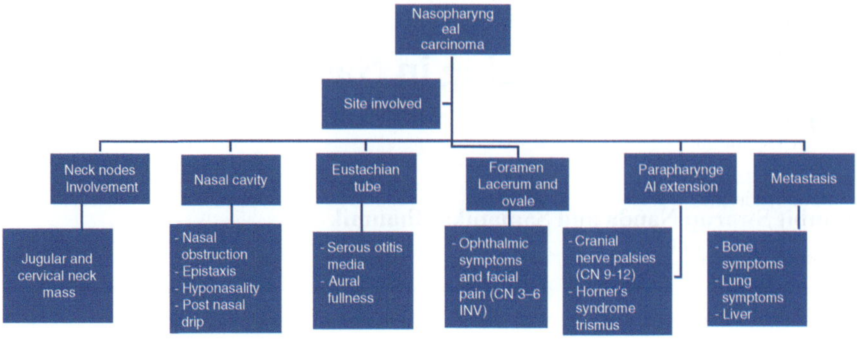

Fig. 6.1 Sitewise symptomatology of NPC [8]

6.3 Clinical Presentation

The clinical features at presentation in a patient with nasopharyngeal carcinoma (NPC) largely depend on the area of involvement of the disease. The most common site of origin is the lateral aspect of the nasopharynx and the fossa of Rosenmuller. The various clinical features according to the sites of involvement are summarized in Fig. 6.1.

6.3.1 Nasal Symptoms

These include nasal obstruction, epistaxis, post-nasal drip, hypo nasal speech, or cacosmia. Nasal obstruction is one of the most common symptoms associated with NPC. The severity of the symptoms is indicative of the size of growth and the extent of local involvement.

6.3.2 Otological Symptoms

Due to the growing mass obstructing the outflow of the eustachian tube, patients may present with symptoms secondary to it, such as conductive hearing loss, middle ear effusion, or aural fullness. An adult with unilateral middle ear effusion must be evaluated by direct visualization of the nasopharynx to exclude a neoplasm. Depending upon the extent of the disease, unilateral or bilateral hearing loss may be the presenting symptom.

6.3.3 Neurological Symptoms

Intracranial extension is prevalent among a small proportion of the patients, and almost 10–20% of NPC may have various cranial nerve palsy as the presenting symptom [4]. Depending upon cranial nerve involvement, patients may present with the associated symptoms like ophthalmoplegia, facial pain, and blurry vision. Extension of NPC to the foramen of lacerum and further to involve the cavernous sinus may involve the oculomotor nerve, the trigeminal nerve, and the ophthalmic and maxillary branches of the trigeminal nerve. Other routes of intracranial extension are through the foramen ovale or direct extension through base of skull erosion. This can lead to impaired vision, reduced facial sensation, and impaired swallowing functions, leading to NPC-related morbidity.

6.3.4 Nodal Involvement

Cervical nodal involvement is one of the most common presentations in NPC. Lymph nodes of the apex of the posterior triangle and the upper jugular are initially most commonly involved, together with retropharyngeal nodes [5].

Out of these symptoms, the most common clinical findings in NPC are a fast-growing neck mass (frequently localized in the posterior neck triangle and upper jugular chain) (63–76%), nasal symptoms (70–73%), aural symptoms (62–73%), and symptoms associated with CN involvement (20–26%) [6, 7].

6.4 Evaluation in the Clinic

Patients with NPC tend to present to an otolaryngologist initially since symptoms are predominantly limited to the head and neck region.

Based on nasal symptoms, differentials like nasal polyp, otitis media, nasal papilloma, nasopharyngeal angiofibroma, or NPC can be considered as differentials. Other infective differentials like rhinosporidiosis, mycobacterial infection, and malignancies like lymphoma could be kept as probable based on initial presentation with enlarged cervical lymphadenopathy.

Patients with cranial neuropathy tend to present to neurologists. Cavernous sinus thrombosis, intracranial bleed, or thrombus remain differentials in patients with such a presentation.

The first step for any patient would be to take a proper history and perform a general examination, followed by a thorough cranial nerve examination as well as nasopharyngoscopy (as the symptoms would dictate). These would include neck palpation to see the neck node levels, their size and numbers, consistency, tenderness, and fixity to adjoining structures. Cranial nerve examination will help in assessing cranial nerve involvement.

In most of the other differentials, the symptoms will be very specific and localized, while a myriad of symptoms involving multiple areas like the neck nodes, cranial nerves, and the ear, all at the same time, should raise most suspicion about a more invasive and extensive differential like malignancy.

Percussion and auscultation of the chest, palpation of the abdomen for possible liver involvement, and percussion of the spine and bones for possible bone metastasis should also be performed, keeping NPC in mind.

Routine blood tests like complete blood count, coagulation profile, viral markers, and liver and kidney function tests need to be done prior to any invasive procedure to establish the baseline fitness and feasibility for biopsy and to get an insight into the presence of any infective foci.

Direct visualization of the disease can help us differentiate between certain differentials upfront based on their characteristic appearances. Procedures as simple as indirect laryngoscopy, or a fiber optic rhinoscopy and nasopharyngoscopy on an outpatient basis, can help in revealing the presence of a mass lesion. Nasopharyngoscopy is the procedure of choice, which not only acts as a great visualization tool but also doubles down as a method to take a biopsy from the visible mass, which will finally prove the diagnosis. This can be performed with local anesthesia in an OPD setting, but biopsy by direct visualization with general anesthesia may be necessary for diagnosis when the tumor is not visible or when the patient cannot cooperate. This can further help in detecting the mucosal extension of the disease, helping to see the vascularity to take a call on the biopsy, as lesions like nasopharyngeal angiofibroma are highly vascular and may lead to excessive bleeding. Direct visualization helps in taking a directed biopsy while avoiding necrotic foci to establish the histopathological confirmation. For suspicious cases of a nasopharyngeal primary tumor with a lack of visible tumor, random biopsies of the most commonly involved sites are warranted: pharyngeal recess (fossa of Rosenmüller) on each of the lateral walls and the superior–posterior wall of the nasopharynx. Fine needle aspiration of a suspicious neck mass may establish the presence of metastatic nasopharyngeal carcinoma in the regional lymphatics.

EBV, which has been associated with NPC as an etiological factor, has been established both as a diagnostic and prognostic factor. The intimate association of EBV with nasopharyngeal carcinoma can serve as a marker for NPC diagnosis. Studies revealed that elevated and sustained EBV-VCA (viral capsid antigen) IgA antibody levels precede the clinical onset of NPC, suggesting that EBV-VCA IgA can be used as an early marker of NPC [9]. In a study conducted by Lin et al., it was found that overall survival ($P < 0.001$) and relapse-free survival ($P = 0.02$) were significantly lower among patients with pretreatment plasma EBV DNA concentrations of at least 1500 copies per milliliter than among those with concentrations of less than 1500 copies per milliliter. Patients with persistently detectable plasma EBV DNA had significantly worse overall survival ($P < 0.001$) and relapse-free survival ($P < 0.001$) than patients with undetectable EBV DNA 1 week after the completion of radiotherapy. Thus, a baseline test of plasma EBV DNA can be used as an indicator for prognosis, and can also work as a surveillance tool in a posttreatment setting [10].

6.5 Imaging

Once the histopathological reports have confirmed the presence of NPC, the next step is to do tumor mapping, which can be done on the basis of radiological tests. The most commonly used radiological investigations are computed tomography (CT) and magnetic resonance imaging (MRI). The CT scan allows better visualization of the lytic and sclerotic components of the anatomical extension of NPC [11]. However, its utility is limited by the ability to detect bone marrow invasion and neural foramina extension, specifically without cortical bone destruction. MRI has better sensitivity in detecting early bone marrow invasion. The MRI interpretation of marrow invasion can be distorted by peritumoral inflammation, which obscures MR images, resulting in false positive findings [12–14].

The sensitivity and specificity of CT and MRI have been under evaluation in NPC. As per the study by Ng et al., the following was the difference between CT and MRI of the head and neck in NPC [15].

Feature detected	Sensitivity	
	MRI (%)	CT (%)
Skull base involvement	60	40
Intracranial involvement	57	36
Retropharyngeal node	58	21
Tumor infiltration of prevertebral muscles (i.e., longus colli muscles) (vs.)	51	22

Due to features like these, MRI is considered the imaging technique of choice, while CT does still make an acceptable alternative.

The rate of systemic metastasis in NPC can go up to 41%, which is significantly higher than other head and neck subsites (5–24%), with bone and lung being the most predominant sites of metastasis [16]. Thus, evaluation not only on the primary site but also on the metastatic site remains pivotal for proper management of NPC. For patients with deranged liver function test values during the routine investigations and those who present with clinical features suggestive of liver or lung metastasis, contrast-enhanced CT thorax and abdomen can help indicate the exact location and size of the lesion. In patients with advanced locoregional disease or symptoms suggestive of bone metastasis or an elevated serum alkaline phosphatase, a bone scan is a useful technique. Traditionally, chest X-ray, CT images, and bone scan have been used to detect metastatic lesions in NPC. However, newer imaging modalities have evolved with better sensitivity and specificity for the same.

Functional imaging like [18^F] fluorodeoxyglucose positron emission tomography (FDG)-PET provides a one-stop solution to evaluate all the metastatic sites in one investigation. 18^FFDG-PET has been found to be better than conventional workup (i.e., chest X-ray, isotope bone scan, and abdominal ultrasound) in the detection of distant metastases. PET scan can offer a sensitivity and specificity of 100% and 90.1%, respectively [17]. A meta-analysis by Chen et al. compared CT, MRI, and PET CT for local and systemic disease detection in NPC. They demonstrated a higher sensitivity of CT (92%) compared to MRI (88%) and PET CT (88%) for cervical nodal detections [18]. NG et al. showed that PET CT has better accuracy than MRI for cervical nodal staging, but did not have contrast resolution to identify retropharyngeal nodes merged with the primary tumor [19]. In the Chen meta-analysis, the sensitivity of PET CT (82%) was higher than that of CT (80%) and MRI (53%) for the detection of distant metastasis. A similar finding of higher sensitivity with PET compared to CT and MRI was observed in the Senft study [20].

Among the newer modalities, whole body MRI and dual energy CT have been under evaluation in NPC. In a recent study, Zhan et al. compared dual-energy CT vis-à-vis simulated single-energy CT and MRI for skull base invasion in NPC. They showed higher sensitivity (90.74%) vs. CT (75%) and MRI (84.26%) (both $P < 0.001$). The specificity also improved from 93.23% (CT) and 93.75% (MRI) to 95.31% in dual-energy CT [21], thus making it a viable alternative to MRI in base of skull invasion. However, its utility is yet to be established on a large scale. Whole body contrast-enhanced MRI has been advocated as a viable alternative to PET CT for detecting distant metastasis. Recently, a meta-analysis by Li et al. evaluated five studies of head and neck cancers and showed similar sensitivity (0.82 vs. 0.81) and specificity (0.97 vs. 0.98) with PET CT versus contrast-enhanced MRI [22]. The use of whole-body contrast-enhanced MRI has been limited by the long time required for the imaging and the motion artifact associated with it. Some early studies have evaluated the clinical application of simultaneous whole-body ^{18}F-FDG PET/MRI as a one-stop imaging modality in the primary staging of NPC, both for primary and distant metastasis. Chan et al. evaluated it in 113 patients with NPC. PET/MR was more apparent than PET CT for primary tumor mapping, specifically for intracranial extension. N staging had higher sensitivity (99.5% vs. 94.2%) and was more useful for retropharyngeal nodes. For detecting metastatic lesions, sensitivity was similar for PET MRI and PET CT [23].

For staging of NPC, the two most commonly used systems are AJCC and Ho's staging system. Both come with advantages and drawbacks of their own and require certain investigations, which, if done at the initial stages of the patient presentation itself, can further expedite the treatment procedure. The following table has a comparison between the two systems [24, 25].

6.6 Staging and imaging recommendations

T/N/M stage	AJCC eighth edition	Ho staging	Investigation of choice
TX	Primary tumor cannot be assessed	–	MRI > CT scan
T0	No tumor identified, but EBV-positive cervical node(s) involvement	–	
Tis	Tumor in situ	–	
T1	Tumor confined to the nasopharynx, or extension to the oropharynx and/or the nasal cavity without parapharyngeal involvement	Tumor confined to the nasopharynx (space behind the choanal orifices and nasal septum, and above the posterior margin of the soft palate in the resting position)	
T2	Tumor with extension to the parapharyngeal space and/or adjacent soft tissue involvement (medial pterygoid, lateral pterygoid, prevertebral muscles)	Tumor extended to the nasal fossa, oropharynx, or adjacent muscles or nerves below the base of the skull	
T3	Tumor with infiltration of bony structures in the skull base, cervical vertebra, pterygoid structures, and/or paranasal sinuses	Tumor extending beyond T2 limits and sub-classified as follows: T3a bone involvement below the base of the skull (including floor of sphenoid sinus) T3b involvement of thc base of the skull T3c involvement of cranial nerve(s) T3d involvement of the orbit, laryngopharynx (hypopharynx) or infratemporal fossa	
T4	Tumor with intracranial extension, involvement of cranial nerves, hypopharynx, orbit, parotid gland, and/or extensive soft tissue infiltration beyond the lateral surface of the lateral pterygoid muscle		
NX	Regional lymph nodes cannot be assessed		
N0	No regional lymph node metastasis	No palpable nodes (excluding nodes thought to be benign)	
N1	Unilateral metastasis in cervical lymph node(s) and/or unilateral or bilateral metastasis in retropharyngeal lymph node(s), 6 cm or smaller in greatest dimension, above the caudal border of cricoid cartilage	Ni node(s) wholly in the upper cervical. Level, bounded below by the neck crease extending laterally and backwards from or just below the thyroid notch (laryngeal eminence)	

T/N/M stage	AJCC eighth edition	Ho staging	Investigation of choice
N2	Bilateral metastasis in cervical lymph node(s), 6 cm or smaller in the greatest dimension, above the caudal border of the cricoid cartilage	N2 palpable node(s) between the crease and the supraclavicular fossa, the upper limit being a line joining the upper margin of the sternal end of the clavicle and the apex of an angle formed by the lateral surface of the neck and the superior margin of the trapezius	
N3	Unilateral or bilateral metastasis in the cervical lymph node(s), larger than 6 cm in greatest dimension, and/ or extension below the caudal border of the cricoid cartilage	N3 palpable nude(s) in the supraclavicular fossa and or skin involvement in the form of carcinoma en cuirasse or satellite nodules above the clavicles	

6.7 Other Investigations

Some other tests that can be done in the initial stages of patient management, once the diagnosis is confirmed, which might come in handy in the later stages, but save some time both for the patient and the physician. For instance, once the diagnosis of NPC is confirmed, it may be anticipated that the patient may land up with ototoxicity at the end of the treatment, either owing to radiation therapy or more so due to the use of cisplatin (ototoxicity seen in around 36% adult patients and 40–60% pediatric patients) [26] as a concurrent chemotherapeutic agent used rather commonly in the treatment of NPC [27]. Hearing loss post radiotherapy through the conventional technique, along with concurrent chemotherapy, can range from 5% to 82% of patients, while with IMRT and concurrent chemo, it ranges from 37% to 42% [28]. Thus, getting a baseline pure tone audiometry (PTA) post the confirmation of NPC, before starting the treatment, is a wise step. Similarly, it is possible that the patient post-treatment for NPC may get endocrine dysfunction, due to the radiotherapy (as commonly as 82% as per some studies) [29, 30]. Thus, getting a baseline hormonal panel including growth hormone, thyroid-stimulating hormone, cortisol, LH, and FSH (for females) and testosterone levels (for males) at the initial stages of patient visit would be helpful in serving as a baseline.

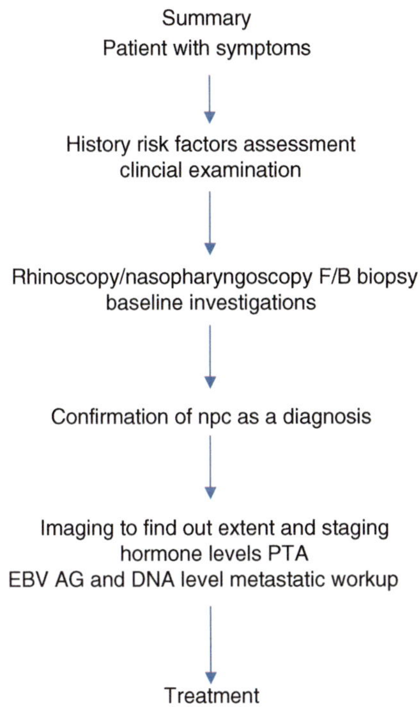

References

1. Chang ET, Ye W, Zeng YX, Adami HO. The evolving epidemiology of nasopharyngeal carcinoma. Cancer Epidemiol Biomarkers Prev. 2021;30(6):1035–47.
2. IARC [Internet]. [cited 2023 Dec 12]. Available from: https://gco.iarc.fr/today/data/factsheets/cancers/4-Nasopharynx-fact-sheet.pdf.
3. American Cancer Society. The requested resource was not found [Internet]. [cited 2023 Jul 2]. Available from: https://www.cancer.org/content/dam/CRC/PDF/Public/8754.00.pdf.
4. Denton AJ, Khunger A, Reyes-Corcho A. Case of nasopharyngeal carcinoma presenting with rare combination of multiple cranial nerve palsies. Cureus. 2021;13(12):e20357.
5. Shah AB, Nagalli S. Nasopharyngeal carcinoma. In: StatPearls [Internet]. Treasure Island: StatPearls Publishing; 2023. Available from: http://www.ncbi.nlm.nih.gov/books/NBK554588/.
6. Sham JST, Poon YF, Wei WI, Choy D. Nasopharyngeal carcinoma in young patients. Cancer. 1990;65(11):2606–10.
7. Wei WI, Sham JS. Nasopharyngeal carcinoma. Lancet. 2005;365(9476):2041–54.
8. Dhingra PL, Dhingra S. Diseases of ear, nose and throat. 6th ed. Elsevier; 2014.
9. Ji MF, Wang DK, Yu YL, Guo YQ, Liang JS, Cheng WM, et al. Sustained elevation of Epstein–Barr virus antibody levels preceding clinical onset of nasopharyngeal carcinoma. Br J Cancer. 2007;96(4):623–30.
10. Lin JC, Wang WY, Chen KY, Wei YH, Liang WM, Jan JS, et al. Quantification of plasma Epstein–Barr Virus DNA in patients with advanced nasopharyngeal carcinoma. N Engl J Med. 2004;350(24):2461–70.

11. Yi W, Liu ZG, Li X, Tang J, Jiang CB, Hu JY, et al. CT-diagnosed severe skull base bone destruction predicts distant bone metastasis in early N-stage nasopharyngeal carcinoma. Onco Targets Ther. 2016;9:7011–7.
12. Olmi P, Fallai C, Colagrande S, Giannardi G. Staging and follow-up of nasopharyngeal carcinoma: magnetic resonance imaging versus computerized tomography. Int J Radiat Oncol Biol Phys. 1995;32(3):795–800.
13. Becker M, Zbären P, Laeng H, Stoupis C, Porcellini B, Vock P. Neoplastic invasion of the laryngeal cartilage: comparison of MR imaging and CT with histopathologic correlation. Radiology. 1995;194(3):661–9.
14. Becker M, Zbären P, Casselman JW, Kohler R, Dulguerov P, Becker CD. Neoplastic invasion of laryngeal cartilage: reassessment of criteria for diagnosis at MR imaging. Radiology. 2008;249(2):551–9.
15. Ng SH, Chang TC, Ko SF, Yen PS, Wan YL, Tang LM, et al. Nasopharyngeal carcinoma: MRI and CT assessment. Neuroradiology. 1997;39(10):741–6.
16. Sham JST, Choy D, Choi PHK. Nasopharyngeal carcinoma: the significance of neck node involvement in relation to the pattern of distant failure. Br J Radiol. 1990;63(746):108–13.
17. Chang JTC, Chan SC, Yen TC, Liao CT, Lin CY, Lin KJ, et al. Nasopharyngeal carcinoma staging by (18)F-fluorodeoxyglucose positron emission tomography. Int J Radiat Oncol Biol Phys. 2005;62(2):501–7.
18. Chen WS, Li JJ, Hong L, Xing ZB, Wang F, Li CQ. Comparison of MRI, CT and 18F-FDG PET/CT in the diagnosis of local and metastatic of nasopharyngeal carcinomas: an updated meta analysis of clinical studies. Am J Transl Res. 2016;8(11):4532–47.
19. Ng SH, Chan SC, Yen TC, Chang JTC, Liao CT, Ko SF, et al. Staging of untreated nasopharyngeal carcinoma with PET/CT: comparison with conventional imaging work-up. Eur J Nucl Med Mol Imaging. 2009;36(1):12–22.
20. Senft A, de Bree R, Hoekstra OS, Kuik DJ, Golding RP, Oyen WJG, et al. Screening for distant metastases in head and neck cancer patients by chest CT or whole body FDG-PET: a prospective multicenter trial. Radiother Oncol. 2008;87(2):221–9.
21. Zhan Y, Wang P, Wang Y, Wang Y, Tang Z. Dual-energy CT for the detection of skull base invasion in nasopharyngeal carcinoma: comparison of simulated single-energy CT and MRI. Insights Imaging. 2023;14(1):95.
22. Li J, Zhou H, Zhang X, Song F, Pang X, Wei Z. A two-way comparison of whole-body 18 FDG PET-CT and whole-body contrast-enhanced MRI for distant metastasis staging in patients with malignant tumors: a meta-analysis of 13 prospective studies. Ann Palliat Med. 2020;9(2):24755–255.
23. Chan SC, Yeh CH, Yen TC, Ng SH, Chang JTC, Lin CY, et al. Clinical utility of simultaneous whole-body 18F-FDG PET/MRI as a single-step imaging modality in the staging of primary nasopharyngeal carcinoma. Eur J Nucl Med Mol Imaging. 2018;45(8):1297–308.
24. Amin MB, et al. AJCC cancer staging manual. 8th ed. Springer; 2018.
25. Ho JHC. Stage classification of nasopharyngeal carcinoma: a review. In: de Thé G, Ito Y, editors. Nasopharyngeal carcinoma: etiology and control. International Agency for Research on Cancer (IARC) Scientific Publication No. 20. Lyon: IARC; 1978. p. 99–113. Google Search [Internet]. [cited 2023 Aug 27].
26. Chattaraj A, Syed MP, Low CA, Owonikoko TK. Cisplatin-induced ototoxicity: a concise review of the burden, prevention, and interception strategies. JCO Oncol Pract. 2023;19(5):278–83.
27. Chan ATC, Grégoire V, Lefebvre JL, Licitra L, Hui EP, Leung SF, et al. Nasopharyngeal cancer: EHNS–ESMO–ESTRO Clinical Practice Guidelines for diagnosis, treatment and follow-up†. Ann Oncol. 2012;23:vii83–5.
28. Isaradisaikul SK, Chowsilpa S. Ototoxicity after chemoradiotherapy for nasopharyngeal carcinoma. Ann Nasopharynx Cancer. 2020;4:9.
29. Lam K, Tse V, Wang C, Yeung R, Ho J. Effects of cranial irradiation on hypothalamic-pituitary function—a 5-year longitudinal study in patients with nasopharyngeal carcinoma. Q J Med. 1991;78(2):165–76.
30. Ratnasingam J, Karim N, Paramasivam SS, Ibrahim L, Lim LL, Tan ATB, et al. Hypothalamic pituitary dysfunction amongst nasopharyngeal cancer survivors. Pituitary. 2015;18(4):448–55.

Chapter 7
Evaluation and Staging of Oropharyngeal, Laryngeal and Hypopharyngeal Cancers

Kanika Sood Sharma and Manisha Himthani

7.1 Introduction

Oropharyngeal cancers are one of the common cancers worldwide, with an annual incidence of 98,400 and mortality of 48,100, whereas the incidence of laryngeal cancer was 184,615 and hypopharyngeal cancer was 84,254 in the year 2020 [1].

7.2 Risk Factors

The risk factors for the development of cancer can be attributed to personal habits such as tobacco smoking and alcohol, which is a primary risk factor for laryngeal cancers. Other etiological agents are betel quid and tobacco chewing. Infection with human papillomavirus is a significant risk factor, particularly in oropharyngeal cancers (OPC). The incidence of HPV+ has rapidly increased over the last few decades, especially in high-income countries. AJCC in its eighth edition has unconnected the HPV+ oropharyngeal squamous cell carcinoma (OPSCC) owing to its improved prognosis [2]. In laryngeal and hypopharyngeal cancers, pack years and initial stage at presentation are important prognostic factors, and p16 has minimal implications on survival in these subsites [3].

K. S. Sharma (✉) · M. Himthani
Dharamshila Narayana Superspeciality Hospital, New Delhi, India

S. Pradhan et al. (eds.), *Evidence Based Handbook on Diagnosis and Staging in Oncology*, https://doi.org/10.1007/978-981-95-9701-7_7

7.3 Evaluation

Clinical features of these cancers are predominantly site-specific, and an elaborate history and physical examination with fiberoptic laryngoscopy is crucial in all patients. While a CT scan is preferred as the initial diagnostic evaluation tool, other modalities like MRI and PET CT offer their own set of advantages. In low-resource nations, CT scan remains the investigation of choice due to its wider availability. p16 testing with IHC is an important investigation for staging, treatment, and prognostication. Sentinel node biopsy can be a reliable test in clinical negative neck.

7.4 Clinical Features

The symptoms depend on the size and location of the primary tumor. Approximately 70% of the OPCs occur in the tonsillar region or base of tongue [4]. The symptoms vary in HPV+ and HPV− cancers.

Some of the common reported symptoms of OPC are [5] also depicted in Fig. 7.1.

(a) Neck mass (most common symptom of HPV+ OPC) (Fig. 7.2)
(b) Pain (most common symptom in HPV− OPC)
(c) Difficulty in swallowing and speech ("hot potato voice")
(d) Sensation of lump in throat

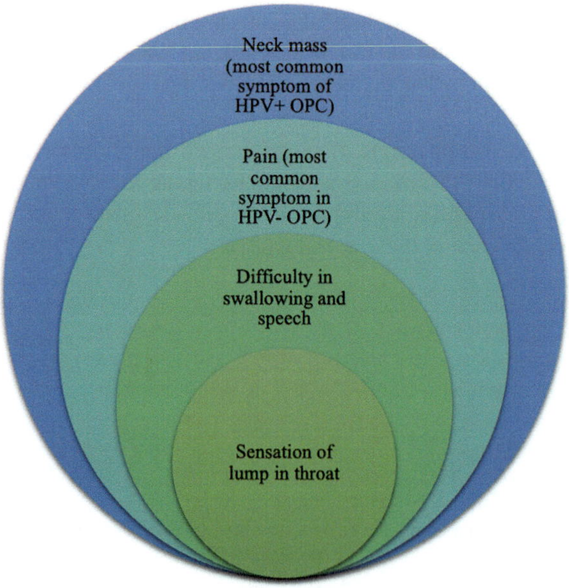

Fig. 7.1 Illustration depicting common symptoms of oropharyngeal cancers. (Original content, copyright protected, cannot be refurnished without consent)

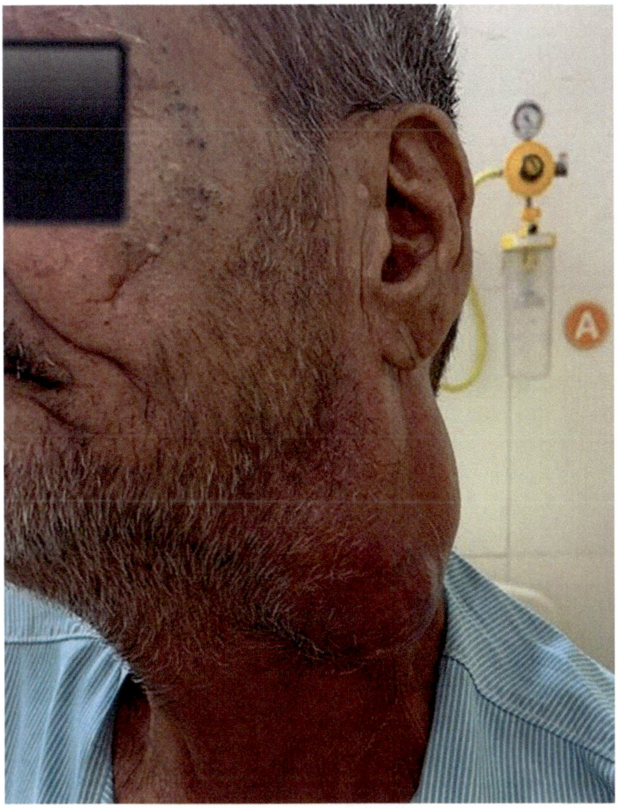

Fig. 7.2 Patient with oropharyngeal cancer presenting with a huge neck mass. (Photo credits: Dr. Amita Prakash Ambasta)

Pain can either present as local pain or a sore throat, and it might also manifest as referred pain to the ear. Other common symptoms with which the patient might present include trismus in advanced cases of OPC, supraglottic, and hypopharyngeal cancers. Halitosis can be a manifesting symptom due to secondary infection and pooling of secretions.

Systemic symptoms are fatigue and unexplained weight loss. Depending on the location of the primary tumor of OPC, symptoms are enumerated in Table 7.1.

Laryngeal and hypopharyngeal cancers commonly present with hoarse voice, coughing, difficulty in swallowing, and noisy breathing as their presenting symptoms. The symptoms, as per different subsites, are elaborated in Table 7.2.

Table 7.1 Clinical presentation according to different subsites of OPC

Subsite	Symptoms
Tonsil	Pain Difficulty in swallowing Loss of weight Otalgia Neck mass
Base of tongue	Pain Difficulty in swallowing Loss of weight Referred pain to the ear Trismus Neck mass Tongue fixation (in advanced cases) Bad breath
Vallecula	Pain Difficulty in swallowing
Soft palate	Pain Difficulty in swallowing Bad breath
Posterior pharyngeal wall (symptomatic in the advanced stage)	Pain Bleeding Difficulty in swallowing Weight loss Neck mass

Table 7.2 Clinical presentation of laryngeal and hypopharyngeal cancers

Subsite	Symptoms
Supraglottic larynx	Pain Difficulty in swallowing Loss of weight Otalgia (recurrent laryngeal nerve involvement) Neck mass
Glottic larynx	Hoarseness of voice and sore throat Difficulty in breathing Noisy breathing Coughing
Subglottic larynx	Pain Difficulty in swallowing due to pressure effects
Hypopharynx	Pain Otalgia Difficulty in swallowing "Hot potato" voice Weight loss Neck mass

7.5 Differential Diagnosis

Certain other diseases that cause symptoms like oropharyngeal cancers are as follows:

1. Tonsillitis
2. Pharyngitis
3. Gastroesophageal reflux disease (GERD)
4. Tuberculosis
5. Benign tumors of the tonsil and pharynx, like squamous papillomas
6. Oral thrush
7. Lymphadenopathy due to other conditions

Conditions that might mimic laryngeal and hypopharyngeal cancers are as follows:

1. Vocal cord nodules and polyps
2. Reflux laryngitis due to GERD
3. Laryngotracheitis due to infections or allergens
4. Zenker's diverticulum
5. Tuberculosis
6. Laryngeal papillomatosis due to HPV infection
7. Neurological disorders or recurrent laryngeal nerve palsy

7.6 Evaluation

7.6.1 History and Clinical Examination

Once the patient presents to the OPD, careful history and physical examination are an indispensable part of clinical evaluation. History should emphasize the first presenting symptom along with its duration to assess the primary location of the tumor.

Examination should include direct visual inspection and indirect laryngoscopy or flexible fiberoptic laryngoscopy. Laryngoscopy helps in determining the extent of the lesion, tumor size, and vocal cord mobility. Palpation of the primary tumor and neck nodes in terms of location and size is vital in clinically staging the disease. Assessment of laryngeal crepitus helps determine fixity to underlying structures, and fullness over the thyroid notch is suggestive of pre-epiglottic space involvement. Clinical evaluation has been summarized in Fig. 7.3.

Complete blood count with basic metabolic panel must be done as a laboratory workup.

Pure tone audiometry is important to rule out referred pain from any primary pathology in the ear and assess the intensity of hearing loss. A complete dental evaluation is a must prior to commencement of treatment.

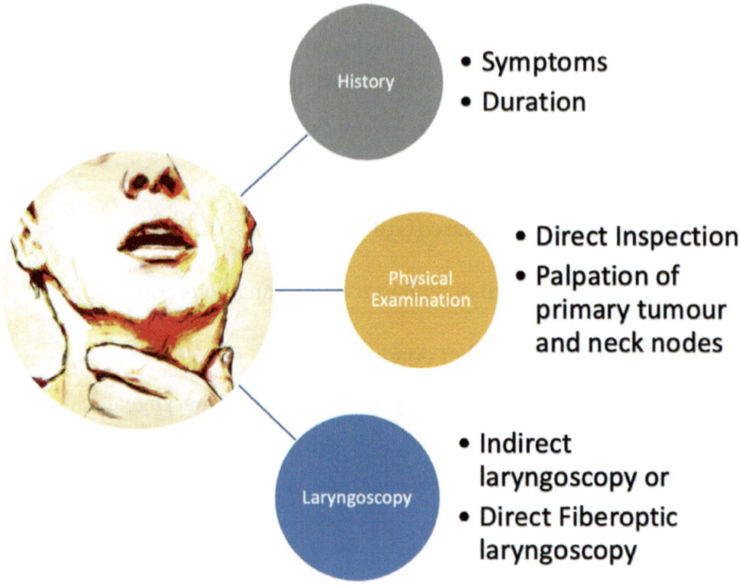

Fig. 7.3 Clinical evaluation of the patient. (Original content, copyright protected, cannot be refurnished without consent)

7.6.2 Radiological Evaluation

CT scan or MRI studies of face and neck with contrast are recommended along with chest imaging [6]. While the former (CT) has the advantages of being a faster imaging option at a lower cost, better assessment of bone and cartilage invasion, the latter helps evaluate soft tissue structures better. CT scan also offers the advantages of availability across centers, especially in a lower-resource nation.

When should MRI be preferred, and when should it not?

- MRI becomes the preferred investigation in cases that involve the orbit or skull base and wherever perineural invasion needs to be evaluated.
- MRI also better analyzes the pre-epiglottic space, base of tongue, paraglottic, and subglottic involvement in laryngeal cancers.
- MRI is least suited for nodal evaluation [7, 8]. The sensitivity and specificity of various techniques for cervical nodal detection are highlighted in Table 7.3.

Besides CT and MRI, PET CT scan is another imaging modality that not only assesses the primary tumor and nodal involvement but also provides information about the metastatic status of the disease.

Nonetheless, imaging plays a crucial role in accurately staging the tumor. Barium swallow can help in identifying tracheo-esophageal fistula in advanced cases of laryngeal and hypopharyngeal cancers.

Nodal involvement can be best assessed on PETCT vis-à-vis CT.

The comparative details of the imaging techniques are summarized in Fig. 7.4.

Table 7.3 Sensitivity and specificity values of various imaging modalities *(CI, confidence interval)*

Modality	Sensitivity (95% CI)	Specificity (95% CI)
CT scan	81% (68–90%)	76% (62–87%)
MRI scan	81% (65–91%)	63% (43–80%)
PET CT scan	79% (72–85%)	86% (83–89%)

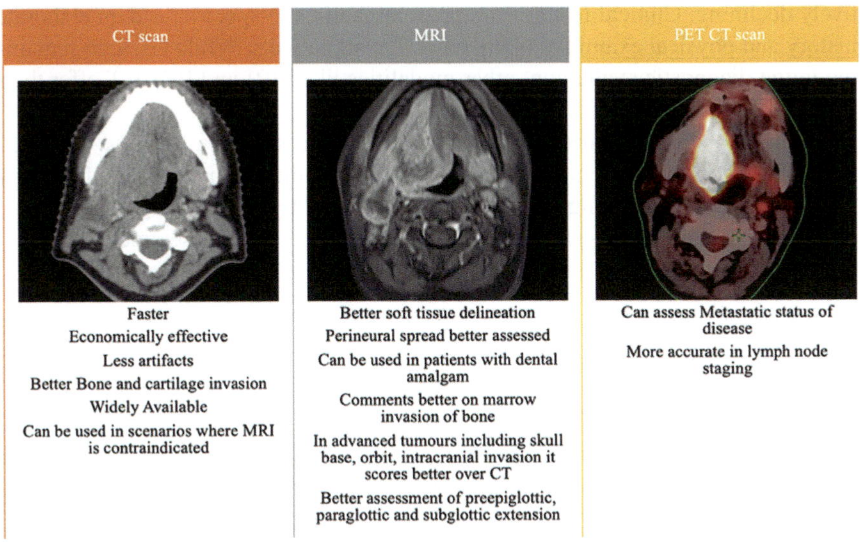

Fig. 7.4 Comparative advantages of various imaging techniques. (Original content, copyright protected, cannot be refurnished without consent)

7.6.3 *Pathological Evaluation*

A biopsy of the disease is mandatory in all cases for confirmation of the diagnosis.

For OPCs, AJCC in its eighth edition has modified the staging for HPV+ and HPV− OPC as HPV+ infection responds better to treatment and has a good prognosis, and there are enormous studies for dose de-escalation. Therefore, p16 evaluation is also paramount for the assessment of HPV infection. HPV DNA is commonly detected via PCR and in situ hybridization (ISH). Its surrogate marker p16 is detected via immunohistochemistry (IHC) on the biopsy specimen [9].

Furthermore, in the eighth edition of AJCC staging, separate pathological staging has also been introduced for OPCs, as the number of nodes was the sole predictor of disease recurrence, whereas other factors like extra nodal extension, laterality of nodes, and size of nodes at presentation were insignificant [10, 11].

Sentinel lymph node biopsy using indocyanine green combined with methylene blue mapping for OPC and ^{99m}Tc-phytate for laryngeal and hypopharyngeal cancer is a relatively new method, which is reasonably reliable [12, 13]. It helps in the detection of occult metastasis in a clinically negative neck, but it is not yet part of the standard of care.

7.7 Conclusion

Oropharyngeal cancers are on the rise, and HPV+ OPCs are more commonly seen in the younger population. The incidence of HPV+ OPC has increased over the last few decades, especially in the Western world. On the other hand, due to increased awareness and tobacco cessation, laryngeal and hypopharyngeal cancers are relatively declining. Clinical features are predominantly site-specific, and an elaborate history and physical examination are crucial in all patients. While CT scan remains the initial diagnostic evaluation, other modalities like MRI and PET CT offer their own set of advantages.

In low-resource countries, contrast-enhanced CT scan remains the preferred imaging choice owing to its good sensitivity and specificity. Biopsy is confirmatory for all cases, and p16 testing is a must in OPCs due to the different staging, response, and prognosis of HPV+ versus HPV− OPCs. Sentinel node assessment is a relatively newer approach to assessing occult nodal metastasis.

References

1. Lorenzoni V, Chaturvedi AK, Vignat J, Laversanne M, Bray F, Vaccarella S. The current burden of oropharyngeal cancer: a global assessment based on GLOBOCAN 2020. Cancer Epidemiol Biomarkers Prev. 2022;31(11):2054–62.
2. Lechner M, Liu J, Masterson L, Fenton TR. HPV-associated oropharyngeal cancer: epidemiology, molecular biology and clinical management. Nat Rev Clin Oncol. 2022;19(5):306–27.
3. Dahm V, Haitel A, Kaider A, Stanisz I, Beer A, Lill C. Cancer stage and pack-years, but not p16 or HPV, are relevant for survival in hypopharyngeal and laryngeal squamous cell carcinomas. Eur Arch Otorrinolaringol. 2018;275:1837–43.
4. Plummer M, de Martel C, Vignat J, Ferlay J, Bray F, Franceschi S. Global burden of cancers attributable to infections in 2012: a synthetic analysis. Lancet Glob Health. 2016;4(9):e609–16.
5. Carpén T, Sjöblom A, Lundberg M, et al. Presenting symptoms and clinical findings in HPV-positive and HPV-negative oropharyngeal cancer patients. Acta Otolaryngol. 2018;138(5):513–8.
6. Forastiere AA, Ang KK, Brizel D, et al. Head and neck cancers. J Natl Compr Cancer Netw. 2008;6(7):646–95.
7. De Bondt RB, Nelemans PJ, Hofman PA, et al. Detection of lymph node metastases in head and neck cancer: a meta-analysis comparing US, USgFNAC, CT and MR imaging. Eur J Radiol. 2007;64(2):266–72.
8. Kyzas PA, Evangelou E, Denaxa-Kyza D, Ioannidis JP. 18F-fluorodeoxyglucose positron emission tomography to evaluate cervical node metastases in patients with head and neck squamous cell carcinoma: a meta-analysis. J Natl Cancer Inst. 2008;100(10):712–20.
9. Cantley RL, Gabrielli E, Montebelli F, Cimbaluk D, Gattuso P, Petruzzelli G. Ancillary studies in determining human papillomavirus status of squamous cell carcinoma of the oropharynx: a review. Pathol Res Int. 2011;2011:138469.
10. Sinha P, Kallogjeri D, Gay H, et al. High metastatic node number, not extracapsular spread or N-classification is a node-related prognosticator in transorally-resected, neck-dissected p16-positive oropharynx cancer. Oral Oncol. 2015;51(5):514–20.

11. Haughey BH, Sinha P, Kallogjeri D, et al. Pathology-based staging for HPV-positive squamous carcinoma of the oropharynx. Oral Oncol. 2016;62:11–9.
12. Peng H, Wang SJ, Niu X, Yang X, Chi C, Zhang G. Sentinel node biopsy using indocyanine green in oral/oropharyngeal cancer. World J Surg Oncol. 2015;13(1):1–7.
13. Tomifuji M, Shiotani A, Fujii H, et al. Sentinel node concept in clinically n0 laryngeal and hypopharyngeal cancer. Ann Surg Oncol. 2008;15:2568–75.

Chapter 8
Evaluation and Staging in Oral Cavity Cancer

Ajay S. Krishnan and Shreya Jain

8.1 Introduction

India contributes to one-third of all global cases of oral cavity cancer, as per the GLOBOCAN database [1]. Oral cavity cancer alone accounts for 30% of all cancer cases in India. The Indian Council of Medical Research (ICMR) reports that oral cavity cancer claims more lives among men than among women [2].

Low-income groups in India face a higher burden because many people chew tobacco, and they lack access to new methods for detecting cancer early. As a result, cases of oral cavity cancer (OCC) are often reported late [3]. OCC leads to an annual productivity loss estimated at $386 million in India [4]. While globally and in the United States, OCC most often originates on the tongue, in India and South Asia, it predominantly starts on the inner lining of the cheeks (buccal mucosa) [5, 6].

8.2 Incidence and Epidemiology

In 2018, a total of 354,864 oral cavity cancer (OCC) cases were reported globally, with age-standardized rates (ASR) of 5.8 per 100,000 for males and 2.3 per 100,000 for females [7]. OCC is the most common cancer in men and the fourth most frequent in women in India, ranking second overall [8, 9].

India reported 119,992 new OCC cases in 2018. Worldwide, OCC caused 177,384 deaths that year, with age-standardized mortality rates of 2.8 per 100,000 for males and 1.2 for females. In India, OCC is the leading cause of cancer-related

A. S. Krishnan (✉) · S. Jain
Department of Radiation Oncology, MPMMCC/HBCH Varanasi, Units of Tata Memorial Centre, and Homi Bhabha National institute, Mumbai, India

S. Pradhan et al. (eds.), *Evidence Based Handbook on Diagnosis and Staging in Oncology*, https://doi.org/10.1007/978-981-95-9701-7_8

deaths, with 72,619 fatalities, making up 9.3% of all cancer deaths in the country [9]. The ASMR for OCC in India was 5.6 in 2018 [8].

8.3 Risk Factors

1. *Age*: Risk increases with age, usually occurring in people over the age of 40 with an average age of 60 at presentation.
2. *Sex*: Men > Women.
3. *Ethnicity*: Racially, black Americans are at higher risk for oral and throat cancer than whites.
4. *Tobacco*: The World Health Organization (WHO) regards smokeless tobacco (SLT) as a carcinogen, though its link to cancer development is still debated [10].
5. Naswar, a type of smokeless tobacco, is placed in the buccal sulcus where it absorbs active agents through the oral mucosa [10].
6. *Smoking*: Cigarette smoke contains compounds, including nicotine, which affect the oral cavity and gastrointestinal tract [11, 12]. Nicotine metabolites such as nitrosamines (NNK and NNN) are carcinogenic, binding to nicotinic acetylcholine receptors to promote cell proliferation and create a tumor-promoting microenvironment [16].
7. *Alcohol*: Alcohol alone does not directly cause cancer but synergizes with tobacco to increase cancer risk [12]. Ethanol in alcohol is metabolized into acetaldehyde, a known carcinogen that promotes oral cancer development [13]. Alcohol also contains carcinogenic impurities like polycyclic aromatic hydrocarbons and nitrosamines [13]. Alcohol may enhance the permeability of oral epithelium to carcinogens, facilitating their penetration into target tissues [14].
8. *Infections*: High acetaldehyde levels, produced by certain bacteria like *Streptococcus* and *Neisseria* species in the mouth, are associated with increased risk of head and neck squamous cell carcinoma (HNSCC) in smokers and heavy drinkers [15]. *Candida* infections may also contribute to acetaldehyde production, further complicating the carcinogenic process [16].
9. *HPV and HIV*: Oral HPV infection is more likely to occur when factors like oral epithelial wounds and poor hygiene are present, as they allow the virus to penetrate from superficial layers to the basal layer [18]. Persistent infection with HPV can lead to progression from pre-malignant lesions to invasive squamous cell carcinoma (SCC) [18]. Smoking enhances the risk of oral HPV infection because of its pro-inflammatory and immunosuppressive effects [19, 20]. HPV plays a crucial role in oral squamous cell carcinoma (OSCC), even among individuals who do not smoke or drink alcohol [21]. The positivity rate for HPV is notably higher in pre-cancerous conditions such as leukoplakia, erythroplakia, and oral submucous fibrosis, as well as in oral cancers [17]. The tongue is the most frequent site, accounting for 50% of HPV-related OSCC cases, whereas the floor of the mouth is affected in about 26.8% of cases [22]. HPV can also cause benign oral lesions like squamous papilloma and focal epithelial

hyperplasia [23]. Generally, HPV-associated oral and oropharyngeal cancers tend to have a better prognosis compared to other oral cancers [24].

10. *Chronic inflammation*: Chronic inflammation significantly contributes to the development of epithelial cancers, such as oral and pharyngeal tumors [25]. The tumor microenvironment, which includes fibroblasts, myofibroblasts, adipose tissue, immune and inflammatory cells, as well as the extracellular matrix (ECM), plays a vital role in tumor formation [26]. Changes in ECM biomechanics promote cell migration, a key event in cancer progression. Moreover, the ECM acts as a reservoir for growth factors like FGFs, HGF, VEGF, BMPs, and TGF-β [26]. Matrix metalloproteinases (MMPs), particularly MMP2 and MMP9, break down ECM components like type IV collagen, aiding cancer invasion [27, 28]. In patients with head and neck squamous cell carcinoma (HNSCC), high levels of MMP9 and MMP2 are associated with lymph node involvement [29, 30]. COX-2, which is overexpressed in 80% of head and neck pre-malignant and malignant tissues, is linked to lymph node metastasis and has been shown to promote carcinogenesis in animal studies [31, 32].
11. *Oral microbiome*: The oral microbiome includes over 700 bacterial species living in the human mouth and plays essential roles in health, such as modulating immune responses, aiding nutrient digestion, and metabolizing carcinogens. Certain microorganisms are associated with various cancers: HPV with cervical and oropharyngeal cancers; EBV with head and neck cancers; hepatitis B/C with hepatocellular carcinoma; *Helicobacter pylori* with gastroduodenal cancer; and *Porphyromonas gingivalis* with aero-digestive cancers [33–38]. Periodontitis, mainly caused by *P. gingivalis*, contributes to conditions like oral leukoplakia and interacts with oral cancer cells [39–42]. Poor oral health is linked to a higher risk of cancers including those of the head, neck, esophagus, stomach, and pancreas, potentially due to chronic inflammation mediated by oral microbiota such as *H. pylori* [43–45].
12. *Genetic predisposition*: Genetic factors significantly impact the development of oral squamous cell carcinoma (OSCC), especially in cases involving the tongue and buccal mucosa [46]. Around 29.5% of first-degree relatives of head and neck cancer patients might develop cancers of the respiratory or upper aero-digestive tract [47]. Identifying genetic or familial risk factors for oral cancer is difficult because of overlapping risk factors such as smoking and alcohol consumption. Variations in genes involved in carcinogen metabolism, like P450 enzymes and xenobiotic metabolizing enzymes (XMEs), are key in determining susceptibility to tobacco-related oral cancers [48]. Loss of tumor suppressor genes such as p53 and pRb causes genomic instability and drives cancer progression by hindering apoptosis and increasing telomerase activity [49]. Additionally, the epithelial-mesenchymal transition (EMT), which fosters cancer stemness and metastasis [50–54], can be triggered by compounds like areca nut extract and arecoline in oral epithelial cells.
13. *Precancerous* lesions are pivotal as approximately 50% of oral cancers develop from them, highlighting the need for early detection and management to prevent progression. However, surgical removal alone may not effectively stop

malignant transformation due to field cancerization, a concept introduced by Slaughter et al. in 1953. This phenomenon involves molecular changes in seemingly normal tissue that can evolve through premalignant stages, such as dysplasia, to full cancer over time [55]. Tobacco smoking greatly increases the risk by causing sustained proliferation of oral epithelial cells even after quitting, which contributes to field cancerization. Genetic changes including loss of chromosomal segments and mutations—especially in genes like TP53—are vital in this process [56–58]. The field effect can span several centimeters around the lesion, containing early genetic alterations that predispose tissues to malignancy [58–60].

8.3.1 Oral Cavity Cancer Screening

Oral visual inspection (OVI) is the screening method of choice in limited resource centers (health and wellness center, primary health center (PHC), and community health center (CHC)). It can be done by any trained healthcare personnel. The target age group is the at-risk population who use tobacco/alcohol/areca nuts, who are more than 15 years of age and screening is done at 5-year intervals. Screening protocols are further explained in the chapter of screening of cancers. No proven benefit of image-based screening tests has been seen.

8.4 Evaluation of Oral Cavity Cancer

8.4.1 Clinical Presentation

Clinical features of oral cavity cancer can vary but typically include the following:

1. Painless ulcers: Persistent ulcers or sores that do not heal, particularly on the tongue, floor of the mouth, or inside the cheek.
2. Red or white patches: Areas of leukoplakia (white patches) or erythroplakia (red patches) that may indicate precancerous lesions or early-stage cancer.
3. Swelling or mass: Development of a lump, thickening, or swelling in the oral cavity, often accompanied by pain or tenderness.
4. Difficulty swallowing: Dysphagia (difficulty swallowing) or a feeling that something is caught in the throat.
5. Persistent sore throat: Chronic sore throat or feeling of irritation that does not resolve with usual treatments.
6. Hoarseness or voice changes: Changes in voice quality or persistent hoarseness.
7. Ear pain: Unexplained pain in the ears, which can be referred pain from the oral cavity.

8. Loose teeth or dentures: Loose teeth or ill-fitting dentures without other dental causes.
9. Bleeding: Unexplained bleeding in the mouth or throat.
10. Weight loss: Unintended weight loss, often associated with advanced stages of cancer.

Differential diagnoses may include the following:

- Oral candidiasis: Fungal infection causing white patches that can resemble leukoplakia.
- Oral lichen planus: Chronic inflammatory condition causing white patches and ulcers.
- Aphthous ulcers: Recurrent, painful ulcers typically smaller than cancerous ulcers.
- Traumatic ulcers: Ulcers caused by mechanical trauma or biting, which can resemble early cancerous lesions.
- Benign oral tumors: Fibromas or papilloma, which are usually painless and slow-growing compared to malignant tumors.

8.4.2 Diagnostic Workup

- History—including tobacco/smoking/alcohol intake
- Weight loss

8.4.3 Physical Examination

- Oral hygiene evaluation
- Oral cavity palpation to assess the extent of disease, bony involvement, tongue fixation, and bimanual assessment for depth of invasion
- Cervical lymph node examination
- Indirect laryngoscopy for oropharyngeal, laryngeal, or hypopharyngeal examination
- Blood investigation: Complete blood count/liver and renal function test/serum electrolytes/viral markers, PT/INR
- Histopathology with biopsy to confirm cancer

8.4.4 Imaging in Oral Cavity Cancer

- For diagnosis and staging (CT/MRI used for loco-regional staging; CT/X-ray for lung evaluation)

- For treatment planning (both surgery and radiotherapy) (panoramic X-ray (orthopantogram) needed for dental evaluation before radiotherapy)
- For response evaluation (CT/PET used along with clinical examination)
- For detection of recurrences (CT/PET used along with clinical examination)

8.5 Imaging in Oral Cavity Cancer

8.5.1 Evaluation of Primary

Contrast-enhanced CT (CECT) face and neck:

CECT is the preferred imaging for local staging in oral cavity lesions except tongue.

CECT with puffed cheek is recommended for evaluating oral cavity lesions, as it helps distinguish margins between normal and diseased mucosa and separates the mucosal surface from the alveolus. This allows for a better assessment of subtle lesions that might be missed with routine imaging.

CECT enables identification of local and regional extent of the tumor, presence of bony erosion, and perineural spread by identifying widening of foramina.

CECT also helps in deciding if surgical resection is possible. Resection is possible with involvement of low infratemporal fossa (ITF) or retro-antral ITF.

The infratemporal fossa is divided into the supranotch and infranotch regions by the sigmoid notch of the mandible. Disease extension into the supranotch compartment is termed high ITF involvement and renders the disease unresectable. Conversely, infranotch disease is considered resectable (Table 8.1).

8.5.2 MRI Face and Neck

CE-MRI is the modality of choice for evaluation of tongue cancer.

MRI is not indicated in other sub-sites of oral cavity due to motion artefact affecting the quality of images.

The MRI imaging protocol for the tongue should comprise the following sequences: STIR and T1-weighted images in the coronal plane, T1- and T2-weighted images in the axial plane, T2-weighted images in the sagittal plane, DWI images in the axial plane, and post-contrast images in all three planes.

Table 8.1 CT protocol for oral cavity evaluation

Intravenous contrast	3–5 mL/s iodinated contrast
Maneuvers	Puffed cheek
Reconstruction	Bone algorithm Multi-planar reconstruction

The slice thickness should be 3 mm with a slice gap of 1 mm.

MRI defines muscles of tongue involvement, midline extension, floor of mouth involvement, neurovascular structure involvement, and posterior third tongue involvement.

MRI is not useful for mandibular involvement (Table 8.2).

8.6 Evaluation of Regional Nodes

Loss of fatty hilum, a rounded appearance, necrosis, and cystic changes can suggest nodal involvement.

Size alone may not be a good criterion for nodal involvement. Interestingly, it is seen that using a 1.5 cm versus 1 cm size criterion changes the specificity from 39% to 84% while decreasing sensitivity from 88% to 55% for neck nodes.

A meta-analysis on cervical lymph node metastasis in cN0 patients compared the sensitivity and specificity of imaging methods such as CT, MRI, PET, and USG. It found no significant differences overall, except that CT was superior to US in specificity (Table 8.3).

Table 8.2 MRI sequences and utility

Sequence	Utility
Pre-contrast T1W	Identify muscular anatomy (muscle: low intensity; intermuscular fat: high intensity)
STIR and T2W	Intermediate/high signal intensity
Coronal STIR and post-contrast T1-W images	Involvement of the neurovascular bundle and invasion of the sublingual and submandibular space, floor of mouth
Three-plane post-contrast T1-W images	Perineural spread, marrow invasion, and nodal involvement

*Depth of invasion (DOI) is not properly measured either by CT or MRI

Table 8.3 Sensitivity and specificity of imaging modalities for nodes

Modality	Sensitivity (%)	Specificity (%)
CT	47	88.9
MRI	56.6	82.5
PET	48.3	86.2
Ultrasound	63.3	79.1

8.7 Evaluation of Metastases

CT scan of thorax is preferred to identify small metastases. X-ray chest will detect only large metastases.

Panoramic X-ray oral cavity is used:

For determining bone invasion (If CT scan is not feasible)

For evaluating teeth and planning dental treatment of oral cavity prior to radiation to reduce subsequent complications

8.8 PET CT

FDG PET CT is not routinely used for staging of OCC.

FDG-PET for detecting residual or recurrent HNSCC shows a sensitivity, specificity, positive predictive value (PPV) and negative predictive value (NPV) of 94%, 82%, 75%, and 95%, respectively.

In case of clinical suspicion of recurrence, PET CT may help in clinching the diagnosis.

References

1. Mohan P, Richardson A, Potter JD, Coope P, Paterson M. Opportunistic screening of oral potentially malignant disorders: a public health need for India. JCO Glob Oncol. 2020;6:688–96.
2. India Against Cancer. Oral cancer. https://cancerindia.org.in/oral-cancer/. Accessed 10 Jul 2022.
3. Sharma S, Satyanarayana L, Asthana S, Shivalingesh KK, Goutham BS, Ramachandra S. Oral cancer statistics in India on the basis of first report of 29 population-based cancer registries. J Oral Maxillofac Pathol. 2018;22:18–26.
4. Amarasinghe H, Jayasinghe RD, Dharmagunawardene D, et al. Economic burden of managing oral cancer patients in Sri Lanka: a cross-sectional hospital-based costing study. BMJ Open. 2019;9:e027661.
5. Gangane N, Chawla S, Anshu, Gupta SS, Sharma SM. Reassessment of risk factors for oral cancer. Asian Pac J Cancer Prev. 2007;8:243–8.
6. Tandon P, Dadhich A, Saluja H, Bawane S, Sachdeva S. The prevalence of squamous cell carcinoma in different sites of oral cavity at our rural health care Centre in Loni, Maharashtra—a retrospective 10-year study. Contemp Oncol. 2017;21:178–83.
7. Bray F, Ferlay J, Soerjomataram I, Siegel RL, Torre LA, Jemal A. Global cancer statistics 2018: GLOBOCAN estimates of incidence and mortality worldwide for 36 cancers in 185 countries. CA Cancer J Clin. 2018;68:394–424.
8. World Health Organization. Global cancer observatory. Geneva: World Health Organization; 2018. https://gco.iarc.fr/. Accessed 11 Jul 2022.
9. Dar M, Sharma K. Burden of cancer in India: GLOBOCAN 2018 estimates incidence, mortality, prevalence and future projections of cancer in India. Burden Cancer India. 2019;6:505–14.
10. Khan Z, Dreger S, Shah SMH, et al. Oral cancer via the bargain bin: the risk of oral cancer associated with a smokeless tobacco product (Naswar). PLoS One. 2017;12:e0180445.

11. Jensen K, Afroze S, Munshi MK, Guerrier M, Glaser SS. Mechanisms for nicotine in the development and progression of gastrointestinal cancers. Transl Gastroint Cancer. 2012;1:81–7.
12. Sheikh MN, Hanif S, Zia M, Qayyum Z. Effects of nicotine on an in vitro reconstituted model oral mucosa in terms of cytokine production. J Ayub Med Coll Abbottabad. 2011;23:80–4.
13. Khan Z, Bisen PS. Oncoapoptotic signaling and deregulated target genes in cancers: special reference to oral cancer. Biochim Biophys Acta. 2013;1836:123–45.
14. Feng L, Wang L. Effects of alcohol on the morphological and structural changes in oral mucosa. Pak J Med Sci. 2013;29:1046–9.
15. Hayes RB, Ahn J, Fan X, et al. Association of oral microbiome with risk for incident head and neck squamous cell cancer. JAMA Oncol. 2018;4:358–65.
16. Neville B, Damm DD, Allen C, Chi A. Oral and maxillofacial pathology. 4th ed. USA: Saunders Elsevier; 2016; St. Louis, Missouri: USA.
17. Yete S, D'Souza W, Saranath D. High-risk human papillomavirus in oral cancer: clinical implications. Oncology. 2018;94:133–41.
18. Dalla Torre D, Burtscher D, Solder E, Rasse M, Puelacher W. The correlation between the quality of oral hygiene and oral HPV infection in adults: a prospective cross-sectional study. Clin Oral Investig. 2019;23:179–85.
19. Sonawane K, Suk R, Chiao EY, et al. Oral human papillomavirus infection: differences in prevalence between sexes and concordance with genital human papillomavirus infection, NHANES 2011 to 2014. Ann Intern Med. 2017;167:714–24.
20. Wang CC, Palefsky JM. Human papillomavirus-related oropharyngeal cancer in the HIV-infected population. Oral Dis. 2016;22(Suppl. 1):98–106.
21. Vargas-Ferreira F, Nedel F, Etges A, Gomes AP, Furuse C, Tarquinio SB. Etiologic factors associated with oral squamous cell carcinoma in non-smokers and non-alcoholic drinkers: a brief approach. Braz Dent J. 2012;23:586–90.
22. Chocolatewala NM, Chaturvedi P. Role of human papilloma virus in the oral carcinogenesis: an Indian perspective. J Cancer Res Ther. 2009;5:71–7.
23. Candotto V, Lauritano D, Nardone M, et al. HPV infection in the oral cavity: epidemiology, clinical manifestations and relationship with oral cancer. Oral Implantol. 2017;10:209–20.
24. Kalavrezos N, Scully C. Mouth cancer for clinicians part 13: life after mouth cancer treatment. Dent Update. 2016;43:672.
25. Shivappa N, Hebert JR, Rosato V, Garavello W, Serraino D, La Vecchia C. Inflammatory potential of diet and risk of oral and pharyngeal cancer in a large case-control study from Italy. Int J Cancer. 2017;141:471–9.
26. Gattazzo F, Urciuolo A, Bonaldo P. Extracellular matrix: a dynamic microenvironment for stem cell niche. Biochim Biophys Acta. 2014;1840:2506–19.
27. Jablonska-Trypuc A, Matejczyk M, Rosochacki S. Matrix metalloproteinases (MMPs), the main extracellular matrix (ECM) enzymes in collagen degradation, as a target for anticancer drugs. J Enzyme Inhib Med Chem. 2016;31(Suppl 1):177–83.
28. Webb AH, Gao BT, Goldsmith ZK, et al. Inhibition of MMP-2 and MMP-9 decreases cellular migration, and angiogenesis in in vitro models of retinoblastoma. BMC Cancer. 2017;17:434.
29. Markwell SM, Weed SA. Tumor and stromal-based contributions to head and neck squamous cell carcinoma invasion. Cancer. 2015;7:382–406.
30. Pietruszewska W, Bojanowska-Pozniak K, Kobos J. Matrix metalloproteinases MMP1, MMP2, MMP9 and their tissue inhibitors TIMP1, TIMP2, TIMP3 in head and neck cancer: an immunohistochemical study. Otolaryngol Pol. 2016;70:32–43.
31. Mohammad S, Ram H, Gupta PN, Husain N, Bhatt M. Overexpression of COX-2 in oral squamous cell carcinoma patients undergoing chemoradiotherapy. Nat J Maxillofac Surg. 2011;2:17–21.
32. McCormick DL, Phillips JM, Horn TL, Johnson WD, Steele VE, Lubet RA. Overexpression of COX-2 in rat oral cancers and prevention of oral carcinogenesis in rats by selective and non-selective COX inhibitors. Cancer Prev Res. 2010;3:73–81.

33. St Laurent J, Luckett R, Feldman S. HPV vaccination and the effects on rates of HPV-related cancers. Curr Probl Cancer. 2018;42:493–506.
34. Fernandes Q, Merhi M, Raza A, et al. Role of Epstein-Barr virus in the pathogenesis of head and neck cancers and its potential as an immunotherapeutic target. Front Oncol. 2018;8:257.
35. Moore MS, Bocour A, Tran OC, et al. Effect of hepatocellular carcinoma on mortality among individuals with hepatitis B or hepatitis C infection in new York City, 2001–2012. Open Forum Infect Dis. 2018;5:ofy144.
36. Vinagre R, Vinagre IDF, Vilar ESA, Fecury AA, Martins LC. *Helicobacter pylori* infection and immune profile of patients with different gastroduodenal diseases. Arq Gastroenterol. 2018;55:122–7.
37. Inaba H, Sugita H, Kuboniwa M, et al. *Porphyromonas gingivalis* promotes invasion of oral squamous cell carcinoma through induction of proMMP9 and its activation. Cell Microbiol. 2014;16:131–45.
38. Woo BH, Kim DJ, Choi JI, et al. Oral cancer cells sustainedly infected with *Porphyromonas gingivalis* exhibit resistance to Taxol and have higher metastatic potential. Oncotarget. 2017;8:46981–92.
39. Irani S. Oral health and related factors: an update. J Int Oral Health. 2016;8:140–4.
40. Irani S. Orofacial bacterial infectious diseases: an update. J Int Soc Prev Community Dent. 2017;7(Suppl 2):S61–7.
41. Katz J, Onate MD, Pauley KM, Bhattacharyya I, Cha S. Presence of *Porphyromonas gingivalis* in gingival squamous cell carcinoma. Int J Oral Sci. 2011;3:209–15.
42. Petersen PE, Bourgeois D, Ogawa H, Estupinan-Day S, Ndiaye C. The global burden of oral diseases and risks to oral health. Bull World Health Organ. 2005;83:661–9.
43. Irani S, Monsef Esfahani A, Bidari Zerehpoush F. Detection of *Helicobacter pylori* in oral lesions. J Dent Res Dent Clin Dent Prospects. 2013;7:230–7.
44. Irani S, Monsef Esfahani A, Sabeti S, Bidari Zerehpoush F. Detection of *Helicobacter pylori* in oral lichen planus and oral lichenoid reaction. Avicenna J Dent Res. 2014;6:e23213.
45. Monsef Esfahani A, Irani S, Sabeti S, Bidari Zerehpoush F. The possible role of *Helicobacter pylori* in the development of Sjogren's syndrome and chronic sialadenitis. Avicenna J Dent Res. 2015;7:e23212.
46. Ali J, Sabiha B, Jan HU, Haider SA, Khan AA, Ali SS. Genetic etiology of oral cancer. Oral Oncol. 2017;70:23–8.
47. Kim KM, Kim YM, Shim YS, et al. Epidemiologic survey of head and neck cancers in Korea. J Korean Med Sci. 2003;18:80–7.
48. Kumar M, Nanavati R, Modi TG, Dobariya C. Oral cancer: etiology and risk factors: a review. J Cancer Res Ther. 2016;12:458–63.
49. Shah A, Malik A, Garg A, Mair M, Nair S, Chaturvedi P. Oral sex and human papilloma virus-related head and neck squamous cell cancer: a review of the literature. Postgrad Med J. 2017;93:704–9.
50. Irani S, Dehghan A. The expression and functional significance of vascular endothelial-cadherin, CD44, and vimentin in oral squamous cell carcinoma. J Int Soc Prev Community Dent. 2018;8:110–7.
51. Irani S, Dehghan A. Expression of vascular endothelial-cadherin in mucoepidermoid carcinoma: role in cancer development. J Int Soc Prev Community Dent. 2017;7:301–7.
52. Irani S, Jafari B. Expression of vimentin and CD44 in mucoepidermoid carcinoma: a role in tumor growth. Indian J Dent Res. 2018;29:333–40.
53. Irani S, Salajegheh A, Smith RA, Lam AK. A review of the profile of endothelin axis in cancer and its management. Crit Rev Oncol Hematol. 2014;89:314–21.
54. Wang TY, Peng CY, Lee SS, Chou MY, Yu CC, Chang YC. Acquisition cancer stemness, mesenchymal transdifferentiation, and chemoresistance properties by chronic exposure of oral epithelial cells to arecoline. Oncotarget. 2016;7:84072–81.
55. Slaughter DP, Southwick HW, Smejkal W. Field cancerization in oral stratified squamous epithelium; clinical implications of multicentric origin. Cancer. 1953;6:963–8.

56. Pitiyage G, Tilakaratne WM, Tavassoli M, Warnakulasuriya S. Molecular markers in oral epithelial dysplasia: review. J Oral Pathol Med. 2009;38:737–52.
57. Braakhuis BJ, Leemans CR, Brakenhoff RH. A genetic progression model of oral cancer: current evidence and clinical implications. J Oral Pathol Med. 2004;33:317–22.
58. Van Houten VM, Tabor MP, van den Brekel MW, et al. Mutated p53 as a molecular marker for the diagnosis of head and neck cancer. J Pathol. 2002;198:476–86.
59. Mohan M, Jagannathan N. Oral field cancerization: an update on current concepts. Oncol Rev. 2014;8:244.
60. Lydiatt WM, Anderson PE, Bazzana T, et al. Molecular support for field cancerization in the head and neck. Cancer. 1998;82:1376–80.

Chapter 9
Evaluation and Staging of Thyroid Cancers

Prashanth Giridhar and Rahul Sisodiya

9.1 Introduction and Epidemiology

Thyroid cancer is ranked the seventh most common cancer and composes 4.1% of all newly diagnosed cases as per the GLOBOCAN 2022 statistics [1] published by the International Agency for Research on Cancer. The incidence rate is three times higher in women than in men. Thyroid cancer ranked 24th in terms of cancer deaths, constituting 0.5% of all cancer deaths. The highest incidence rates in both sexes are found in Eastern Asia, where the rate is two times higher than that seen in the second-ranking Northern America [1].

The incidence rate of thyroid cancer among women is increasing [2]. Thyroid cancer is highly vulnerable to overdiagnosis, a phenomenon in which many clinically inapparent tumors are identified without leading to a measurable decrease in disease-specific mortality [3]. This occurs because subclinical thyroid disease is relatively common and diagnostic tools are widely available and highly sensitive, enabling the detection of lesions that would otherwise remain asymptomatic.

Most thyroid malignancies are well-differentiated tumors that arise from follicular cells and are categorized as papillary thyroid carcinoma (PTC) or follicular thyroid carcinoma (FTC). Papillary carcinoma is the predominant subtype, accounting for approximately 79% of cases, whereas follicular carcinoma represents about 13%. Hürthle cell carcinoma (HCC), which is now considered a distinct entity rather than a variant of FTC, comprises around 5% of follicular cell–derived thyroid cancers. Medullary thyroid carcinoma (MTC), originating from parafollicular C cells, accounts for roughly 4% of all thyroid malignancies. Anaplastic thyroid carcinoma (ATC) is an undifferentiated and aggressive form, making up approximately 2% of cases. Poorly differentiated thyroid carcinoma (PDTC) is a rare subtype that

P. Giridhar (✉) · R. Sisodiya
Department of Radiation Oncology, MPMMCC & HBCH Varanasi, Units of Tata Memorial Centre and affliated with Homi Bhabha National Institute, Mumbai, India

S. Pradhan et al. (eds.), *Evidence Based Handbook on Diagnosis and Staging in Oncology*, https://doi.org/10.1007/978-981-95-9701-7_9

Table 9.1 Risk factors for thyroid cancer

High risk	Low risk
1. Radiation exposure (head and neck region) 2. Chromosomal (genetic) alterations 3. Hereditary conditions Hereditary medullary thyroid cancer Non-syndromic familial non-medullary thyroid cancer Syndromic familial non-medullary thyroid cancer	1. Thyroid imaging with iodine 131 2. Iodine deficiency 3. High thyroid-stimulating hormone (TSH) level 4. Autoimmunity 5. Thyroid nodule 6. Environmental pollutants 7. Lifestyle and diet 8. High BMI

occupies an intermediate biological position between PTC/FTC and ATC, with reported incidence rates ranging from 2% to 15% of thyroid cancers [4].

9.2 Risk Factors

Female sex, a family history of thyroid cancer, and radiation exposure of the thyroid gland during childhood are the major risk factors associated with differentiated thyroid cancer [5] (Table 9.1).

9.3 Chromosomal (Genetic) Alterations

The mitogen-activated protein kinase (MAPK) and phosphoinositide 3 kinase–AKT (PI3K–AKT) signaling cascades are thought to contribute to the development and progression of thyroid cancer. In papillary thyroid carcinoma, activation of the MAPK pathway is observed in nearly 70% of cases [6]. In follicular thyroid carcinoma, abnormal cellular proliferation is promoted by genetic alterations such as RAS oncogene mutations and the PAX8/PPARγ fusion protein resulting from chromosomal translocation, which are present in approximately 40% and 30% of patients, respectively [7].

Medullary thyroid carcinoma (MTC) arises from parafollicular C cells rather than follicular epithelial cells. These neural crest–derived cells are responsible for the secretion of calcitonin. Most MTC cases occur sporadically (about 80%), while the remainder are associated with inherited multiple endocrine neoplasia syndromes, including MEN2A, MEN2B, and familial MTC. The implementation of RET mutation screening has led to increased identification of hereditary MTC at very young ages, including infancy and early childhood. Current genotype-based guidelines recommend prophylactic thyroidectomy between 5 and 6 years of age for individuals with RET mutations linked to MEN2A and familial MTC. In contrast, patients from MEN2B families are advised to undergo thyroidectomy during infancy due to the earlier onset and more aggressive nature of MTC in this group [8] (Table 9.2).

Table 9.2 Clinical and genetic characteristics of familial thyroid follicular cell cancer

Syndrome	Chromosome linkage/gene	Characteristics
Papillary thyroid cancer with papillary renal neoplasia	1q21	Autosomal dominant with partial penetrance
Familial non-medullary thyroid cancer	2q21 and 19p13	Two genetic loci identified Autosomal dominant with partial penetrance
Familial thyroid tumors with cell oxyphilia	19p13.2	Characteristics of oxyphilic cells Autosomal dominant with partial penetrance
Familial adenomatous polyposis	5q21-22/APC	Papillary thyroid cancer (cribriform morular variant) Colorectal cancer, ampullary cancer, hepatoblastoma, medulloblastoma Autosomal dominant
Cowden syndrome	10q23.3/PTEN	Follicular and papillary thyroid cancer Multiple hamartomas, breast, and endometrial cancer Autosomal dominant
Carney complex 1	17q/PRKAR1A	Follicular and papillary thyroid cancer Skin pigmentation and cardiac, endocrine, cutaneous, and neural myxomatous tumors Autosomal dominant

9.4 Clinical Features

The most frequent initial manifestation of thyroid malignancy is a neck mass, which may be noticed by the patient or identified during clinical examination. Thyroid nodules are also commonly discovered incidentally on imaging studies performed for unrelated reasons. Associated symptoms may include hoarseness, difficulty swallowing, shortness of breath, loss of appetite, fever, and unintended weight loss. On neck examination, features such as a firm or fixed thyroid nodule and the presence of cervical lymphadenopathy should raise concern for malignancy and prompt additional diagnostic workup.

Anaplastic thyroid carcinoma often presents as a swiftly enlarging cervical mass accompanied by the rapid onset of compressive symptoms involving the upper aerodigestive tract.

9.5 Histopathology

Pathologic classification of thyroid cancer is based on the cell of origin, cytologic characteristics, and tumor growth pattern. With the exception of medullary thyroid carcinoma (MTC), which originates from parafollicular C cells, all thyroid carcinomas arise from follicular epithelial cells. The diagnosis of papillary thyroid carcinoma (PTC) relies exclusively on characteristic nuclear features and does not

Table 9.3 Histopathology classification of thyroid cancer

Types of thyroid cancer	Origin/subtype	Characteristics/variants	Incidence (%)
Well-differentiated thyroid cancer (DTC)	Papillary thyroid cancer (PTC)	Classic, follicular variant Oncocytic variant Unfavorable variants include diffuse sclerosing, tall cell, columnar cell, and hobnail	79
		Classic	
	Follicular thyroid carcinoma (FTC)		13
	Hurthle cell carcinoma	A variant of FTC, more aggressive	5
Poorly differentiated thyroid cancer		Insular carcinoma	2–15
Undifferentiated thyroid cancer	Anaplastic carcinoma	Highly aggressive, undifferentiated	2
Parafollicular C cell	Medullary carcinoma	Arises from parafollicular C cells	4

require evidence of tissue invasion. In contrast, follicular carcinoma (FC) is defined by the demonstration of capsular and/or vascular invasion [9] (Table 9.3).

9.6 Evaluation of Thyroid Nodule

A thyroid nodule is a discrete lesion in the gland that is radiologically distinct from the surrounding parenchyma [10]. It is very common with increasing age, particularly in women. It may not only be detected by palpation but may also be found incidentally on imaging studies. Approximately 10% of the nodules are malignant [11].

Differential Diagnosis of Thyroid Nodules

1. Non-neoplastic nodules
   (a) Hyperplastic
      - Spontaneous
      - Compensatory after partial thyroidectomy

   (b) Inflammatory
      - Acute bacterial thyroiditis
      - Subacute thyroiditis
      - Lymphocytic (Hashimoto's) thyroiditis

2. Benign neoplasms
    (a) Non-functioning (cold nodules)
        - Solid (or mixed): adenoma
        - Cystic
    (b) Functioning (hot nodules)
        - Adenoma
3. Malignant neoplasms
    - Papillary carcinoma
    - Follicular carcinoma
    - Anaplastic carcinoma
    - Medullary carcinoma
    - Thyroid lymphoma
    - Thyroid metastasis from other primaries

9.7 Diagnostic Methods Used in the Evaluation of Thyroid Cancer

9.7.1 Clinical Examination

- History of benign thyroid disease
- History of head and neck irradiation
- Family history of thyroid cancer
- Physical examination

Features suggestive of increased potential of malignancy in a patient with a thyroid nodule.

Patient history or characteristics	Physical examination
Family history of MEN, MTC, and PTC	Firm nodule Nodule fixed to adjacent structures
History of head and neck irradiation	Large nodules (>4 cm)
History of Hodgkin and non-Hodgkin lymphoma	Growth of nodules, especially during L-thyroxine therapy suppression therapy
Age <20 or >70 years	Symptoms of compression: hoarseness, dysphagia, dysphonia, dyspnea, cough
Male sex	Abnormal cervical lymphadenopathy, paralysis of the vocal cord

9.8 Laboratory Investigations

- TSH
- Anti-TPO/anti-Tg antibody
- Serum calcitonin (selected cases)

All individuals presenting with thyroid nodules should undergo serum thyroid-stimulating hormone (TSH) testing, along with baseline laboratory investigations, including liver function tests, renal function tests, and a complete blood count. Routine assessment of antithyroid antibodies, such as anti-thyroid peroxidase and anti-thyroglobulin antibodies, is not required during the initial evaluation of thyroid nodules. In contrast, measurement of thyroglobulin levels in conjunction with anti-thyroglobulin antibody titers plays a critical role in post-treatment surveillance, as these markers are used to detect disease recurrence following total thyroidectomy and radioactive iodine ablation. Calcitonin serves as a highly sensitive and specific biomarker for medullary thyroid carcinoma (MTC) and is valuable for diagnosis, monitoring, and prognostication [12].

9.9 Ultrasound and Ultrasound-Guided Fine-Needle Aspiration

High-resolution neck ultrasound, including Doppler assessment, together with ultrasound-guided fine-needle aspiration, constitutes the standard diagnostic strategy for evaluating thyroid nodules, whether clinically palpable or incidentally identified on imaging studies. Ultrasound also serves as a key staging modality by enabling the detection of cervical lymph node involvement. Sonographic features suggestive of nodal metastasis include enlarged lymph nodes, microcalcifications, and irregular or diffuse intranodal vascularity [13]. Reported sensitivity and specificity of ultrasound for identifying nodal metastases are approximately 90% and 82%, respectively [14]. Identification of nonpalpable metastatic lymph nodes on cervical ultrasound has been shown to influence the surgical management in 14–24% of patients with papillary thyroid carcinoma (PTC) [13].

Fine-needle aspiration cytology (FNAC) is the most sensitive and predictive single diagnostic test for thyroid nodules. It is a minimally invasive, cost-effective, and efficient technique that facilitates differentiation between benign lesions, thereby avoiding unnecessary surgery, and malignant nodules that require operative intervention. To standardize reporting and improve diagnostic consistency, the Bethesda System for Reporting Thyroid Cytopathology (TBSRTC) was established in 2007 [15] (Table 9.4).

Table 9.4 The Bethesda System for Reporting Thyroid Cytopathology with implied risk of malignancy

Diagnostic category	Risk of malignancy (%)
Non diagnostic or unsatisfactory-I	1–4
Benign-II	0–3
AUS or FLUS-III	5–15
Follicular neoplasm or suspicious for a follicular neoplasm-IV	15–30
Suspicious for malignancy-V	60–75
Malignant-VI	97–99

Table 9.5 Sensitivity and specificity of CT and MRI for extrathyroid invasion [17–19]

Structure	Imaging modality	Sensitivity	Specificity
Trachea	CT	59	91
	MRI	100	84
Esophagus	CT	29	82
	MRI	96	84
Recurrent laryngeal nerve	CT	78	94
	MRI	90	82
Carotid artery	CT	75	100
	MRI	99	88

9.10 Computed Tomography and Magnetic Resonance Imaging

CT and MRI commonly detect otherwise clinically occult thyroid nodules. However, there are specific clinical symptoms and physical examination findings that suggest local invasion beyond the thyroid capsule and should prompt cross-sectional imaging. The major role of CT or MRI in this scenario is to evaluate critical surrounding structures for involvement that may affect prognosis and/or surgical planning. MRI is superior to CT for establishing the local extent, as it will more clearly show esophageal or tracheal invasion [16] (Table 9.5).

In general, iodinated contrast is avoided in the workup of DTC because the large iodine load can persist for several weeks and reduce radioactive iodine uptake at the time of ablation. Therefore, non-contrast CT or MRI is usually the preferred cross-sectional imaging study when the postoperative treatment may include I-131 therapy (Table 9.5).

9.11 PETCT

PETCT is not recommended for preoperative evaluation of DTC. However, it can be useful for initial staging in larger, poorly differentiated, or undifferentiated tumors when distant metastases are highly suspected. It may also be useful in the initial staging of invasive or metastatic Hurthle cell carcinoma [20]. PETCT imaging has become part of the surveillance algorithm in patients with a rising thyroglobulin, whose other imaging studies, including MRI, US, and 131-I whole-body scan, do not reveal the sites of disease [21]. The utility of FDG PET in patients with elevated TG and negative WBS has been demonstrated in several studies, with sensitivities ranging from 70% to 95% [22]. PETCT is most useful for MTC detection after thyroidectomy if calcitonin levels remain >150 pg/mL, suggesting distant metastatic disease.

9.12 Diagnostic Whole-Body Scan

An iodine-131 (I-131) scan is a noninvasive radionuclide imaging procedure used to visualize the functionality of thyroid tissue, detect metastatic thyroid cancer, and assess the remaining thyroid tissue after thyroidectomy. I-131 has a half-life of approximately 8.2 days, decays through beta emission, and is more cost-effective and widely accessible. I-131 is primarily utilized for imaging in cases of thyroid cancer [23].

Staging of thyroid cancer is done with the updated AJCC staging system.

References

1. Bray F, Laversanne M, Sung H, et al. Global cancer statistics 2022: GLOBOCAN estimates of incidence and mortality worldwide for 36 cancers in 185 countries. CA Cancer J Clin. 2024;74(3):229–63.
2. Mathew IE, Mathew A. Rising thyroid cancer incidence in Southern India: an epidemic of overdiagnosis. J Endocr Soc. 2017;1:480–7.
3. Nabhan F, Ringel MD. Thyroid nodules and cancer management guidelines: comparisons and controversies. Endocr Relat Cancer. 2017;24(2):R13–26.
4. Lim H, Devesa SS, Sosa JA, Check D, Kitahara CM. Trends in thyroid cancer incidence and mortality in the United States, 1974–2013. JAMA. 2017;317:1338–48.
5. Siegel RL, Miller KD, Jemal A. Cancer statistics, 2015. CA Cancer J Clin. 2015;65(1):5–29.
6. Bonnefond S, Davies TF. Thyroid cancer-risks and causes. Oncol Hematol Rev. 2014;10(2):14451. https://doi.org/10.17925/OHR.2014.10.2.144.
7. Cheng G, Lewis AE, Meinkoth JL. Ras stimulates aberrant cell cycle progression and apoptosis in rat thyroid cells. Mol Endocrinol. 2003;17(3):450–9. https://doi.org/10.1210/me.2002-0344.
8. Wells SA Jr, Asa SL, Dralle H, Elisei R, Evans DB, Gagel RF, Lee N, Machens A, Moley JF, Pacini F, Raue F, Frank-Raue K, Robinson B, Rosenthal MS, Santoro M, Schlumberger M, Shah M, Waguespack SG. American Thyroid Association Guidelines Task Force on medullary thyroid carcinoma. Revised American Thyroid Association guidelines for the management of medullary thyroid carcinoma. Thyroid. 2015;25(6):567–610.
9. Ghossein R. Update to the College of American Pathologists reporting on thyroid carcinomas. Head Neck Pathol. 2009;3(1):86–93.

10. Haugen BR, Alexander EK, Bible KC, et al. 2015 American Thyroid Association management guidelines for adult patients with thyroid nodules and differentiated thyroid cancer: the American Thyroid Association Guidelines Task Force on thyroid nodules and differentiated thyroid cancer. Thyroid. 2016;26(1):1–133.
11. Yassa L, Cibas ES, Benson CB, et al. Long-term assessment of a multidisciplinary approach to thyroid nodule diagnostic evaluation. Cancer. 2007;111(6):508–16.
12. Ladenson PW. Optimal laboratory testing for diagnosis and monitoring of thyroid nodules, goiter, and thyroid cancer. Clin Chem. 1996;42:183–7.
13. Gomez NR, Kouniavsky G, Tsai HL, et al. Tumor size and presence of calcifications on ultrasonography are pre-operative predictors of lymph node metastases in patients with papillary thyroid cancer. J Surg Oncol. 2011;104(6):613–6.
14. Gorges R, Eising EG, Fotescu D, et al. Diagnostic value of high-resolution B-mode and power-mode sonography in the follow-up of thyroid cancer. Eur J Ultrasound. 2003;16(3):191–206.
15. Melo-Uribe MA, Sanabria Á, Romero-Rojas A, Pérez G, Vargas EJ, Abaúnza MC, et al. The Bethesda system for reporting thyroid cytopathology in Colombia: correlation with histopathological diagnoses in oncology and non-oncology institutions. J Cytol. 2015;32:12–6.
16. Mancuso AA, Mendenhall WM, Vaysberg M. Thyroid: nodules and malignant tumors. In: Mancuso AA, editor. Head and neck radiology. Philadelphia: Lippincott Williams & Wilkins; 2010. p. 1457–81.
17. Wang JC, Takashima S, Takayama F, et al. Tracheal invasion by thyroid carcinoma: prediction using MR imaging. Am J Roentgenol. 2001;177:929936.
18. Wang J, Takashima S, Matsushita T, Takayama F, Kobayashi T, Kadoya M. Esophageal invasion by thyroid carcinomas: prediction using magnetic resonance imaging. J Comput Assist Tomogr. 2003;27:1825.
19. Seo YL, Yoon DY, Lim KJ, et al. Locally advanced thyroid cancer: can CT help in prediction of extrathyroidal invasion to adjacent structures? Am J Roentgenol. 2010;195:W240244.
20. Cooper DS, Doherty GM, Haugen BR, et al. Revised American Thyroid Association management guidelines for patients with thyroid nodules and differentiated thyroid cancer. Thyroid. 2009;19:1167–214.
21. Dietlein M, Scheidhauer K, Voth E, et al. Fluorine-18 fluorodeoxyglucose positron emission tomography and iodine-131 whole-body scintigraphy in the follow-up of differentiated thyroid cancer. Eur J Nucl Med. 1997;24:1342–8.
22. Abraham T, Schoder H. Thyroid cancer—indications and opportunities for positron emission tomography/computed tomography imaging. Semin Nucl Med. 2011;41:121–38.
23. Choudhury PS, Gupta M. Differentiated thyroid cancer theranostics: radioiodine and beyond. Br J Radiol. 2018;91(1091):20180136.

Chapter 10
Evaluation and Staging of Paranasal Sinus Cancer

Ninad Patil and Chaturbhaj Khandelwal

10.1 Introduction and Epidemiology

Paranasal sinus malignancies are relatively uncommon, representing less than 1% of all malignancies and approximately 3% of head and neck cancers [1]. Studies conducted in India have revealed that the annual incidence of sinonasal malignancies in the Indian population is approximately 1 per 100,000 individuals [2]. Sinonasal malignancies typically manifest in individuals in their sixth decade of life or later, with a higher incidence observed in the white population. The male-to-female ratio for these malignancies is approximately 1.8:1 [3].

10.2 Anatomical Distribution

In paranasal sinus malignancies, the anatomical distribution of tumors shows a notable predominance in the maxillary sinus, accounting for approximately 77% of cases. Following this, about 22% originate from the ethmoid sinus, while only 1% arise from the sphenoid and frontal sinuses combined [3].

N. Patil (✉) · C. Khandelwal
Department of Radiation Oncology, MPMMCC/HBCH Varanasi, Units of Tata Memorial Centre, and Homi Bhabha National Institute, Mumbai, India

S. Pradhan et al. (eds.), *Evidence Based Handbook on Diagnosis and Staging in Oncology*, https://doi.org/10.1007/978-981-95-9701-7_10

10.3 Histopathological Types

The predominant histological subtypes observed in India are squamous cell carcinoma and adenocarcinoma, collectively comprising the majority of cases. Squamous cell carcinoma represents approximately 50% of sinonasal tumors, while adenocarcinoma accounts for around 13% [4]. Less frequent histological types documented in Indian studies include sarcoma, undifferentiated carcinoma, teratocarcinosarcoma, malignant melanoma, adenoid cystic carcinoma, lymphoma, olfactory neuroblastoma, and neuroendocrine carcinoma [4].

10.4 Risk Factors

Woodworkers: Experience a 500–900 times increased risk of intestinal-type adenocarcinoma, and a 20 times increased risk of squamous cell carcinoma. Risks escalate with prolonged exposure exceeding 20 years [4, 5].

Exposure to leather dust, glues, formaldehyde, chrome, nickel, flour, textiles, and organic solvents is associated with sinonasal carcinomas, mostly squamous cell carcinoma [4–6].

Smoking: Smoking raises squamous cell carcinoma risk by two to three times. Its association with sinonasal carcinoma is weaker compared to other head and neck cancers [4, 5].

Human Papillomavirus (HPV): HPV types 16 and 18 link to about 30% of squamous cell carcinoma cases. Squamous cell carcinomas positive for HPV often show a better prognosis [4, 5].

Schneiderian Papilloma: Squamous cell carcinoma may arise from the three variants of Schneiderian papillomas: the exophytic type, which is exceedingly rare; the inverted papillomas, the most common, with 10% (up to 27% in certain reports) progressing to squamous cell carcinoma; and the oncocytic type, where 4–17% develop into squamous cell carcinoma [4, 5].

10.5 Clinical Presentation

Paranasal malignancies typically manifest with nonspecific clinical symptoms, including the following:

- Nasal obstruction.
- Facial pain.
- Persistent rhinorrhea or epistaxis.
- In advanced stages, patients may present with proptosis, diplopia, or other neurological symptoms.

10.6 Workup

10.6.1 History

Patients presenting with sinonasal malignancies may exhibit nonspecific symptoms including nasal obstruction, discharge, epistaxis, facial pain or swelling, anosmia, and proptosis. A meticulous inquiry into the duration and progression of each symptom is essential. Due to the ambiguous and often subtle nature of early-stage manifestations, diagnosis may be delayed. Hence, persistent or prolonged symptoms should prompt a thorough investigation to exclude malignancy.

10.6.2 Clinical Examination

Although the paranasal sinuses are not directly visible, examination of the external nasal structures for deformities, asymmetry, or signs of inflammation is crucial. In suspected cases of sinonasal expansile mass, a complete clinical examination necessitates nasal endoscopy using flexible and/or rigid endoscopes.

In cases of suspected maxillary sinus malignancy, comprehensive examination should also include assessment of the oral cavity. Examination of the oral cavity is essential to evaluate for signs such as loosening of teeth, which may indicate involvement of the alveolar process of the maxilla. Additionally, maxillary sinus tumors may manifest as a submucosal swelling at the level of the cheek or gingiva-buccal sulcus.

In suspected cases of ethmoid or maxillary sinus malignancies, comprehensive cranial nerve examination (CN I-VI) is essential. These tumors can lead to alterations in eyeball positioning, manifesting as proptosis with or without diplopia, due to orbital invasion, compression, or muscle involvement. Additionally, lesions extending into the pterygopalatine fossa may affect the infraorbital nerve, causing cheek sensory disturbances. Involvement of structures like the cavernous sinus or orbital apex may result in visual disturbances from optic nerve infiltration [7].

10.6.2.1 Investigations

Nasal Endoscopy

Nasal endoscopy provides direct visualization of the lesion, aiding in the differentiation between inflammatory polyps (characterized by a smooth surface and translucent appearance) and neoplasms, whether benign or malignant. A unilateral expansile mass exhibiting irregular surface morphology, necrotic areas, and contact bleeding should raise suspicion for malignancy. Endoscopic assessment, especially in cases where the mass does not fully occupy the nasal fossa, may facilitate identification or inference of the lesion's likely origin site, local extent, and the presence of satellite lesions [7].

Biopsy

Endoscopic biopsy, conducted under direct visualization using nasal endoscopy, is favored for lesions accessible via the nasal cavity or sinuses. This minimally invasive approach allows for targeted sampling while minimizing trauma to adjacent tissues [8]. Image-guided biopsy employs advanced imaging modalities like CT or MRI to precisely localize the lesion and guide the biopsy needle to the target site. This method is particularly advantageous for deep-seated or challenging-to-access lesions [9] (Table 10.1).

Staging

Computer Tomography

Contrast-enhanced CT scan of the face and neck is the gold standard for evaluation. If nodal disease or advanced primary disease is present, CT imaging of the thorax is also indicated. CT imaging is highly sensitive in detecting bony erosions and sinus opacifications associated with sinonasal malignancies. Key areas to carefully evaluate on CT are the bony orbital walls, cribriform plate, foveolae ethmoidales, posterior wall of the maxillary sinus, pterygopalatine fossa, pterygoid plates, sphenoid sinus, and the posterior table of the frontal sinus. Studies have reported sensitivity values ranging from approximately 80% to over 95% for CT scans in detecting paranasal sinus malignancies. However, specificity values have been reported to be slightly lower, typically ranging from 80% to 90% [10, 11].

Magnetic Resonance Imaging

MRI is complementary to CT in the assessment of soft tissue extent and extent beyond bones. MRI helps to delineate tumor extent, assess infiltration of adjacent structures, and identify involvement of critical areas such as the orbit and brain.

Table 10.1 IHC markers for common PNS malignancies

Type	IHC stain
Squamous cell carcinoma	AE1/AE3, CK5/6, p40 positive
Intestinal-type adenocarcinoma	Pan CK positive, intestinal markers CK20, CDX2, villin, SATB2, MUC2 positive
NUT carcinoma	NUT1 diffuse speckled pattern, INI1 retained
Sino-nasal undifferentiated carcinoma	SMARCB1 (INI1), and SMARCA4 (BRG1) retained

Table 10.2 Imaging features to identify different benign and malignant tumors of PNS

Type	Location	Features
Osteoma (benign)	Frontal sinus	Dense cortical bone and ground-glass appearance Difficult to differentiate from fibrous dysplasia
Fibrous dysplasia (benign)		Ground glass appearance Radiological findings show three patterns: pagetoid, sclerotic, and cystic; the pagetoid form, with bone expansion and mixed areas of sclerosis and cystic areas, is the most common
Sino-nasal papilloma (benign)	Ethmo-maxillary sinus	CT shows unilateral ethmo-maxillary sinus opacification that demineralizes the bone with medial bulging into the nasal septum
Juvenile nasopharyngeal angiofibroma (benign)	Pterygoid plates at adolescence	Characteristic imaging pattern at CT: Broadening of the pterygopalatine fossa with enlargement of the sphenopalatine foramen medially and the Vidian canal posteriorly
Squamous cell carcinoma/ adenocarcinoma	Maxillary sinuses followed by the ethmoid sinuses	Bone destruction may be seen on CT and may extend beyond the bones
Chondrosarcoma	Skull base	CT shows a multi-lobulated, heterogeneous lesion with peripheral and scattered central calcifications
Adenoid cystic carcinoma	Maxillary or ethmoid sinuses	Low-grade ACC may present as an ethmoid polyp that remodels bone and mimics a simple polyp at both CT and MR imaging High-grade ACC may present as a large, irregular mass with bone destruction and irregular density ACC has a tendency for peri-neural spread along cranial nerves. MRI is therefore necessary
Neuro-endocrine tumors (SNUC, SNEC)		Mimics SCC. Diagnosed by biopsy

MRI exhibits high sensitivity in detecting paranasal sinus malignancies, with sensitivity often reported to range from 85% to 100% [12]. The specificity of MRI is also significant, typically reported to be between 85% and 95% [13]. MRI is better for assessing skull base invasion, soft tissue intracranial, or intra-orbital extension, differentiating retained secretions from tumor and perineural spread (Table 10.2).

PET CT

PET CT is not considered part of standard imaging for the initial evaluation of PNS malignancy. It may be useful in follow-up after radiotherapy to look for response or evaluate residual/recurrent disease.

Staging of paranasal sinus tumors has to be done according to the AJCC 9th edition.

References

1. Dutta R, Dubal PM, Svider PF, Liu JK, Baredes S, Eloy JA. Sinonasal malignancies: a population-based analysis of site-specific incidence and survival. Laryngoscope. 2015;125(11):2491–7.
2. Sahoo AK, Nair RR, Mishra UP, Behera G, Sidam S, Gupta V. Malignancy of nose and paranasal sinuses: an institutional study in Central India. Cureus. 2024;16(1):e52074.
3. Turner JH, Reh DD. Incidence and survival in patients with sinonasal cancer: a historical analysis of population-based data. Head Neck. 2012;34(6):877–85.
4. Goncalves N, Burnell LA, Motakef S, Modi PC. Primary ethmoid sinus squamous cell carcinoma in a young adult man. S Afr Med J. 2016;106(9):893–4.
5. Bracigliano A, Tatangelo F, Perri F, et al. Malignant sinonasal tumors: update on histological and clinical management. Curr Oncol. 2021;28(4):2420–38.
6. Llorente JL, López F, Suárez C, Hermsen MA. Sinonasal carcinoma: clinical, pathological, genetic and therapeutic advances. Nat Rev Clin Oncol. 2014;11(8):460–72.
7. Sharma D, Sharma N, Sharma V, Sharma D, Sharma N, Sharma V. Sinonasal cancers: diagnosis and management. In: Challenging issues on paranasal sinuses [Internet]. IntechOpen; 2019. [cited 2024 Jun 9]. Available from: https://www.intechopen.com/chapters/64095.
8. Wormald PJ, Wormald PJ. Endoscopic sinus surgery: anatomy, three-dimensional reconstruction, and surgical technique. Thieme; 2005. p. 176.
9. Singh A, Kumar R, Thakar A, Sharma SC, Bhalla AS. Role of image guided navigation in endoscopic surgery of paranasal sinuses: a comparative study. Indian J Otolaryngol Head Neck Surg. 2020;72(2):221–7.
10. Diagnostic efficacy of computerized tomography and magnetic resonance imaging in sinonasal tumors: a comparative study. J Oral Maxillofac Pathol. 17(3):329.
11. Imaging in head and neck cancer: United Kingdom National Multidisciplinary Guidelines. J Laryngol Otol. 126(S2):S17–26.
12. Som PM, Curtin HD. Head and neck imaging. Radiology. 2000;216(2):342–4.
13. Hermans R. Imaging of sinonasal tumors. Semin Ultrasound CT MR. 2004;25(6):437–61.

Chapter 11
Evaluation and Staging of Salivary Gland Malignancy

Ashutosh Mukherji and Narapareddy Venkata Dinesh Reddy

11.1 Introduction

Salivary glands are exocrine glands that produce around 0.5–1.5 L of saliva daily, which is essential for facilitating mastication, swallowing and speech, lubrication of the oral cavity, and improving taste perception. It contains enzymes, lipases, and amylases, which help in the digestion of triglycerides and starch. Salivary gland malignancies are relatively rare tumors with varied histological types. They represent less than 5% of all head and neck malignancies. Despite having a higher malignancy risk in tumors of sublingual and submandibular glands, the majority of salivary gland malignancies arise from the parotid gland [1]. Of the tumors of the parotid gland, 75% are benign, and 25% are malignant. While nearly 40% of submandibular glands are malignant. Tumors of the sublingual gland are almost always malignant, unless proven otherwise.

There are no strong risk factors for salivary gland malignancies. Radiation exposure and viruses (including EBV and HIV), immunosuppression, and occupational exposure to rubber or nickel are a few of the proposed etiologies of salivary gland malignancies. Unlike cancers of the oral cavity and oropharynx, there is no strong association of tobacco and alcohol consumption with salivary gland malignancies [2]. However, there is an increased risk of Warthin's tumor of the parotid with smoking [3].

A. Mukherji (✉) · N. Venkata Dinesh Reddy
Department of Radiation Oncology, MPMMCC & HBCH, Varanasi, Units of Tata Memorial Centre and affiliated with Homi Bhabha National Institute, Mumbai, India

S. Pradhan et al. (eds.), *Evidence Based Handbook on Diagnosis and Staging in Oncology*, https://doi.org/10.1007/978-981-95-9701-7_11

Table 11.1 Percentage of nodal involvement with T stage, histology, and location of primary

T+ H score	Parotid	Submandibular	Oral cavity	Other locations
2	4	0	4	0
3	12	33	13	29
4	25	57	19	56
5	33	60	–	–
6	38	50	–	–

T Scoring: based on stage T1 = 1; T2 = 2; T3–4 = 3; *H Scoring:* acinic/adenoid cystic/pleomorphic adenoma = 1; mucoepidermoid = 2; squamous/undifferentiated = 3

11.2 Natural History

Based on the location and type of histology, salivary gland malignancies have local spread, skin invasion for parotid tumors in 10%, and fixation to structures in 20% cases. Nerve palsies occur in malignant salivary tumors in 18–25% cases [4]. Neck nodal involvement is noted in around 14%, and occult pathological positive nodes in 25% cases, as per a study done by the Dutch Head and Neck Oncology group. Based on T stage and histology, the percentage of nodal positivity for salivary gland malignancies varies with the location of the primary, which is represented in Table 11.1 [5].

Around 3–4% of patients with salivary gland malignancies present with distant metastasis [6]. Chances of distant metastases increase if histology is of adenoid cystic, salivary duct, squamous cell, or undifferentiated. Common sites of distant metastases include the lung, bone, and liver. Distant metastases occur late in the course of the adenoid cystic type, generally after 10 years of follow-up in around 40% patients [7].

11.3 Histology

Malignant tumors		*Benign tumors*
Mucoepidermoid carcinoma Adenoid cystic carcinoma Acinic cell carcinoma Polymorphous adenocarcinoma Clear cell carcinoma Basal cell carcinoma Intraductal carcinoma Adenocarcinoma, NOS Salivary duct carcinoma	Myoepithelial carcinoma Carcinoma ex pleomorphic adenoma Secretory carcinoma Sebaceous adenocarcinoma Carcinosarcoma Poorly differentiated carcinoma Lymphoepithelial carcinoma Squamous cell carcinoma Oncocytic carcinoma Sialoblastoma	Pleomorphic adenoma Myoepithelioma Basal cell adenoma Warthin tumor Oncocytoma Lymphadenoma Cystadenoma Sialadenoma Ductal papillomas Sebaceous adenoma Canalicular adenoma

Non-neoplastic epithelial lesions	*Benign soft tissue lesions*	*Hematolymphoid tumors*
Sclerosing polycystic adenosis Nodular oncocytic hyperplasia Lymphoepithelial sialadenitis Intercalated duct hyperplasia	Hemangioma Lipoma/sialolipoma Nodular fasciitis	Extranodal marginal zone lymphoma of mucosa-associated lymphoid tissue [MALT lymphoma]

Histological examination is crucial for accurate diagnosis. Salivary gland tumours constitute a diverse group of neoplasms with varying histological and clinical features. Mucoepidermoid carcinoma is the most common parotid malignancy, and its grade is prognostic. Adenoid cystic carcinoma is commonly associated with perineural invasion and tracks along cranial nerves. The percentage of the solid component compared to tubular and cribriform patterns is a poor prognostic factor for the adenoid cystic variety. Salivary duct carcinomas are more common in males (four times) than in females. It is an aggressive, high-grade tumour with androgen receptors and HER2 amplifications.

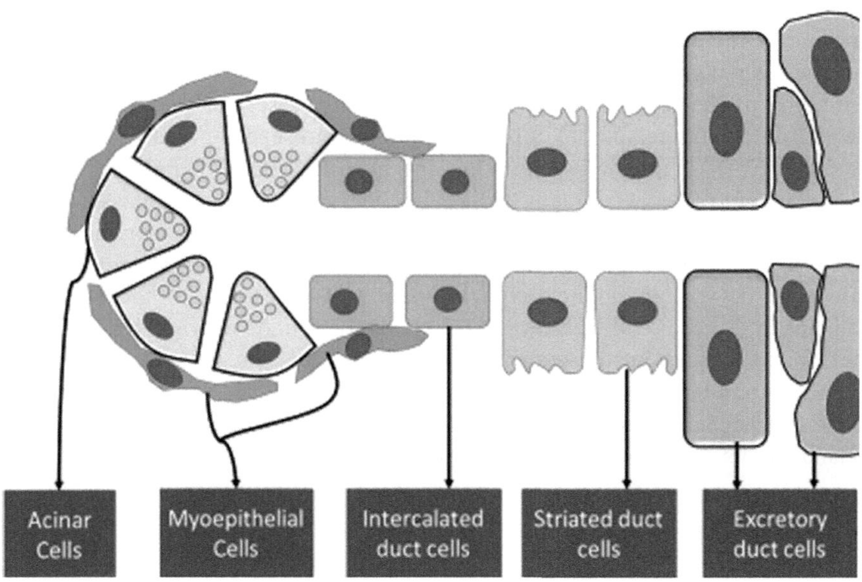

Cell of origin	Tumors
Acinar cells	Acinic cell carcinoma
Myoepithelial cells	Myoepithelioma Myoepithelial carcinoma
Intercalated cells/myoepithelial cells	Adenoid cystic tumors Myoepithelial carcinoma Epithelial-myoepithelial carcinoma Pleomorphic adenoma
Striated duct cells	Warthin's tumor Oncocytic carcinoma
Excretory duct cells	Mucoepidermoid carcinoma Salivary duct carcinoma Adenocarcinoma

11.4 Clinical Presentation

Most often, patients with salivary gland tumors present with a painless enlarging mass. Most patients present with complaints of a firm mass in the preauricular region, i.e., parotid region. However, if the deep lobe of the parotid is primarily involved, the mass is impalpable but displaces the tonsil and soft palate, causing breathing difficulty during sleep, an altered voice, and dysfunction of the eustachian tube. Benign lesions present as painless swelling with rapid enlargement of an indolent mass present for years. Malignant tumors grow rapidly in 3–6 months and are often painful. Pain appears on involvement of deeper structures like the pterygoid muscles or masseter. Few tumors cause salivary flow obstruction, leading to swallowing difficulty. Sublingual salivary gland tumors present as asymptomatic swelling at the floor of the mouth, associated with pain and numbness of the tongue if advanced disease. Unlike major salivary glands, minor salivary gland tumors are found throughout the upper aerodigestive tract, and signs and symptoms depend upon the anatomical site involved.

A few signs and symptoms are helpful in suggesting malignancy of salivary gland tumors, which include the following:

1. Pain and paresthesia
2. Rapid growth
3. Facial/other nerve palsies
4. Fixity
5. Skin involvement/ulceration
6. Associated lymphadenopathy

Apart from benign and malignant salivary tumors, patients presenting with a salivary gland mass can have other differentials, including benign cysts, sialadenitis, sialolithiasis, lymphadenopathy, tuberculosis, mononucleosis, lymphoepithelial cysts, or metastases from other body sites.

11.5 Evaluation

11.5.1 Clinical Examination

The workup of a patient presenting with salivary gland swelling starts with physical examination. The size of the tumor, involvement of overlying skin, lymphadenopathy, and cranial nerve palsies will help in distinguishing malignant from benign types of salivary gland tumors. However, histopathological diagnosis is a must for prognosis and management. Clinical examination and imaging alone without FNAC cannot distinguish benign from malignant lesions.

11.5.2 Role of FNAC and Indication of Biopsy

Fine needle aspiration cytology has a specificity and sensitivity of 85% and 95%, respectively [8], to differentiate between malignant and benign tumors. But if cytological features show suspicion of lymphoma, a biopsy is warranted. Open biopsies are contraindicated unless it is an ulcerated lesion, a minor salivary gland tumor, or FNAC is suggestive of lymphoma.

11.6 Imaging

Plain radiographs are less informative for the diagnosis of malignancy, but give an idea of the presence of bone invasion, and sialography can exclude obstructive disease. USG helps in distinguishing intrinsic from extrinsic tumors and also helps in differentiating solid from cystic masses in the salivary glands. Moreover, USG is used extensively in guiding FNA or core biopsy to increase their diagnostic accuracy. CT excludes recurrent, inflammatory masses and also helps in identifying involved lymph nodes and extension into the deep lobe. MRI, with a sensitivity of 89%, is the imaging modality of choice for salivary gland malignancies [9]. It helps in better delineation of the tumor, along with identifying perineural invasion of cranial nerves. 18FDG PET-CT helps in ruling out distant metastases [10]. FDG PET-CT also helps in post-treatment settings, for monitoring and detecting recurrences. CECT Thorax may be used in place of PET CT to rule out lung metastases in high-grade salivary gland malignancy.

References

1. Green B, Rahimi S, Brennan PA. Salivary gland malignancies–an update on current management for oral healthcare practitioners. Oral Dis. 2016;22(8):735–9.
2. Horn-Ross PL, Ljung BM, Morrow M. Environmental factors and the risk of salivary gland cancer. Epidemiology. 1997;8(4):414–9. https://doi.org/10.1097/00001648-199707000-00011.
3. Kotwall CA. Smoking as an etiologic factor in the development of Warthin's tumour of the parotid gland. Am J Surg. 1992;164(6):646–7.
4. Van de Poorten V, Hart A, Vauterin T, et al. Prognostic index for patients with parotid carcinoma. Cancer. 2009;115:540–50.
5. Terhaard C, Lubsen H, Rasch C, et al. The role of radiotherapy in the treatment of malignant salivary gland tumours. Int J Radiat Oncol Biol Phys. 2005;61:103–11.
6. Bjørndal K. Salivary gland carcinoma in Denmark 1990–2005: outcome and prognostic factors. Results of the Danish Head and Neck Cancer Group (DAHANCA). https://doi.org/10.1016/j.oraloncology.2011.09.005.
7. Spiro RH. Distant metastasis in adenoid cystic carcinoma of salivary origin. Am J Surg. 1997;174(5):495–8. https://doi.org/10.1016/S0002-9610(97)00153-0.
8. Rameeza A, Hemalata M. Fine-needle aspiration cytology of salivary gland lesions. J Oral Maxillofac Pathol. 2022;26(1):52–6.
9. Liu Y, Li J, Tan Y-R, Xiong P, Zhong L-P. Accuracy of diagnosis of salivary gland tumours with the use of ultrasonography, computed tomography, and magnetic resonance imaging: a meta-analysis. https://doi.org/10.1016/j.oooo.2014.10.020.
10. Roh J-L, et al. Clinical utility of ^{18}F-FDG PET for patients with salivary gland malignancies. J Nucl Med. 2007;48:240.

Chapter 12
Rare Tumors of Head and Neck

Lincoln Pujari and Chandrima Mukherjee

12.1 Introduction

As with other sites, rare tumors of the head and neck pose a diagnostic dilemma. The void in the literature regarding the nature of the diseases and their response to conventional treatment further adds to the challenges in their treatment. These mostly include non-epithelial tumors of the head and neck. This chapter aims to shed light on how to diagnose these rare tumors and differentiate them from their epithelial counterparts.

- Paraganglioma
- Mucosal melanoma
- Esthesioneuroblastoma
- Chordoma
- Hemangiopericytoma
- Lethal midline granuloma
- Nasopharyngeal angiofibroma
- SNUCs

12.2 Paraganglioma

Paraganglioma (PGLs) or glomus tumors (GTs) are rare neuroendocrine tumors that arise from the parasympathetic ganglia of glossopharyngeal and vagal nerves. Embryologically, they come from neural crest cells and have large epithelioid cells

L. Pujari (✉) · C. Mukherjee
Department of Radiation Oncology, MPMMCC/HBCH Varanasi, Units of Tata Memorial Centre; Also affliated with Homi Bhabha National Institute, Mumbai, India

S. Pradhan et al. (eds.), *Evidence Based Handbook on Diagnosis and Staging in Oncology*, https://doi.org/10.1007/978-981-95-9701-7_12

with fine granular cytoplasm with rich capillary network. They can be found anywhere in the body, from the base of the skull to the pelvis [1]. These tissues are responsive to changes in oxygen and carbon dioxide tensions and pH. PGs are named after the structure they arise from. For example:

Site of origin	Name of GT
Carotid artery bifurcation	Carotid body tumors
Middle ear	Glomus tympanicum
Jugular bulb	Glomus jugulare
Vagus nerve	Vagal PGL

Among head and neck paraganglioma, 44–48% are carotid body tumors, 16–24% are glomus jugulare, 20% are glomus tympanicum, and 8% are glomus vagale [x5].

PG Ls may occur at any age; however, the majority manifest between the third and the sixth decade. Median age of carotid body tumors (CBTs) and glomus tympanicum has been reported 45 years and 52 years, respectively [2].

Male:Female ratio—3:1

35–40% hereditary—associated with SDHx gene mutation [3].

12.3 Clinical Features

HNPGLs are mostly parasympathetic PGLs. The majority of parasympathetic PGLs are non-functional. <5% HNPGLs secrete catecholamine.

Most HNPGLs present as painless masses [1].

They mostly present as pressure symptoms as per their location [X, X1].

For example, middle ear—start with discomfort and mild earache and gradually proceed to pulsatile tinnitus, hearing loss, and even may lead to cranial nerve palsy because of invasion of base of skull.

Invading middle cranial fossa—temporo-parietal headache, retro-orbital pain, proptosis, paresis of nearby nerves, e.g., CN V and VI.

Posterior cranial fossa—occipital headache, ataxia, and paresis of CN V, VI, VII, IX, XII.

Jugular foramen—paresis of CN—IX, X, IX.

When glomus tumor of the carotid body enlarges, it may be visible as a pulsatile swelling on the neck.

Very rarely these tumors may turn malignant with metastasis on about 5% of patients.

12.4 Diagnostic Workup

Clinical Examination—in majority of patients of middle ear glomus, a red or bluish white mass is seen which may look like cholesteatoma. There is conductive hearing loss on audiometry.

Pulsatile neck swelling with a bruit may be seen in jugular glomus.

12.4.1 Radiological Imaging

They are invaluable in diagnosis of these rare tumors as tissue diagnosis from these tumors at critical locations are not done in fear of hemorrhage.

Simple X-ray of the PNS and mastoid done for evaluation of headache may not reveal the soft tissue mass but may reveal the mastoiditis (clouding of mastoid air cells).

High-resolution computed tomography (HRCT) with contrast gives good information about the tumor located in the middle ear or jugular bulb. They enhance on contrast but hardly erode the bone rather negotiate the bony structures and grow around it. This is in contrast to cholesteatoma of middle ear which usually erodes the bone [x2] *[image of glomus vs. cholesteatoma]*.

Magnification CT angiography is sensitive and specific for detection of middle ear and carotid glomus tumor. It shows a hyper-vascular middle ear mass that appears in the middle to late arterial phase, persists through the capillary phase, and a rapid wash out in the venous phase without demonstrating early draining veins.

Patients with suspected PPGLs should undergo plasma-free or 24-h urinary-fractionated metanephrine screening (sensitivities >90% for secreting PPGLs).

MRI shows presence of peripheral capsule. Paraganglioma shows heterogeneous T1-weighted signal with vascular flow voids. On T2-weighted imaging, they appear hyperintense [4]. Three subtypes of glomus tumors (vascular, solid, and myxoid) may be identified on the basis of relaxation times and enhancement characteristics on MRI [X3] *(MR image)*.

12.4.2 Octreotide Scintigraphy

Octreotide is a somatostatin analog that, when coupled to a radioisotope, produces a scintigraphic image of neuroendocrine tumors (NETs) expressing somatostatin type 2 receptors. In a retrospective study, Bustillo et al. compared the histopathologic diagnosis of 74 patients with head and neck NETs to the findings of octreotide scintigraphy. Octreotide scintigraphy was correctly positive in 36 of the 37 patients with paraganglioma and correctly negative in 19 of the 23 patients who did not display paraganglioma of the 60 patients receiving assessment for suspected paraganglioma (sensitivity of 97% and specificity of 82%) [5].

As glomus tumors show high level of somatostatin receptor (SSTR) subtype 2 and 5, metabolic imaging directed for this can be used for diagnostics and to guide the target delineation for radiotherapy treatment. ^{68}Ga DOTATOC (*DOTA-d-Phe(1)-Tyr(3)-octreotide*) PET, ^{68}Ga-DOTANOC (*^{68}Ga-DOTA-Nal3-octreotide*) PET, or ^{68}Ga-DOTATATE (*^{68}Ga-DOTA-Tyr3-octreotate*) PET may be used for metabolic and functional imaging. ^{68}Ga DOTATOC and ^{68}Ga-DOTATATE have high affinity for SSTR2 but ^{68}Ga-DOTANOC has broad range affinity for SSTR2, SSTR3, and SSTR5 [x4] *(PET Image).*

Arteriography to determine bilateral involvement and collateral cerebral blood flow (optional).

Staging of Glomus Tumor
"Glasscock-Jackson Classification of Glomus Tumors" [33]

12.5 Glomus Tympanicum

I. Small mass limited to promontory
II. Tumor completely filling middle ear space
III. Tumor filling middle ear and extending into the mastoid
IV. Tumor filling middle ear, extending into the mastoid or through tympanic membrane to fill the external auditory canal; may extend anterior to carotid

12.6 Glomus Jugulare

I. Small tumor involving the jugular bulb, middle ear, and mastoid
II. Tumor extending under internal auditory canal; may have intracranial canal extension
III. Tumor extending into the petrous apex; may have intracranial canal extension
IV. Tumor extending beyond the petrous apex into the clivus or infratemporal fossa; may have intracranial canal extension

Modification of McCabe and Fletcher Classification of Chemodectomas [34].

12.7 Group I: Tympanic Tumors

Absence of bone destruction on X-rays of the mastoid bone and jugular fossa

Absence of facial nerve weakness

Intact eighth nerve with conductive deafness only

Intact jugular foramen nerves (cranial nerves IX, X, and XI)

12.8 Group II: Tympanomastoid Tumors

X-ray evidence of bone destruction confined to the mastoid bone and not involving the petrous bone

Normal or paretic seventh nerve

Intact jugular foramen nerves

No evidence of involvement of the superior bulb of the jugular vein on retrograde venogram

12.9 Group III: Petrosal and Extra-Petrosal Tumors

Destruction of the petrous bone, jugular fossa, and/or occipital bone on X-rays

Positive findings on retrograde jugulography

Evidence of destruction of the petrous or occipital bones on carotid arteriogram

Jugular foramen syndrome (paresis of cranial nerves IX, X, or XI)

Presence of metastasis

12.10 Mucosal Melanomas

Mucosal melanomas, a subtype of the non-cutaneous melanoma, arise from the sun-protected mucous membranes. Melanomas can develop due to uninhibited proliferation of melanocytes (melanin-producing cells). It affects the mucosal surfaces of the body, including oral, nasal, anorectal, genitourinary, and vulvovaginal region.

MMHN—less than 1% of melanoma cases in the United States [5, 6].

Mostly occur in fifth-seventh decade of life with a M:F ratio of 1:1 [7].

In a review by Batsakis et al., analysis of 204 mucosal melanomas revealed 56.4% originated in the upper respiratory tract, while 44% came from the oral cavity and pharynx. Melanomas in nasal cavity or paranasal region were rare (less than 1%) among malignant melanomas, accounting for 2–9% of head and neck cases [8].

12.10.1 Clinical Features

Early oral mucosal melanoma lesions are painless and irregularly shaped. They appear as brown to black macules or papules. Lesions can enlarge and transform into nodules or exophytic masses. Gradually, they become more deeply pigmented.

Advanced lesions are painful, ulcerated, and fragile, prone to bleeding. Pigmentation is non-uniform, displaying shades of gray, dark blue, brown, or black [9–11].

12.10.2 Pathology

Three common microscopic patterns of oral mucosal melanomas are seen: in situ, invasive, and combined. In the initial stages, there is radial proliferation of atypical melanocytes in the basal cell layer of the epithelium followed by vertical growth of invasive nodular aggregates of atypical melanocytes in the lamina propria [9].

These cells can be polyhedral, round, fusiform, epithelioid, spindle-shaped, or pleomorphic in shape. Their size varies and their nuclei contain one or more eosinophilic nucleoli: mitotic activity is a prominent feature. They form either solid, loosely cohesive, pseudoalveolar, or organoid patterns [10].

12.10.3 Staging and Workup [12]

- Hopkin's/fiber-optic examination as a part of clinical examination.
- Biopsy: Depending on the site, a punch biopsy/knife biopsy or an excisional biopsy may be required. Stains like HMB-45, S-100, Melan-A can be used.
- Contrast-enhanced CT scan on the head and neck to determine the anatomic extent of disease.
- Metastatic workup may include FDG-PET/CT or CT of thorax abdomen and pelvis (depending on the availability).
- AJCC TNM staging is used in mucosal melanoma. T1, T2 stage is omitted due to poor prognosis of even small and superficial lesions. T3, T4 stages are explained in the following table.

Stage	Description	Comments
T3	Tumor limited to mucosa or immediately underlying soft tissue	
T4	Moderately or very advanced local disease	
T4a	Moderately advanced local disease	
T4b	Very advanced local disease that makes surgery difficult or inoperable	

12.11 Esthesioneuroblastoma

Esthesioneuroblastoma (ENB) is a rare and aggressive malignant nasal tumor, arising from the olfactory neuroepithelium in the upper nasal cavity [13]. Also known as olfactory neuroblastoma, this rare malignancy accounts for only a small fraction of all nasal tumors.

Represents about 5–10% of all malignant sinonasal tumors and has no sex predilection [14].

Bimodal age distribution with peaks at 11–20 years and 40–60 years.

It can spread via hematogenous and lymphatic spread—metastases being reported in 10–30% cases. Most common site being cervical lymph nodes [15].

12.11.1 Clinical Features

ENBs can present with a wide range of clinical features, which can sometimes overlap with other nasal tumors or inflammatory conditions. Common symptoms include the following:

- Nasal obstruction
- Epistaxis (nosebleeds) (tumor is friable and bleeds easily)
- Anosmia (loss of sense of smell)
- Facial pain

As the tumor grows, it may lead to headache, visual disturbances, rhinorrhea, proptosis (bulging of the eye), diplopia (double vision), and even intracranial extension, potentially causing neurological deficits.

12.11.2 Diagnosis

On visual inspection, the red mass can be seen in the nasal cavity. However, the ocular and nasopharyngeal mass are present even in early lesions.

CT scan with contrast is one of the initial investigations which gives a good idea about the extent of the disease and gives information about bony destruction.

MRI with gadolinium contrast may give additional information about soft tissue involvement and intracranial extension.

This tumor also expresses SSTR2. Hence, ^{68}Ga DOTATATE PET CT is of major help in the diagnosis and demarcation of the lesion, and it helps in evaluation of recurrence and metastatic setting as well [16]. Bone scan is useful in detecting the bone metastasis as well.

Although they secrete catecholamines, measurement of urine vanillylmandelic acid (VMA) has not been proven to be clinically useful.

12.11.3 Pathology

Pathological landmark of ENB is the aggregation of tumor cells into rosettes, pseudorosettes, sheets, or clusters separated by a fibromuscular stroma. Chromaffin granules may be seen which arises from the primitive neural crest cells. At times it is confused with SNUC (sinonasal undifferentiated carcinoma), but SNUC lacks rosettes and intercellular fibrils [17].

12.11.4 Staging

Kadish et al. first introduced a three-tier classification of ENBs in 1976 based on local extent of disease.

Kadish classification for staging of tumors

Stages	Description	Comment
Stage A	Tumor confined to nasal cavity	
Stage B	Tumor involved the nasal cavity along with 1 or more sinuses	
Stage C	Extension of tumor beyond the sinonasal cavities and into the paranasal sinuses. Involvement of the cribriform plate, orbit, skull base, and intracranial extension	Contrast-enhanced MRI needed to rule out intracranial extension
Stage D	Cervical LN involvement or distant metastasis	Both loco-regional and distant metastases grouped in the same category

12.12 Chordoma

12.12.1 Introduction

Chordoma arises from the remnant of the primitive notochord in the axial skeleton. Approximately 50% originate in the sacrococcygeal region. Around 35% originate intracranially, often affecting the clivus. The remaining 15% emerge along the midline, following the notochord path, mainly impacting cervical vertebrae.

Most chordomas occur during the fourth decade of life, with a male-to-female ratio of 2 to 1.

12.12.1.1 Clinical Features and Presentation

Chordomas are locally invasive, and basi-sphenoidal chordoma becomes symptomatic relatively early due to its critical location. These base of skull chordomas present with headache and ocular symptoms like diplopia, bi-temporal hemianopia, pituitary insufficiency, nasal stuffiness, and cranial nerve palsy. Metastases from the disease may reach up to 25% with commonest site being lung followed by liver and bone.

12.12.2 *Imaging*

On contrast-enhanced computed tomography (CT), chordomas are typically visualized as destructive midline lesions, allowing accurate delineation of local disease extent. Intratumoral calcifications are commonly identified. The lesions demonstrate variable attenuation values and generally show enhancement following contrast administration [18].

Magnetic resonance imaging (MRI) provides superior tissue characterization. Chordomas usually appear hypointense to isointense on T1-weighted images and show striking hyperintensity on T2-weighted sequences, a feature attributed to the high fluid content within vacuolated tumor cells. Small areas of T1 hyperintensity may be observed due to intratumoral hemorrhage or protein-rich material, while fibrous septa may appear as focal hypointense bands on T2-weighted images. Following gadolinium administration, moderate contrast enhancement is typically seen, although tumors with extensive necrosis may demonstrate only minimal enhancement. MRI is also valuable in evaluating complications such as spinal cord compression and invasion of adjacent neural and vascular structures [18].

Given the midline location and locally aggressive nature of chordomas, involvement or encasement of critical neurovascular structures is common. When vascular encroachment is suspected, CT angiography or MR angiography may be required to assess vessel patency and involvement [18].

Distant metastasis is uncommon but may occur. Functional imaging modalities such as bone scintigraphy and positron emission tomography (PET) can be utilized during metastatic evaluation. However, these modalities have limited utility in assessing primary chordomas due to variable tracer uptake and the availability of more cost-effective and accessible imaging techniques [18].

12.12.2.1 Histopathology

Grossly, chordomas appear as soft, lobulated masses with a white to gray gelatinous consistency. The cut surface often reveals dense fibrous trabeculae interspersed with mucoid material, along with areas of necrosis, hemorrhage, calcification, and sequestrated bone fragments. A pseudocapsule may surround the soft tissue component, formed by compressed adjacent tissues rather than representing a true capsule [19].

Chordomas are classified into three histological subtypes: *classical (conventional)*, *chondroid*, and *dedifferentiated*. Among these, classical chordoma is associated with the most favorable prognosis, followed by the chondroid variant. Dedifferentiated chordoma, accounting for less than 4% of cases, demonstrates the most aggressive behavior and has a predilection for pediatric patients [19].

All variants display marked cytological heterogeneity. The characteristic tumor cells include large vacuolated cells containing mucopolysaccharide-rich material, known as *physaliphorous cells*, along with smaller non-vacuolated stellate cells.

Histologically, chordomas show a heterogeneous architecture with areas of necrosis, mucoid degeneration, cartilage formation, and connective tissue elements.

Immunohistochemistry plays a crucial role in diagnosis. Chordomas typically express *S-100 protein*, *vimentin*, *low-molecular-weight cytokeratins*, and *epithelial membrane antigen (EMA)*. Differentiation between chondroid chordoma and chondrosarcoma may be challenging due to overlapping morphology and shared S-100 positivity [19]. Recent studies have identified *brachyury*, a T-box transcription factor, as a highly sensitive and specific marker that aids in distinguishing chordoma from its histological mimics [20, 21].

12.12.3 Hemangiopericytoma

12.12.3.1 Introduction

These rare tumors are derived from the pericytes surrounding the blood vessels. These pericytes are believed to be the supporting cells which maintain the structural support and have contractile functions. These are rare tumors accounting for about 5% of all soft tissue tumors. Among them up to 30% of all hemangiopericytoma occur in head and neck region, and the sinonasal area is the most common site in head and neck region [22, 23].

12.12.3.2 Clinical Features and Presentation

These tumors are firm, slow-growing painless, and well localized. In sinonasal area, they may present as soft polypoidal mass with epistaxis and obstruction. Orbital lesions may present as proptosis. All symptoms are mainly related to the mass effect of the tumor. In brain they resemble meningioma. The incidence of metastasis in hemangiopericytoma reach up to 50–80%, and late metastasis even after 10 years is not uncommon. The most common site for extracranial metastasis is bone followed by lung and liver [24].

12.12.4 Imaging

On plain radiographs, hemangiopericytoma (HPC) typically presents as a soft-tissue density mass within the nasal cavity or other regions of the head and neck. Remodeling or pressure erosion of adjacent bony structures may be observed, whereas calcification is uncommon. On contrast-enhanced computed tomography (CT), the lesion appears as a well-circumscribed mass demonstrating intense, homogeneous enhancement, reflecting its marked vascularity.

Magnetic resonance imaging (MRI) further characterizes the lesion. The tumor usually exhibits signal intensity similar to or slightly higher than skeletal muscle on both T1- and T2-weighted sequences. A distinctive feature is the presence of multiple tortuous intratumoral flow voids, seen on both T1- and T2-weighted images, representing high-velocity blood flow. In larger tumors, particularly those exceeding 2 cm in diameter, these punctate flow voids are visible on T2-weighted images against a relatively hyperintense background, producing the classic *"salt-and-pepper" appearance*. Prominent flow voids from enlarged feeding vessels may also be seen along the tumor periphery.

Angiography typically demonstrates the hallmarks of a hypervascular neoplasm, including enlarged feeding arteries, dense tumor blush, and early venous drainage. Hypervascularity remains the most consistent and defining imaging characteristic of HPC.

In intracranial locations, the principal radiological differential diagnosis is meningioma. However, features favoring HPC include the absence of calcification, minimal peritumoral edema, ring-like contrast enhancement, and higher apparent diffusion coefficient (ADC) values on diffusion-weighted imaging. Both CT and MRI play complementary roles in accurately defining tumor extent and anatomical relationships [25].

12.12.5 Histopathology

Histologically, hemangiopericytomas are composed of a dense proliferation of pericytic cells arranged concentrically around endothelial-lined vascular channels. These vessels vary widely in caliber, ranging from small capillary-sized channels to large, irregular, sinusoidal spaces. The tumors are generally well circumscribed and may be partially or completely enclosed by a pseudocapsule.

Distinguishing benign from malignant HPC can be challenging on morphological grounds alone. However, features such as increased mitotic activity (greater than four mitoses per high-power field), areas of tumor necrosis, and heightened cellularity are suggestive of malignant behavior [26].

12.12.6 Lethal Midline Granuloma

12.12.6.1 Introduction

This rare disease is also known as Stewart's granuloma, polymorphic reticulosis, and T/NK cell lymphomas. LMG is characterized by ulcerative destruction of the facial tissue in the midline of the body, mainly upper aero-digestive tract. The patient presents with complaints of rhinorrhea, epistaxis, nasal obstruction, and pain.

12.12.6.2 Clinical Features and Presentation

Patients most commonly present in their 50s and is more common in male. Most common sites of involvement are nasal cavity (including destruction of the septum) and the paranasal sinuses (particularly maxillary antrum). The local extension of the lesion may extend into the orbits, the oral cavity (palate, gingiva), and even the pharynx [27].

12.12.6.3 Histology

Pathologically, PMR is characterized by an atypical mixed lymphoid infiltration of the submucosa with extensive areas of necrosis. The lesion has variable zones of small lymphocytes and plasma cells. PMR has been considered a lymphoproliferative disorder, as well as most cases are peripheral T-cell lymphomas [28].

12.12.6.4 Imaging

The role of imaging studies is mainly to know the exact extension of the disease which is mainly characterized by destruction of the adjacent structures. They are invaluable during radiotherapy planning and treatment [29].

12.12.7 Nasopharyngeal Angiofibroma

12.12.7.1 Introduction

Nasopharyngeal angiofibroma is a rare highly vascular tumor within the posterior nasal cavity found almost exclusively in adolescent boys. Though histologically benign, it may invade locally into nasal cavity, nasopharynx, and pterygopalatine fossa, with larger lesions extending into other para nasal sinuses. They can also involve inferior orbital fissure, and masticator space through the infratemporal fossa. They may even have orbital and intracranial involvement, seen in approximately 10–37% of cases [30].

12.12.7.2 Clinical Features and Presentation

Patients present most commonly with nasal obstruction, epistaxis, nasal voice, nasal discharge, cheek swelling, proptosis, diplopia, hearing loss, and headaches as per their size and sites of invasion. A firm, friable, reddish, or reddish-purple mass within the nasal cavity is seen on clinical examination and nasal endoscopy.

12.12.7.3 Investigations

Biopsies are to be considered with caution because of the potential for severe hemorrhage. But it may be required when the clinical picture (sex, age, location, and behavior of the lesion) is not consistent with JNPAF. Some lesions may turn out to be sarcomas or chronic sinusitis.

On contrast-enhanced CT scan, it is avidly enhancing mass in nasal cavity with its local extension. Bone window in CT scan can demonstrate adjacent bony destructions. MRI can give better soft tissue resolution and can help in better delineation of the lesion. On non-contrast sequences, nasopharyngeal angiofibroma is heterogeneous, with intermediate T1-weighted, and intermediate to high T2-weighted signal intensity. Diffusion-weighted imaging (DWI) with associated apparent diffusion coefficient (ADC) values tend to show facilitated diffusion, with elevated ADC values [30].

12.12.8 Sinonasal Undifferentiated Carcinoma (SNUC)

Sinonasal undifferentiated carcinoma (SNUC) is a high-grade epithelial malignancy that demonstrates epithelial differentiation while lacking morphologic or immunophenotypic features of squamous, glandular, neuroectodermal, mesenchymal, melanocytic, or other specific lineages. It is a highly aggressive tumor, thought to arise from the Schneiderian mucosa or the embryologic nasal ectoderm lining the paranasal sinuses. Clinically, SNUC typically presents as a rapidly expanding mass involving multiple regions of the sinonasal tract, frequently extending beyond the confines of the nasal cavity and paranasal sinuses at the time of diagnosis [31].

Patients commonly present with symptoms such as nasal obstruction, epistaxis, proptosis, periorbital swelling, diplopia, facial or periorbital pain, and cranial nerve deficits. These tumors demonstrate aggressive local growth with extensive destruction of the sinus walls and often involve multiple paranasal sinuses simultaneously. Orbital and intracranial extension is not uncommon, and posterior spread to the nasopharynx may also be observed.

Immunohistochemically, SNUC shows strong positivity for pan-cytokeratin markers such as AE1/AE3 and low-molecular-weight cytokeratin (CAM 5.2). Cytokeratin 7 (CK7) expression is observed in approximately half of cases. Neuroendocrine markers, including synaptophysin and chromogranin, as well as squamous differentiation markers such as CK5/6, p63, and p40, are typically negative. In addition, SNUC lacks expression of markers associated with sarcomas (e.g., CD99, desmin, myogenin), lymphomas (CD45), and melanocytic tumors (Melan-A, HMB-45). Molecular studies have identified mutations in IDH1 or IDH2 in more than 80% of cases, with IDH2 R172 mutations being the most frequently encountered alteration [31].

On computed tomography (CT), SNUC appears as a non-calcified soft-tissue mass demonstrating variable contrast enhancement, often with areas of central necrosis. Magnetic resonance imaging (MRI) typically shows the lesion to be isointense on T1-weighted images and iso- to hyperintense on T2-weighted images, with heterogeneous enhancement following gadolinium administration. These radiological features are nonspecific, making it challenging to reliably distinguish SNUC from other epithelial malignancies of the nasal cavity and paranasal sinuses based on imaging alone [32].

References

1. Head and neck paragangliomas: physiology and biochemistry - PubMed [Internet]. [cited 2023 Aug 10]. Available from: https://pubmed.ncbi.nlm.nih.gov/11557442.
2. Larson TC, Reese DF, Baker HL, McDonald TJ. Glomus tympanicum chemodectomas: radiographic and clinical characteristics. Radiology. 1987;163(3):801–6.
3. Galan SR, Kann PH. Genetics and molecular pathogenesis of pheochromocytoma and paraganglioma. Clin Endocrinol. 2013;78(2):165–75.
4. Güneyli S, Ceylan N, Bayraktaroğlu S, Acar T, Savaş R. Imaging findings of vascular lesions in the head and neck. Diagn Interv Radiol. 2014;20(5):432–7.
5. Soto-Montenegro ML, Peña-Zalbidea S, Mateos-Pérez JM, et al. Meningiomas: a comparative study of 68Ga-DOTATOC, 68Ga-DOTANOC and 68Ga-DOTATATE for molecular imaging in mice. PLoS One. 2014;9(11):e111624.
6. Chang AE, Karnell LH, Menck HR. The National Cancer Data Base report on cutaneous and noncutaneous melanoma: a summary of 84,836 cases from the past decade. The American College of Surgeons Commission on Cancer and the American Cancer Society. Cancer. 1998;83(8):1664–78.
7. McLaughlin CC, Wu XC, Jemal A, Martin HJ, Roche LM, Chen VW. Incidence of noncutaneous melanomas in the U.S. Cancer. 2005;103(5):1000–7.
8. Batsakis JG. Tumors of the head and neck: clinical and pathological considerations. 2nd ed. Baltimore: Williams & Wilkins Co; 1979. p. 573, illus. $49.50 - Davidson - 1980 - Head &; Neck Surgery - Wiley Online Library [Internet]. [cited 2023 Aug 20]. Available from: https://onlinelibrary.wiley.com/doi/abs/10.1002/hed.2890030117.
9. Chatzistefanou I, Kolokythas A, Vahtsevanos K, Antoniades K. Primary mucosal melanoma of the oral cavity: current therapy and future directions. Oral Surg Oral Med Oral Pathol Oral Radiol. 2016;122(1):17–27.
10. Update on primary head and neck mucosal melanoma - López - 2016 - Head & Neck - Wiley Online Library [Internet]. [cited 2023 Aug 20]. Available from: https://onlinelibrary.wiley.com/doi/10.1002/hed.23872.
11. Smith MH, Bhattacharyya I, Cohen DM, et al. Melanoma of the oral cavity: an analysis of 46 new cases with emphasis on clinical and histopathologic characteristics. Head Neck Pathol. 2016;10(3):298–305.
12. NCCN [Internet]. [cited 2023 Aug 12]. Guidelines detail. Available from: https://www.nccn.org/guidelines/guidelines-detail.
13. McCormack LJ, Harris HE. Neurogenic tumors of the nasal fossa. JAMA J Am Med Assoc. 1955;157(4):318–21.
14. Neuroblastomas and neuroendocrine carcinomas of the nasal cavity: a proposed new classification - PubMed [Internet]. [cited 2023 Aug 12]. Available from: https://pubmed.ncbi.nlm.nih.gov/7139532/.
15. Davis RE, Weissler MC. Esthesioneuroblastoma and neck metastasis. Head Neck. 1992;14(6):477–82.

16. Roytman M, Tassler AB, Kacker A, et al. [68Ga]-DOTATATE PET/CT and PET/MRI in the diagnosis and management of esthesioneuroblastoma: illustrative cases. J Neurosurg Case Lessons. 2021;1(2):CASE2058.
17. Batsakis JG. Tumors of the head and neck: clinical and pathological considerations. 2nd ed. Baltimore: Williams & Wilkins; 1979.
18. Lee SH, Kwok KY, Wong SM, et al. Chordoma at the skull base, spine, and sacrum: a pictorial essay. J Clin Imaging Sci. 2022;12:44.
19. Santegoeds RGC, Temel Y, Beckervordersandforth JC, et al. State-of-the-art imaging in human Chordoma of the skull base. Curr Radiol Rep. 2018;6(5):16.
20. Vujovic S, Henderson S, Presneau N, et al. Brachyury, a crucial regulator of notochordal development, is a novel biomarker for chordomas. J Pathol. 2006;209(2):157–65. [PubMed] [Google Scholar].
21. Oakley GJ, Fuhrer K, Seethala RR. Brachyury, SOX-9, and podoplanin, new markers in the skull base chordoma vs chondrosarcoma differential: a tissue microarray-based comparative analysis. Mod Pathol. 2008;21(12):1461–9.
22. Digumarthy SR, Peri N, Malladi UD, Jinna JMR, Sundaram C. Haemangiopericytoma of the internal jugular vein: an unusual neck mass. Clin Radiol Extra. 2003;58:45–7.
23. Fareed MM, Al Amro ASM, Akasha R, et al. Parapharyngeal space hemangiopericytoma treated with surgery and postoperative radiation- a case report. Head Neck Oncologia. 2012;4:10.
24. Ratneswaren T, Hogg FRA, Gallagher MJ, et al. Surveillance for metastatic hemangiopericytoma-solitary fibrous tumors-systematic literature review on incidence, predictors and diagnosis of extra-cranial disease. J Neuro-Oncol. 2018;138(3):447–67.
25. El-Abtah ME, Murayi R, Lee J, Recinos PF, Kshettry VR. Radiological differentiation between intracranial meningioma and solitary fibrous tumor/hemangiopericytoma: a systematic literature review. World Neurosurg. 2023;170:68–83.
26. Enzinger FM, Weiss SW. Hemangiopericytoma. In: Enzinger FM, Weiss WS, editors. Soft tissue tumors. 2nd ed. St. Louis: Mosby; 1988. p. xi–989.
27. Mallya V, Singh A, Pahwa M. Lethal midline granuloma. Indian Dermatol Online J. 2013;4(1):37–9.
28. Prasad KC, Harshitha N, Harshita TR, Pillai DAR, Brindha HS. Lethal midline granuloma: an enigma in diagnosis-a rare case report. Indian J Otolaryngol Head Neck Surg. 2019;71(Suppl 3):2140–2.
29. Milford CA, Drake-Lee AB, Lloyd GA. Radiology of the paranasal sinuses in non-healing granulomas of the nose. Clin Otolaryngol Allied Sci. 1986;11(3):199–204.
30. Tork CA, Simpson DL. Nasopharyngeal angiofibroma. [Updated 2023 Jun 26]. In: StatPearls [Internet]. Treasure Island: StatPearls Publishing; 2023.
31. Goel R, Ramalingam K, Ramani P, Chandrasekar T. Sino nasal undifferentiated carcinoma: a rare entity. J Nat Sci Biol Med. 2012;3(1):101–4.
32. Kawaguchi M, Kato H, Tomita H, Mizuta K, Aoki M, Hara A, Matsuo M. Imaging characteristics of malignant sinonasal tumors. J Clin Med. 2017;6(12):116.
33. Jackson CG, Glasscock ME 3rd, Harris PF. Glomus tumors: diagnosis, classification, and management of large lesions. Arch Otolaryngol. 1982;108(7):401–10.
34. Wang ML, Hussey DH, Doornbos JF, et al. Chemodectoma of the temporal bone: a comparison of surgical and radiotherapeutic results. Int J Radiat Oncol Biol Phys. 1988;14(4):643–8.

Chapter 13
Presentation and Evaluation of Lung Cancer

Avradeep Datta, Arvind Chavhan, and Ashutosh Mukherji

13.1 Introduction

Lung cancer is the most common cancer to affect humanity as of today, ranking first in cancers among men and second in women. Although it accounts for around 12% of cancer incidence, it has a much higher share of the mortality, reaching close to 19% [1].

Lung cancer is broadly classified into small cell lung cancer (SCLC) (15–20%) and non-small cell lung cancer (NSCLC (80–85%) based on clinico-histopathological features. Further, NSCLC is subdivided broadly into squamous cell and adenocarcinoma subtypes. Large cell, bronchoalveolar, and mixed histologies are rarely reported.

13.2 Etiology

Lung cancer was not a common cancer at the beginning of the twentieth century. Only with the advent of smoking tobacco have the rates of lung cancer seen an astronomical rise over the years, causing more than 80% of all lung cancer cases at

A. Datta · A. Mukherji (✉)
Department of Radiation Oncology, MPMMCC & HBCH, Varanasi, Units of Tata Memorial Centre and affliated with Homi Bhabha National Institute, Mumbai, India

A. Chavhan
Department of Radiation Oncology, MPMMCC & HBCH, Varanasi, Units of Tata Memorial Centre and affliated with Homi Bhabha National Institute, Mumbai, India

Department of Radiodiagnosis, MPMMCC / HBCH, Varanasi, Units of Tata Memorial Centre and affliated with Homi Bhabha National Institute (HBNI), Mumbai, India

S. Pradhan et al. (eds.), *Evidence Based Handbook on Diagnosis and Staging in Oncology*, https://doi.org/10.1007/978-981-95-9701-7_13

present. Due to various sociocultural connotations of smoking, the rates of lung cancer in men have been dropping since the 1990s, whereas they have yet to do so in women.

Before we go further, it would be wise to review a few salient points about lung cancer and smoking tobacco:

- A person who has smoked less than 100 cigarettes a day in his/her entire life is considered a non-smoker. Anyone smoking more than that is considered a smoker.
- Both first-hand and second-hand smoke are known to cause lung cancer.
- Third-hand smoke is the particles and residues of cigarette smoke left on surfaces, whereas fourth-hand smoke is the lingering smoke around smokers.
- Nicotine is not carcinogenic but addictive. But tar, acrolein, benzene, acetaldehyde, and traces of various heavy metals present in tobacco smoke cause lung cancer.
- Smoking causes field carcinogenesis.

Other than smoking tobacco, occupational exposure to arsenic, asbestos, and polycyclic aromatic hydrocarbons (PAH) has been implicated in lung cancer.

Air pollution, both indoor and outdoor, causes lung cancer. While radon exposure is the culprit in indoor pollution, it is the result of the ever-increasing presence of particulate matter in the air in major cities are leading to increased rates of lung cancer.

Indoor pollution in the form of radon exposure and outdoor air pollution in the form of particulate matter in the air are both responsible for the ever-increasing incidence of lung cancer in major cities of the world.

13.3 Clinical Signs and Symptoms

The following signs and symptoms should arouse suspicion of lung cancer and warrant further investigation:

Presentation	
Cough	Mostly unproductive, rule out tuberculosis (TB) or other infectious etiology. Background of COPD in most smokers
Hemoptysis	Rule out TB. Generally, small amounts of blood. Massive hemoptysis is fatal in >50% patients
Dyspnea	Due to atelectasis, effusion, and obstructive pneumonia. Rule out exacerbation of COPD and any cardiac comorbidity
Chest pain	Due to direct extension, obstructive pneumonitis, and pulmonary embolism
Hoarseness of voice	Due to the involvement of the recurrent laryngeal nerve
Superior vena cava syndrome	Facial edema, shortness of breath, headache, chest pain, engorged neck, and chest veins
Pancoast syndrome	Triad of shoulder and arm pain, wasting of hand muscles, and ipsilateral Horner syndrome

Presentation	
Horner syndrome	Triad of ptosis (drooping eyelids), miosis (constricted pupil), and anhidrosis (loss of sweating)
Pain in the back/ extremities	Due to bone metastasis to the vertebrae and bones, rule out any impending compression of the spinal cord
Features of raised intracranial pressure	Due to brain metastasis, headache, vomiting, hemiparesis, seizure, cranial nerve defects, and visual field loss
Paraneoplastic syndrome	See below

Paraneoplastic syndromes are more common with lung cancers than with any other cancer. They are caused by the misfiring of the body's immune response towards cancer cells. The following paraneoplastic syndromes are associated with lung cancer:

Paraneoplastic syndrome	Features
Cushing syndrome	Muscle weakness, weight loss, hypertension, hirsutism, and osteoporosis
SIADH (syndrome of inappropriate anti-diuretic hormone secretion)	Headache, muscle cramps, anorexia, decreased urine output, and cerebral edema
Hypercalcemia	Anorexia, nausea, vomiting, constipation, lethargy, polyuria, polydipsia, and dehydration. Renal failure (late)
Lambert-Eaton myasthenia syndrome	Muscle weakness of limbs that improves on repeated testing. Proximal muscles affected. Cannot rise from the chair or climb stairs
Hypertrophic osteoarthropathy	Clubbing, pain in ankles, knees, wrists, and elbows (joint pain)

13.4 Examination

While examining a suspected case of lung cancer, a thorough examination of the respiratory system is warranted.

In examining the respiratory system, special emphasis is to be paid to check for air entry in both lungs and individually in all lobes. During examination, we must keep in mind that most of these patients are long-term smokers and would have already developed some long-term sequelae of chronic obstructive pulmonary disease (COPD).

Reduced broncho-vesicular breath sounds point to reduced air entry, which in turn may point to atelectasis and collapse. It may also point to pleural effusion if found localized to the lower lobes.

A thorough palpation of the superficial nodal regions, especially the supraclavicular, is required to rule out any palpable nodes suspicious of malignancy.

Other important systems that need to be examined are the cardiovascular system to detect any abnormality that may be contributing to the presenting symptoms of shortness of breath, and also may hinder fitness for further treatment.

The neurological system needs a thorough examination to rule out any signs of intracranial disease or any metastasis to the spine. It may also help localize the primary if a patient presents with symptoms of Horner's syndrome.

13.5 Differential Diagnosis

Differential	Investigations
Primary malignancy of the lung	See below
Primary of the other site with metastasis to the lung	Check for localizing symptoms in other body parts/organ systems and proceed with histopathology ± (IHC) from the suspected primary
Tuberculosis of the lung	Sputum for acid-fast bacilli, X-ray of the chest, Mantoux testing, and interferon gold
Exacerbation of COPD	Pulmonary function test to look at FEV1 and FVC
Pneumonia	Sputum for gram stain and culture/sensitivity

13.5.1 Histology

When a case of lung cancer is suspected, a biopsy with adequate tissue to run complete Immunohistochemistry (IHC) panels is required. If metastasis is suspected, then a biopsy or at least a fine-needle aspiration cytology (FNAC) sample from the metastatic site should be obtained. The only exception may be when the patient presents with grossly disseminated disease, which is visibly metastatic on cross-sectional imaging. If pleural effusion is present, then it must be aspirated and sent for malignant cytology, as it may upstage the disease and change the treatment pathway and goals.

While obtaining a tissue sample, the following salient points need to be considered:

- Relatively non-invasive procedures, such as image-guided or endoscopic ones, are preferred over surgical ones, like thoracoscopy.
- In case of a peripheral surgically amenable suspected disease where mediastinal nodal involvement has been ruled out, upfront resection may be the choice of intervention rather than a biopsy.

- Endobronchial ultrasound (EBUS)-guided biopsies are preferred for central lesions, whereas computed tomography (CT)-guided biopsies are preferred for peripherally placed lesions.
- If the primary biopsy has been inconclusive or the tissue harvested is inadequate for IHC, then a surgical modality is preferred for the repeat biopsy.
- To properly stage according to TNM, the following schema may be kept handy.

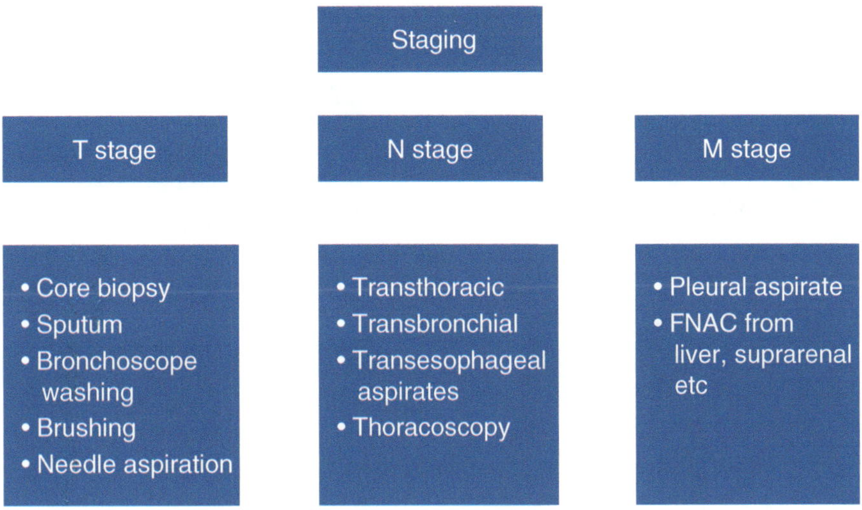

Adenocarcinoma under the microscope should show intracytoplasmic mucin or neoplastic gland formation. The presence of keratin and or intracellular desmosomes characterizes squamous cell carcinomas. Small cell carcinomas have small, round, blue cells with rosette formation and a high nuclear to cytoplasmic ratio.

The following IHC markers are positive in the three major types of lung cancer described above:

Adenocarcinoma	Squamous cell carcinoma	Small cell carcinoma
Thyroid transcription factor (TTF1)	p40	Synaptophysin
Mucin	p63	CD 56
Napsin A	CK 5/6	Chromogranin
Surf A		Neuron-specific enolase
Surf B		
Periodic acid Schiff (PAS) D		
Cytokeratin (CK) 7		

The following schematic shows the path followed in distinguishing between the subtypes of lung cancer:

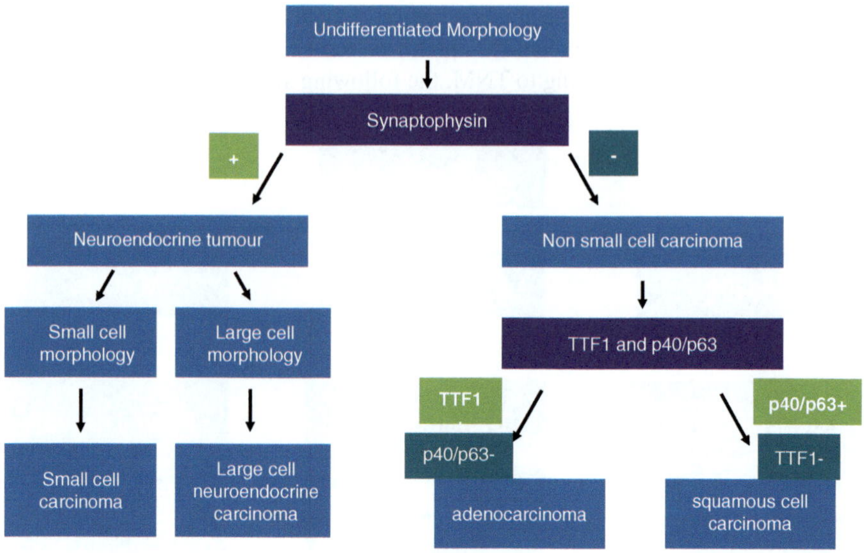

13.6 Imaging

In the clinic, the very first imaging that is ordered when a patient walks in with symptoms suggestive of lung cancer is a chest skiagram or X-ray. Although it may miss a lesion in around a quarter of all cases, the following features should warrant further imaging:

- Any gray-white mass in X-ray
- Widening of mediastinal or hilar shadow
- Pleural effusion
- Any white-out lung field

A chest X-ray may also help in ruling out hydro-pneumothorax in these patients, especially after a diagnostic or therapeutic drainage of pleural effusion has been attempted. A chest X-ray or images taken in a fluoroscopic simulator may be used as a part of conventional radiotherapy planning.

Any suspicion of malignancy in a chest X-ray should ideally be investigated by a CT scan. The following features in a CT scan are suggestive of malignancy:

- Any lesion greater than 3 cm that is new
- Any lesion with speculated margins
- Any endobronchial lesion
- Any area of consolidation not responding to treatment for pneumonia
- Thick-walled cavitary lesions when TB or other infections have been ruled out

- Multiple small nodules spread out in the lung fields
- Pleural effusion, especially unilateral
- Pleural-based nodules or plaques

A CECT will always give better information, especially since mediastinal nodal involvement is common in lung cancer. Contrast can safely be given if the glomerular filtration rate (GFR) is >30. If GFR is between 30 and 44, contrast should be administered, followed by IV fluids. A CECT with respiratory gating to account for the movement of the tumor over breathing cycles is generally conducted separately as a part of modern radiotherapy planning.

Even if an FDG PET (fluorodeoxy-glucose positron emission tomography) CT is being planned for the patient, a chest CECT at baseline gives important information that may not be available with a lower resolution CT that generally accompanies the PET. These include conditions such as atelectasis and post-obstructive pneumonia, any coexisting lung disease such as COP, and any subpleural or other lung nodule with little or no tracer uptake.

PET CT is rapidly replacing CECT as the investigation of choice in lung cancer for its superior sensitivity (80% vs. 55%) as well as specificity (81% vs. 88%) while detecting involved mediastinal lymph nodes. It also has a better probability of picking up small metastatic disease and thus helps in proper staging and prevents futile treatment. For the primary lesion, PET can distinguish between a collapsed lung and disease and thus helps in delineation in radiotherapy planning.

PET CT may also give false positive results, especially in inflammations, infections, and granulomatous diseases. It has a poor sensitivity in picking up brain lesions as well.

A specific point of discussion is the case of mediastinal lymph node evaluation. While the gold standard for the detection of mediastinal lymph node positivity is still thoracoscopy-guided sampling of suspicious nodes, it is an invasive process. While PET CT is non-invasive with a high sensitivity of around 90%, it lacks specificity. Further complicating matters is the presence of underlying infections and granulomatous diseases in regions endemic for the same. Non-standardization of SUVmax values to be considered as a cutoff also poses significant challenges in declaring a node positive/negative [2].

All locally advanced NSCLC and all cases of SCLC, irrespective of stage, should undergo a Magnetic Resonance Imaging (MRI) scan of the brain, preferably with contrast to rule out brain metastasis. An MRI scan of the spine may also be ordered if bone metastasis of the vertebra is suspected to be causing spinal cord compression. It may also be useful in planning for ablative radiotherapy in oligo-metastatic disease of the brain or vertebral column.

Blood investigations should include a complete blood count, renal and liver function tests for basic therapeutic fitness of the patient. Liver function derangement may also point towards the possibility of liver metastasis if not already detected. A coagulogram is necessary for further biopsies to take place without any untoward events. Serum alkaline phosphatase (ALKP) is an important marker that points towards liver or bone mets. Serum gamma-glutamyl transferase (GGT), when elevated along with ALKP, indicates liver metastasis, whereas a normal GGT value with raised ALKP indicates bone metastasis.

Other important investigations that help plan treatment and guide therapy are a 2D echocardiogram for fitness for chemotherapy, as well as to document baseline cardiac function before radiation or surgery. A baseline pulmonary function test is also generally performed before surgery or radical radiotherapy. Any patient planned for radical surgery with lobectomy should have a post-surgery FEV1 (forced expiratory volume in 1 s) and DLCO (diffusing capacity for carbon monoxide) value of >60% post-surgery in ideal conditions. Any value less than 30% is a contraindication for lobectomy. The stair climbing test or shuttle walk test may also guide therapy in cases where FEV1 and DLCO values are between 30% and 60%. Similar criteria are used for patients planned for upfront ablative radiotherapy to small lung primaries in patients refusing surgery or not medically fit for surgery due to other underlying comorbidities.

13.7 Staging

Lung cancer is currently staged according to the AJCC (American Joint Committee on Cancer) 8th edition. The overall stage ranges from I to IV (denoted by roman numerals) and is a composite of T (tumor), N (nodal), and M (metastasis) stages of the tumor. If the patient undergoes an upfront surgery, then a prefix of 'p' denoting pathological precedes the T, N, and M stages. If the patient has received any neoadjuvant therapy before surgery, then a prefix of 'yp' is used.

The following is a discussion on the AJCC staging. The reader is suggested to read the International Association for the Study of Lung Cancer (IASLC) lymph node stations for a better understanding of which groups of lymph nodes constitute N1, N2, and N3 [3].

Although AJCC recommends the use of the TNM staging for all subtypes of lung cancer, for small-cell lung cancer, a much simpler approach can be considered. A modified version of the Veterans' Affairs Lung Study Group (VALSG) stage for SCLC, introduced in the 1950s, is a simple approach to guide clinical decisions. According to it, SCLC can be divided into:

Limited Stage Disease: Tumor limited to the ipsilateral lung and nodal regions, and possible to be covered by a single tolerable radiotherapy field (from stages I to IIB according to AJCC staging).

Extensive Stage Disease: Tumors beyond limited stage disease, including all tumors with any associated effusion or metastasis. Also includes tumors with contralateral hilar and/or supraclavicular nodes.

AJCC Staging system 9th edition is presently used for the staging of lung cancers.

13.8 Prognostic Factors

Prognostication of any malignancy is an attempt to predict the outcomes of the future, whereas it is based on data of the past. For a cancer like lung where the treatment options are ever evolving, it is always a balancing act to prognosticate these malignancies. However, the following points may shed some light on the prognosis of the disease at hand:

1. Condition of the patient:
   - Performance status (generally recorded by ECOG (Eastern Cooperative Oncology Group) or KPS (Karnofsky Performance Status)
   - Presence of any comorbidities, such as cardiac or lung dysfunction, that might limit the use of therapeutic options
   - Personal choices of treatment
2. Condition of the tumor
   - TNM stage
   - Specific location of the primary, such as tumors causing SVCO or Pancoast tumors
   - Histologic type
   - Growth rate
   - Mutations
3. Sociocultural
   - Access to healthcare
   - Quality of care
   - Variability of care due to regional differences in the standard of care
   - Ethnic and racial differences

13.9 Biomarkers

The treatment of lung cancer has been revolutionized in recent years with the identification of several druggable targets. Unfortunately, for now, these targets can only be found in adenocarcinomas of the lung.

Tissue obtained from a biopsy of the primary is generally used for mutational testing. While next-generation sequencing (NGS) is being more commonly used with each passing day due to its ability to process multiple DNA sequences at once, other methods in use are direct sequencing, real-time-PCR, high-resolution melting analysis, and denaturing high-performance liquid chromatography (DHPLS). If tissue biopsy samples are not available, liquid biopsy, which searches for mutated cells in patients' blood, can be used.

The following table lists common biomarkers and their targeted agents in lung cancer:

Mutations	Targeted agents
EGFR	Erlotinib, Geftinib, Afatinib, Osimertinib
KRAS	Trametinib
BRAF	Dabrafenib, Vemurafenib
Her2	Trastuzumab, Afatinib
MET	Crizotinib, Cabozantinib

Gene fusions	Targeted agents
ALK	Crizotinib, Ceritinib, Alectinib
ROS1	Crizotinib, Ceritinib
RET	Cabozantinib, Vandetanib, Alectinib
NTRK1	Entrectinib
FGFR1/3	Erdafitinib, Pemigatinib, Futibatinib
NRG1	Afatinib, Dacomitinib

Gene fusions	Targeted agents
FGFR1	As mentioned previously
EGFR	
MET	
Her2	

PD1 and PDL1 proteins are also tested in lung cancer and provide useful indications as to patient selection for immune checkpoint inhibitors. Examples of immune checkpoint inhibitors approved for use in lung cancer are as follows:

- Nivolumab and Pembrolizumab (PD1 inhibitor)
- Atezolizumab and Durvalumab (PDL1 inhibitor)

13.10 Conclusion

Lung cancer continues to be a deadly disease even with the significant strides made in the past few decades in the form of immune checkpoint inhibitors and targeted agents, along with the traditional triad of radiation, chemotherapy, and surgery. Most cases are still present in an advanced stage and are incurable. Screening programs have yet to meet with any significant success, and efforts must thus be concentrated towards prevention by regulation of tobacco and its abuse. Only then can the burden of lung and other tobacco-related cancers be eased on the public health infrastructure of countries.

References

1. Bray F, Laversanne M, Sung H, Ferlay J, Siegel R, et al. Global cancer statistics 2022: GLOBOCAN estimates of incidence and mortality worldwide for 36 cancers in 185 countries. CA Cancer J Clin. 2024;74:229–63.
2. Cordeiro de Lima VC, Baldotto CS, Mascarenhas E, Gelatti A, Mathias C, et al. EP.05A.09 the accuracy of CT, 18FDG-PET/CT, and mediastinoscopy for staging in NSCLC - a systematic review and meta-analysis. J Thor Oncol. 2024;19(10 Supplement):S486.
3. El-Sherief AH, Lau CT, Wu CC, Richard L, et al. Rice International Association for the Study of Lung Cancer (IASLC) lymph node map: radiologic review with CT illustration. Radiographics. 2014;34(6):1680–91.

Chapter 14
Screening for Cancers

Ajay Kumar Choubey and Pritam Mondal

14.1 Definition

The World Health Organization (WHO) defines disease screening as "the presumptive identification of unrecognized disease in an apparently healthy, asymptomatic population using tests, examinations, or other procedures that can be applied rapidly and easily to the target population."

14.2 WHO Principles of Screening

1. Condition should be an important health problem.
2. The natural history of the condition should be adequately understood.
3. There should be a recognizable latent or early symptomatic stage.
4. There should be a suitable test or examination.
5. The test should be acceptable to the population.
6. A facility for diagnosis and treatment should be available.
7. An acceptable treatment option should exist for patients with a recognized disease.
8. There should be an agreed policy on who to treat as a patient.
9. The cost of case finding (including diagnosis and treatment) should be economically balanced.
10. Case finding should be a continuing process.

A. K. Choubey (✉) · P. Mondal
Department of Radiation Oncology, MPMMCC/HBCH Varanasi, Units of Tata Memorial Centre and also affliated with Homi Bhabha National Institute, Mumbai, India

S. Pradhan et al. (eds.), *Evidence Based Handbook on Diagnosis and Staging in Oncology*, https://doi.org/10.1007/978-981-95-9701-7_14

14.3 Common Cancer Screening

I. *Breast cancer screening*: Breast cancer is the most common cancer in India. According to "GLOBOCAN 2020," the incidence of breast cancer is 13.5% among all cancers. An effective treatment option is available; early treatment can alter the prognosis.

14.4 Guidelines for Breast Cancer Screening

14.4.1 USPSTF (United States Preventive Services Task Force) Guidelines [1]

14.4.1.1 Age-Wise Recommendation for Women

- For 40- to 49-year-old women, screening decisions are individualized.
- For 50- to 74-year-old women, biennial conventional mammography is recommended.
- For ≥75 years women, no recommendation for screening. (Insufficient evidence).

14.4.1.2 Tests Advised

- Recommendation against breast self-examination (BSE).
- Clinical breast examination (CBE) has insufficient evidence.
- Evidence is insufficient for additional benefit or harm of breast ultrasound, MRI, and digital mammography.
- Recommend medication use to reduce risk and genetic screening for BRCA1 and BRCA2.

14.4.2 American Cancer Society (ACS) Guidelines [2]

ACS categorized the target population into two groups: "average-risk" and "high-risk."

Average risk women (lifetime risk of developing breast cancer: 10–15%)

Who has

(a) No personal or family history of breast cancer
(b) No BRCA1, BRCA2 mutation
(c) No chest wall irradiation before 30 years of age

Screening guidelines for "average-risk" women

- Women between 40 and 44 years choose to start screening with mammography every year.
- Women between 45 and 54 years should go for screening mammography every year.
- Women 55 years and older can switch to alternate-year mammography.
- No bar for stopping screening. Screening should continue as long as a woman is in good health or expected to live more than 10 years.
- Clinical breast examination (CBE) is not recommended.

High-risk women (lifetime risk of developing breast cancer is 20–25%)
Who has

(a) Known BRCA1, BRCA2 mutation
(b) A first-degree relative with a BRCA1 or BRCA2 mutation
(c) Received radiation therapy to the chest wall between 10 and 30 years of age
(d) A personal history of breast cancer and ductal carcinoma in situ
(e) Li-Fraumeni, Cowden Syndrome, or Bannayan-Riley-Ruvalcaba syndrome, or first-degree relatives having one of these syndromes
(f) Extremely heterogeneous dense breasts on mammography

Screening guidelines for "High-risk" women

- Screening with yearly breast MRI and mammography, starting at the age of 30 years (MRI not used as a supplement to mammography)
- Continue screening as long as good health or the family physician's decision

14.4.3 National Cancer Grid (NCG) of India Guidelines

For limited resource settings (i.e., health and wellness centers, primary health centers (PHC), community health centers (CHC))

- Clinical breast examination (CBE) is the screening method of choice.
- It can be done by any trained healthcare personnel.
- The target age group is 40- to 65-year-old women, and after 75 years, patients may exit from screening.
- At least one to three times screening is to be done in this period.

For optimally enhanced resource setting (i.e., health and wellness centers, primary health centers (PHC), community health centers (CHC))

- Clinical breast examination (CBE) is the screening method of choice in optimally enhanced resource centers.
- It can be done by a trained physician or nurse.
- The target age group is 40- to 65-year-old women.
- After 75 years, the patient may exit from screening.
- Screening is to be done at every 2-year interval.

For high-resource setting centers (district hospitals, medical colleges, and private sectors)

- Clinical breast examination (CBE) and conventional mammography are the screening methods of choice.
- It can be done by trained physicians, surgeons, or nurses.
- The target age group is 40- to 65-year-old women.
- After 75 years, the patient may exit from screening.
- Screening is to be done at every 2-year interval.

14.5 Indian Council of Medical Research (ICMR) Guidelines [3]

ICMR does not recommend population-based mammography screens for any age group. It emphasizes health education, periodic check-ups by trained health workers, and self-breast examination (SBE).

14.6 Conclusion

In India, there is no level 1 evidence of breast cancer screening, and no guideline recommends population-based mammography screening for breast cancer at any age group. Emphasis on health education and self-breast examination (SBE) may be helpful in a country like India.

14.7 Cervical Cancer Screening

14.7.1 USPSTF (United States Preventive Services Task Force) Guidelines [4]

High-risk features for the development of cervical cancer are (a) sexually active women aged 21 to 65 years, (b) HIV infection, (c) in-utero exposure to diethylstilboestrol, (d) high-grade precancerous lesion in cervix treated previously, (e) personal history of cervical cancer.

Screening guidelines for women with high-risk features

- Women aged 21–29 years
  Screening with cervical cytology alone every 3 years
- Women aged 30–65 years

If screening is done with cervical cytology alone, then every 3 years, or if screening is done with hrHPV (high-risk HPV) testing or co-testing (both cervical cytology and HPV-DNA), then every 5 years.
- Women <21 years or >65 years are not recommended for screening.

14.7.2 American Cancer Society (ACS) Guidelines [5]

- Screening for cervical cancer should begin at 25 years of age.
- For women of 25–65 years of age, an HPV-DNA test is done 5 yearly, or a combined HPV-DNA test and Pap smear is done 5 yearly, or only a Pap smear is done 3 yearly.
- Above 65 years of age, who have had a normal screen in the last 10 years or no history of CIN2 (cervical intraepithelial neoplasm 2) or more diagnosed in the last 25 years, may stop screening.
- Women having undergone a total hysterectomy (uterus and cervix) may stop screening (unless the hysterectomy is done for treatment of cervical carcinoma).
- If a supra cervical hysterectomy is done, continue screening as above.
- Women vaccinated against HPV should also follow the same screening guidelines.

14.7.3 National Cancer Grid (NCG) Guidelines

For limited resource settings (i.e., health and wellness centers, primary health centers (PHC), or community health centers (CHC)).

- Visual inspection with acetic acid (VIA) is the screening method of choice.
- It can be done by any trained healthcare personnel.
- The target age group is women aged 30–65 years.
- Exit from screening is resource-dependent.
- At least one to three times screening should be done in the target age group.

For optimally enhanced resource settings (i.e., health and wellness centers, primary health centers (PHC), and community health centers (CHC)).

- HPV DNA is the screening method of choice.
- Can be done by a trained physician or nurse.
- Target age group: 30- to 65-year-old women.
- Done 10 yearly if 2 consecutive negative tests at 5-year intervals.
- May exit from screening at ≥65 years if consistent negative results for the last 15 years.

For high resource settings (i.e.,, district hospitals, medical colleges, private sectors)

- HPV DNA is the screening method of choice.
- Can be done by trained physicians, surgeons, or nurses.
- Target age group—25- to 65-year-old women.
- Should be done 5 yearly.
- Patients may exit from screening at ≥65 years if consistent negative results for the last 15 years.

14.8 Conclusion

In India, there is no level 1 evidence against cervical cancer screening, and no guideline recommends population-based HPV-DNA or cervical cytology screening for cervical cancer at any age group. Emphasis on health education and hygiene practice may be helpful in a country like India. In case of high suspension or high-risk population may go for cervical cytology (Pap smear), visual inspection with acetic acid (VIA) screen. ICMR is also against population-based screening for cervical cancer.

14.9 Oral Cancer Screening

14.9.1 National Cancer Grid (NCG) Guidelines

For limited resource settings (health and wellness centers, primary health centers (PHC), and community health centers (CHC))

- Oral visual inspection (OVI) is the screening method of choice.
- Can be done by any trained healthcare personnel.
- Target age group—population using tobacco/alcohol/areca nut, and ≥15 years of age.
- At least one to three times screening can be done in their lifetime.

For optimally enhanced resource setting (i.e., health and wellness centers, primary health centers (PHC), and community health centers (CHC))

- Oral visual inspection (OVI)—the screening method of choice.
- Can be done by any trained healthcare personnel.
- Target age group—population using tobacco/alcohol/Areca nuts, ≥15 years of age.
- Should be done at 5-year intervals, and there is no bar to stop screening.

For high resource settings (i.e., district hospitals, medical colleges, private sectors)

- Oral visual inspection (OVI) is the screening method of choice.
- Can be done by trained physicians, dentists, and surgeons.
- Target age group—population using tobacco/alcohol/ areca nut, and ≥15 years of age.
- Should be done at 2-year intervals, and there is no bar to stop screening.

14.10 Conclusion

As oral cancers are most prevalent in India and tobacco use is the most common aetiology, strengthening health education and tobacco-free campaigns are most impactful for oral cancer prevention. People at risk (i.e., using tobacco/alcohol/ areca nuts) should undergo screening at least 1–3 times in their lifetime. Oral Visual inspection (OVI) is a very low-cost, easy, and socially acceptable screening tool that should be promoted in developing countries like India.

14.11 Colorectal Cancer Screening

PLCO (prostate, lung, colorectal, and ovarian cancer screening trial) [6] is a US-based randomized trial by the National Cancer Institute to evaluate the effect of cancer screening on cancer mortality in the age group of 55–74 years. This study suggests that in the case of colorectal cancer, flexible colonoscopy screening significantly decreased colorectal cancer incidence (both proximal and distal colon cancer) and mortality (distal colon only).

14.11.1 American Cancer Society (ACS) Guidelines [7]

14.11.1.1 "Average-Risk" Population

Who do not have

- Personal history of colorectal cancer.
- Family history of colorectal cancer.
- Personal history of ulcerative colitis or Crohn's disease.
- Confirmed hereditary colorectal cancer syndromes (i.e., familial adenomatous polyposis, Lynch syndrome, or hereditary non-polyposis colon cancer).
- Prior radiation history to the abdomen or pelvic area.

Screening

- Start regular screening at 45 years and continue till 75 years.
- Stool-based test
  - Fecal immunochemical test (FIT) every year.
  - Guaiac-based fecal occult blood test (g FOBT) every year.
  - Multi-target stool DNA with a fecal immunochemical test every 3 years).
- Visual test
  - Colonoscopy every 10 years.
  - CT colonoscopy every 5 years, or sigmoidoscopy every 5 years.

14.11.1.2 "High-Risk" Population

Who have

- Personal history of colorectal cancer.
- Family history of colorectal cancer.
- Personal history of ulcerative colitis or Crohn's disease.
- Confirmed hereditary colorectal cancer syndromes (i.e., familial adenomatous polyposis, Lynch syndrome, or hereditary non-polyposis colon cancer).
- Prior radiation history to the abdomen or pelvic area.

Screening

- Start screening earlier, before the youngest family member is diagnosed with colorectal cancer (possibly before 45 years of age).
- Colonoscopy at 3-year intervals in people with a history of polyp removal.
- Colonoscopy every year in people with h/o colorectal cancer.
- Colonoscopy/stool-based test starts at least 8–10 years after abdominal or pelvic irradiation.
- Colonoscopy 1–3 yearly after 8 years of diagnosis of inflammatory bowel disease.
- Patients with hereditary colorectal cancer syndromes—start screening with colonoscopy more frequently in their teenage years.
- Screening continues till 75 years of age.

14.11.2 USPSTF Recommendations [8]

USPSTF recommends screening for colorectal cancer to start at 45 years and up to 75 years of age.

Screening strategies are

(a) Guaiac-based fecal occult blood test or fecal immunochemical test (FIT) every year.

(b) Stool DNA-FIT every 1–3 years.
(c) CT colonoscopy or flexible sigmoidoscopy every 5 years.
(d) Flexible sigmoidoscopy every 10 years with yearly FIT.
(e) Colonoscopy every 10 years.

The highest benefit of colorectal cancer screening is shown in the age group of 50–75 years, with moderate benefit in adults aged 45–49 years and very little benefit in those aged >75 years.

14.12 Conclusion

In India, there is no evidence for screening for colorectal cancer. No Guideline recommends screening routinely in Indian populations.

14.13 Lung Cancer Screening Guideline

14.13.1 National Lung Cancer Screening Trial (NLST) [9]

- US-based trial that compared low-dose helical CT (LDCT) with standard chest X-rays for lung cancer screening.
- LDCT screening decreased mortality by 15–20% compared to X-ray screening.

PLCO (prostate, lung, colorectal, and ovarian cancer screening trial) [6].

- US-based randomized trial by the National Cancer Institute to evaluate the effect of cancer screening on cancer mortality in the age group of 55–74 years.
- In lung cancer, there was no benefit of regular screening with low-dose CT (LDCT) on the reduction of cancer-related mortality.

American Cancer Society (ACS) [10] recommends lung cancer screening of the 50- to 80-year-old population with low-dose CT (LDCT), having at least 20 pack-years smoking history.

USPSTF [11] also recommends that

- Adults aged 50–80 years with a history of 20-pack-year smoking and who currently smoke or have quit within the past 15 years should be screened with a low-dose CT scan.
- Discontinue screening if there is no smoking history for 15 years or if developed health issues that limit life expectancy itself.

14.14 Conclusion

In India, there is no level 1 evidence of population-based screening for lung cancer. ICMR (Indian Council of Medical Research) does not recommend population-based screening for any age group.

14.15 Prostate Cancer Screening

PLCO (prostate, lung, colorectal, and ovarian cancer screening trial) [6] suggests that in prostate cancer, there was no benefit of regular screening on the reduction of cancer-related mortality.

But the European-based *ERSPC* trial [12, 13] suggests that early PSA screening in the age group of 55–69 years of the male population significantly reduces prostate cancer mortality.

American Cancer Society (ACS) recommends that [14]

Screening population

- Men of 50 years of age or more who are expected to live at least 10 years.
- Men of 45 years of age with a high risk of prostate cancer development (i.e., African American men and if one first-degree relative had been diagnosed with prostate cancer below 65 years of age).
- Men of 40 years of age with a high risk of prostate cancer development (>one first-degree relative had been diagnosed with prostate cancer below 65 years of age).

14.15.1 Screening Tests

- Blood prostate-specific antigen test (PSA), and digital rectal examination (DRE).
- If the PSA value is <2.5 ng/ml, screen every 2 years, or if PSA $\geq$2.5 ng/ml, screening should be done yearly.

USPSTF [15] recommends PSA screening in men aged 55–69 years and against PSA screening in men aged 70 or above.

The American Urological Association [16] recommends that

- For average-risk people, start a PSA screen at 45 years of age and screen 2 yearly.
- High-risk people start a PSA screen at the age of 40–45 years and screen yearly.
- Recommendation against PSA screening for those below 40 years of age.

The European Association of Urology [17] recommends that

- PSA screening should be considered only for people with a life expectancy of at least 10–15 years.

- Average-risk patients start screening at the age of 50 years.
- High-risk patients start screening at age 45 years.
- Men with a known BRCA2 mutation start screening at age 40 years.

14.16 Conclusion

In India, there is no level 1 evidence of population-based screening for prostate cancer. ICMR (Indian Council of Medical Research) does not recommend population-based PSA screening for any age group.

14.17 Screening for Other Cancers

For other cancers like skin cancers, thyroid cancers, bladder cancers, and endometrial cancers, there are no population-based screening recommendations.

References

1. Siu AL, U.S. Preventive Services Task Force. Screening for breast cancer: U.S. preventive services task force recommendation statement. Ann Intern Med. 2016;164(4):279–96.
2. ACS Breast Cancer Screening Guidelines | American Cancer Society Available from: https://www.cancer.org/cancer/types/breast-cancer/screening-tests-and-early-detection/american-cancer-society-recommendations-for-the-early-detection-of-breast-cancer.html.
3. Guidelines | Indian Council of Medical Research | Government of India Available from: https://main.icmr.nic.in/guidelines?field_select_disease_tid=91.
4. US Preventive Services Task Force, Curry SJ, Krist AH, Owens DK, Barry MJ, Caughey AB, et al. Screening for cervical cancer: US preventive services task force recommendation statement. JAMA. 2018;320(7):674–86.
5. New ACS Cervical Cancer Screening Guideline - NCI. Available from: https://www.cancer.gov/news-events/cancer-currents-blog/2020/cervical-cancer-screening-hpv-test-guideline.
6. Prostate, Lung, Colorectal, and Ovarian Cancer Screening Trial (PLCO) | Division of Cancer Prevention. Available from: https://prevention.cancer.gov/major-programs/prostate-lung-colorectal-and-ovarian-cancer-screening-trial-plco.
7. Colorectal Cancer Guideline | How Often to Have Screening Tests | American Cancer Society. Available from: https://www.cancer.org/cancer/types/colon-rectal-cancer/detection-diagnosis-staging/acs-recommendations.html.
8. US Preventive Services Task Force. Screening for colorectal cancer: US preventive services task force recommendation statement. JAMA. 2021;325(19):1965–77.
9. National Lung Screening Trial (NLST) - NCI. Available from: https://www.cancer.gov/types/lung/research/nlst.
10. Lung Cancer Screening Guidelines | American Cancer Society. Available from: https://www.cancer.org/health-care-professionals/american-cancer-society-prevention-early-detection-guidelines/lung-cancer-screening-guidelines.html.

11. Marshall RC, Tiglao SM, Thiel D. Updated USPSTF screening guidelines may reduce lung cancer deaths. J Fam Pract. 2021;70(7):347–9.
12. Hugosson J, Roobol MJ, Månsson M, Tammela TLJ, Zappa M, Nelen V, et al. A 16-yr follow-up of the European randomized study of screening for prostate cancer. Eur Urol. 2019;76(1):43–51.
13. Schröder FH, Hugosson J, Roobol MJ, TLJ T, Zappa M, Nelen V, et al. The European randomized study of screening for prostate cancer – prostate cancer mortality at 13 years of follow-up. Lancet. 2014;384(9959):2027–35.
14. American Cancer Society Recommendations for Prostate Cancer Early Detection. Available from: https://www.cancer.org/cancer/types/prostate-cancer/detection-diagnosis-staging/acs-recommendations.html.
15. US Preventive Services Task Force, Grossman DC, Curry SJ, Owens DK, Bibbins-Domingo K, Caughey AB, et al. Screening for prostate cancer: US preventive services task force recommendation statement. JAMA. 2018;319(18):1901–13.
16. Wei JT, Barocas D, Carlsson S, Coakley F, Eggener S, Etzioni R, et al. Early detection of prostate cancer: AUA/SUO guideline part I: prostate cancer screening. J Urol. 2023;210(1):46–53.
17. Mottet N, van den Bergh RCN, Briers E, Van den Broeck T, Cumberbatch MG, De Santis M, et al. EAU-EANM-ESTRO-ESUR-SIOG guidelines on prostate cancer-2020 update. Part 1: screening, diagnosis, and local treatment with curative intent. Eur Urol. 2021;79(2):243–62.

Chapter 15
Evaluation of Benign Masses in Thorax

Ajay Kumar Choubey, Arvind Chavhan, and Samapika Bhaumik

15.1 Introduction

The area enclosed between the abdomen inferiorly and the root of the neck superiorly is the thorax. It comprises the thoracic wall, its superficial structures (breast, muscles, and skin), and the thoracic cavity [1]. The compartment that extends throughout the length of the thoracic cavity between the pleural sacs of the lungs is the mediastinum. Longitudinally, it extends from the thoracic inlet to the superior surface of the diaphragm [2].

15.2 The Mediastinum

The mediastinum houses many vital structures, including the heart, great vessels, trachea, and essential nerves. It also functions as a protected pathway for structures traversing from the neck, superiorly, and into the abdomen, inferiorly. Although there are no physical barriers between compartments other than the pericardium, the mediastinum is typically discussed based on subdivisions. As per the Fujimoto et al. of the Japanese Association for Research on the Thymus (JART), the four-compartment model of mediastinum was proposed based on transverse CT images, which divides the mediastinum into the superior portion of mediastinum, anterior mediastinum (pre-vascular zone),

A. K. Choubey (✉) · S. Bhaumik
Department of Radiation Oncology, MPMMCC/HBCH Varanasi, Units of Tata Memorial Centre and also affliated with Homi Bhabha National Institute, Varanasi, India

A. Chavhan
Department of Radio-Diagnosis, MPMMCC/HBCH Varanasi, Units of Tata Memorial Centre and also affliated with Homi Bhabha National Institute, Mumbai, India

S. Pradhan et al. (eds.), *Evidence Based Handbook on Diagnosis and Staging in Oncology*, https://doi.org/10.1007/978-981-95-9701-7_15

middle mediastinum (peri-tracheoesophageal zone), and posterior mediastinum (paravertebral zone) [3]. Each of these regions of the mediastinum is bordered by the following boundaries: the superior mediastinum is defined by its superior border being the thoracic outlet, its inferior border being the transverse thoracic plane (the plane of Ludwig) or sternal angle, its lateral border being the medial border of the pleural sacs, its anterior border being the dorsal surface of the sternum, and its posterior border being the ventral surface of the first four thoracic vertebral bodies. The anterior mediastinum is delineated by the pericardium posteriorly, the medial border of the pleural sacs laterally, and the sternum, transversus thoracis muscles, and the fifth, sixth, and seventh left costal cartilages anteriorly. The middle mediastinum is created by the pericardial sac's frontal and rear boundaries, extending to the inner edges of the pleural sacs on both sides, the upper transverse thoracic plane, and the thoracic surface of the diaphragm below. The posterior mediastinum is surrounded by the pericardium to the front, the thoracic surface of the diaphragm below, the upper transverse thoracic plane above, the bodies of the fifth to the twelfth thoracic vertebrae to the rear, and the pleural sacs to the sides [2]. The mediastinum is also clinically significant due to a variety of physical anomalies and pathologies that can occur in this region.

15.3 Tumors in the Thorax

A variety of tumors arise from the thorax—both mediastinal and non-mediastinal, including benign and malignant. Some of the malignant thoracic lesions are lung cancers (small cell and non-small cell type), esophageal cancers, thymic cancer, mesothelioma, and tracheal malignancies.

15.4 Classification of Benign Masses of the Thorax

Benign masses of the thorax, on the other hand, can include a huge variety of tumors, which can be subdivided based on their organ and location of origin (Figs. 15.1, 15.2, 15.3, and 15.4).

Thymoma is the most common mediastinal tumor.

15.4.1 The Incidence of These Benign Masses Varies

Among the lung masses, the most common benign mass is a hamartoma, accounting for 55% of all benign lung tumors and about 8% of all lung tumors [4].

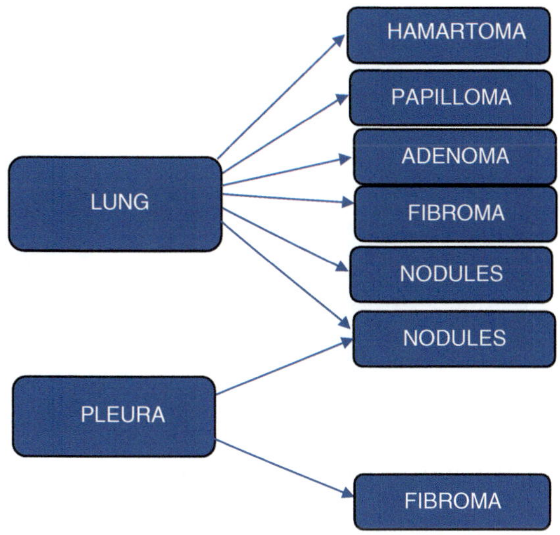

Fig. 15.1 Benign Mediastinal masses as per organ of origin

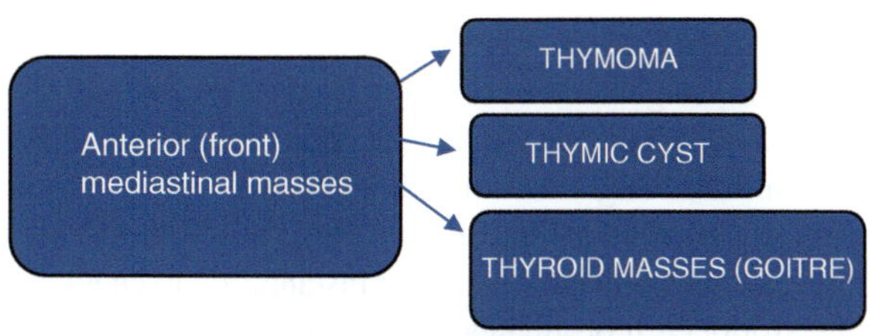

Fig. 15.2 Anterior Mediastinal benign masses of thorax

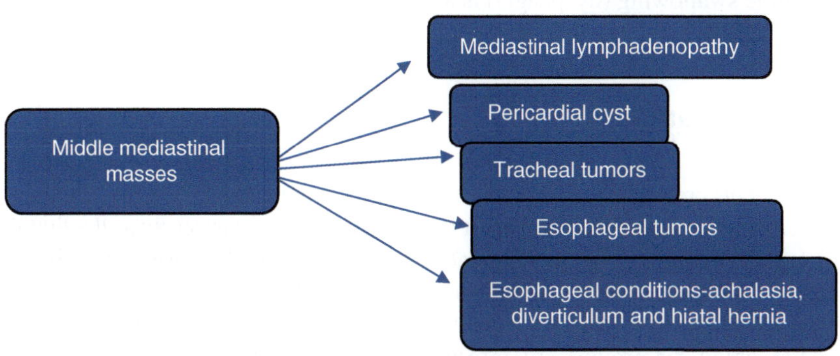

Fig. 15.3 Middle Mediastinal benign masses of the thorax

The most frequent lesions encountered in the mediastinum are thymoma, neurogenic tumors, and benign cysts, together representing 60% of patients with mediastinal masses [5].

About 30–40% of the mediastinal masses occur in the posterior mediastinum, of which approximately 90% are neurogenic in origin, arising from the sympathetic chain present along the vertebral bodies [6].

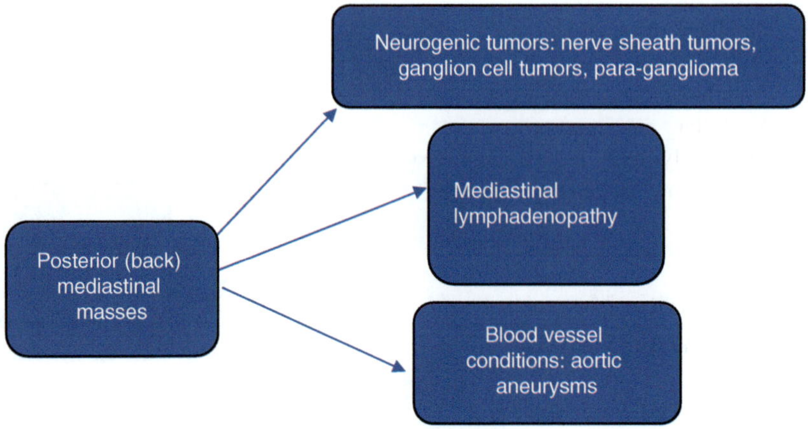

Fig. 15.4 Posterior Mediastinal benign masses of thorax

15.5 Clinical Presentation

Due to the huge number of differentials, thoracic masses can present with a myriad of symptoms, depending on the site. Lung masses may present with symptoms ranging from a mild cough to shortness of breath (dyspnea), chest discomfort, wheezing, or hemoptysis. Mediastinal masses can present with various symptoms depending on their site and nature of origin, for instance, hoarseness, high-pitched, and noisy breathing (stridor) if it originates and/or displaces the tracheobronchial tree.

Trouble swallowing (dysphagia) is associated with the esophagus.

15.6 Evaluation

When patients present with these clinical features, the initial imaging study of choice is a posteroanterior (PA) and lateral chest radiograph. Chest X-ray serves as the first-line radiologic investigation for mediastinal masses and forms the basis for subsequent imaging evaluation. It allows preliminary detection and compartmental localization of the mass while offering limited insight into its size, morphology, and extent [7].

After obtaining preliminary information regarding the lesion's location and approximate dimensions, cross-sectional imaging is employed to further characterize the abnormality and better define its extent. Computed tomography (CT) is generally regarded as the primary cross-sectional modality for assessing mediastinal masses due to its widespread availability, extensive clinical experience, and well-established diagnostic accuracy. Although magnetic resonance imaging (MRI) is increasingly utilized, its role remains secondary to CT in this context because of inferior spatial resolution, longer acquisition times, and higher cost. Comparative studies evaluating pulmonary nodules have demonstrated that CT has significantly greater sensitivity (odds ratio [OR] for MRI vs CT: 0.91; 95% CI: 0.85–0.98; $P = 0.010$) and specificity (OR: 0.82; 95% CI: 0.69–0.97; $P = 0.019$) than MRI [8].

15.6.1 Radiological Findings

15.6.1.1 Hamartoma

On CT imaging, hamartomas typically appear as well-circumscribed lesions containing focal areas of fat or a mixture of fat and calcifications, classically described as "popcorn" calcifications [9].

15.6.1.2 Sarcoidosis

Sarcoidosis is a chronic, multisystem inflammatory disorder characterized by noncaseating granulomas. Thoracic involvement commonly manifests as mediastinal, paratracheal, and bilateral hilar lymphadenopathy on CT imaging. Pulmonary nodules, when present, are usually distributed along the fissures or within the peribronchovascular regions [9].

15.6.1.3 Wegener Granulomatosis

The most frequent thoracic presentation of Wegener granulomatosis consists of multiple bilateral lung nodules without a zonal predominance. These nodules generally range from 2 to 4 cm in size, and approximately 25% of lesions larger than 2 cm may exhibit cavitation with thin or thick walls. The disease can closely resemble tuberculosis, metastatic disease, lung abscesses, or septic emboli. Hemorrhagic nodules may demonstrate a halo sign, characterized by surrounding ground-glass opacity [10].

15.6.1.4 Intrapulmonary Lymph Nodes

Intrapulmonary lymph nodes are typically oval-shaped and located in subpleural lymphatic distributions. They usually measure around 6 mm, may have sharply demarcated triangular margins, appear homogeneous, and lack calcification [11].

15.6.1.5 Pleural Fibroma

Pleural fibromas may appear rounded, elongated, or lobulated and are most commonly found in dependent areas of the thorax. Large lesions tend to displace adjacent structures rather than invade them. Non-contrast CT demonstrates soft-tissue attenuation, while MRI shows intermediate to low signal intensity on both T1- and T2-weighted images. Due to their rich vascular supply, marked contrast enhancement is typical. Associated cystic changes or hemorrhagic necrosis may be present [9].

15.6.1.6 Pleural Lipoma

Pleural lipomas can grow to substantial sizes and are often asymptomatic, though some patients may experience nonproductive cough, exertional dyspnea, chest discomfort, or back pain. On CT imaging, they demonstrate homogeneous fat attenuation (approximately -100 HU). Liposarcomas, which may arise from thoracic adipose tissue, can be differentiated by their heterogeneous appearance on CT or MRI, with irregular enhancing soft-tissue components suggesting malignancy. ^18F-fluorodeoxyglucose positron emission tomography (FDG-PET) can aid in distinguishing benign lipomas from liposarcomas [12].

15.6.1.7 Thymoma

Thymomas are strongly associated with myasthenia gravis; approximately 10–20% of patients with myasthenia gravis have a thymoma, while 30–50% of individuals with thymoma develop myasthenia gravis. Chest radiographs typically reveal a well-defined, lobulated anterior mediastinal mass that may contain calcifications. CT imaging shows a soft-tissue attenuation mass located between the sternum and the great vessels, and mediastinal lymphadenopathy may be observed in 13–44% of cases [9].

15.6.1.8 Thymic Cyst

Thymic cysts may be found in either the cervical region or mediastinum and are classified as congenital (commonly unilocular) or acquired (often multilocular). Acquired cysts may occur following interventions such as thoracotomy, chemotherapy, or radiotherapy, or as a result of inflammation. CT imaging may reveal lobulated lesions with areas of soft-tissue attenuation, while MRI typically demonstrates cystic characteristics without internal enhancement [13].

15.6.1.9 Extramedullary Hematopoiesis

Thoracic manifestations of extramedullary hematopoiesis most commonly include bilateral paraspinal masses with rounded or lobulated contours. Associated findings may include expansion of medullary bone with trabecular resorption. These lesions do not calcify or erode bone and typically demonstrate low attenuation with mild contrast enhancement on CT. Less frequent thoracic presentations include interstitial lung disease, pleural masses, or hemothorax. Splenomegaly or absence of the spleen may also be noted. Diagnosis can be confirmed through percutaneous fine-needle aspiration or biopsy.

15.6.1.10 Goiter

For suspected thyroid enlargement, neck ultrasound with Doppler evaluation is the preferred initial imaging modality. It can identify diffuse gland enlargement, nodularity, colloid content, and potential retrosternal extension. CT imaging is useful for assessing the degree of intrathoracic involvement in large goiters, which often show contrast enhancement and may contain calcifications.

Following initial imaging, once the differential diagnosis has been narrowed based on lesion location and radiologic characteristics, tissue sampling is performed to exclude or confirm malignancy.

15.6.2 Tissue Diagnosis with Biopsy

Before the biopsy, some baseline investigations are done in initial visits to ensure the patient's fitness of the patient. They commonly include a complete blood count, liver function test, renal function test, coagulation profile, blood grouping, and viral markers. Once the tissue diagnosis is confirmed, one can go ahead with the definitive treatment and the investigations as the protocol dictates.

15.6.3 Images Showing Benign Thoracic Masses (Figs. 15.5, 15.6, 15.7, 15.8, 15.9, 15.10, 15.11, and 15.12)

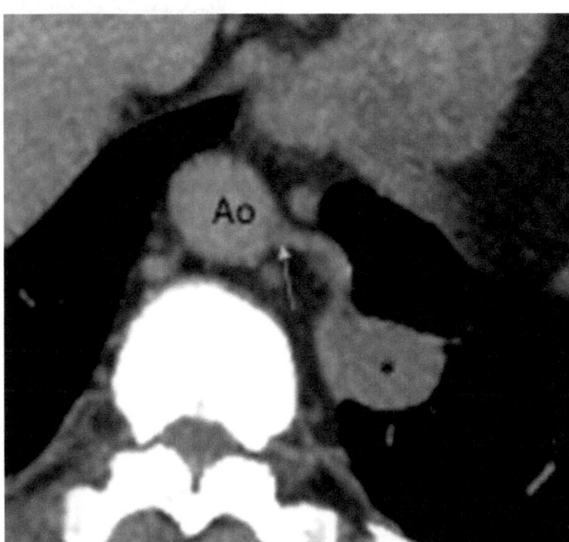

Fig. 15.5 Axial CECT lung mediastinal window in a 55 year male patient with known primary malignancy of Ca buccal mucosa with axial thoracic CT scan done for routine metastatic workup showing soft tissue lesion (*) in the left lower lode of lung with arterial feed (arrow) directly arising from the left lateral wall of descending thoracic aorta (Ao)- The imaging features are characteristic for *Pulmonary sequestration (Intralobar type)*

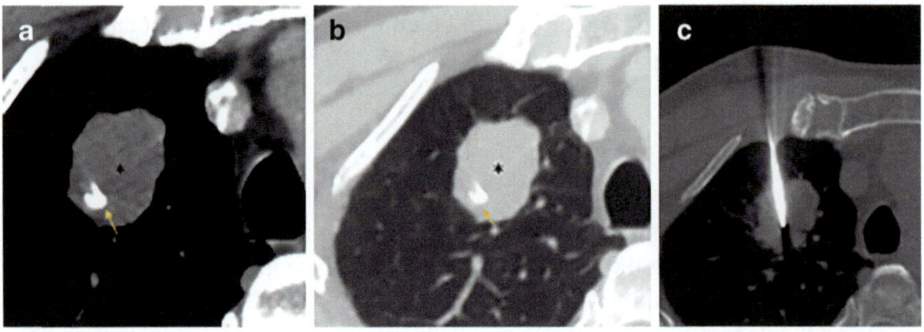

Fig. 15.6 Axial CT (**a**) mediastinal window and (**b**) lung window images in a 65 year male known patient of ca right upper alveolus with axial thoracic CT scan done for routine metastatic workup revealing a well defined lobulated mass (*) which shows calcification (short arrow) within it. Suspecting metastases in a known primary, however presence of coarse calcification warranted HPR confirmation to prove metastases. (**c**) CT guided biopsy image showing needle tip within the lesion to obtain biopsy core. Histopathological report revealing the diagnosis of benign pathology -*Pulmonary harmartoma*

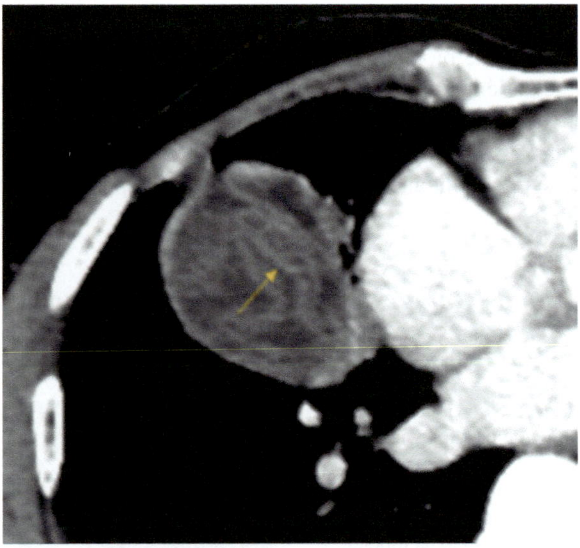

Fig. 15.7 Showing axial CECT lung images in a 45 year male patient complaining of hemoptysis and history of eating unprepared pork revealing a well defined cystic lesion with undulating membranes (arrow) within it. *The imaging appearance are typical of Pulmonary Hydatid cyst*

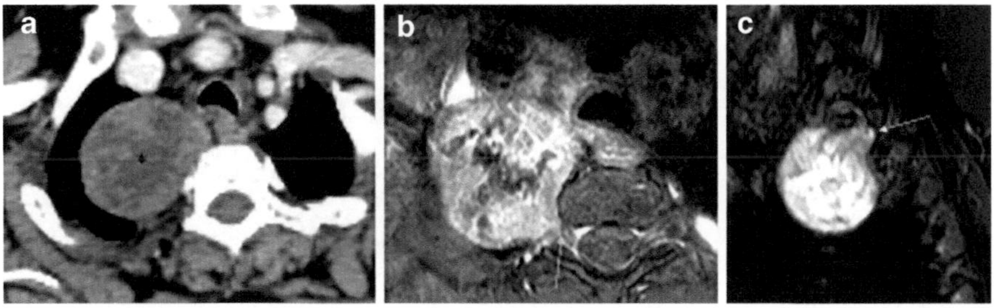

Fig. 15.8 (**a**) Axial CECT image in a 56 year female with complains of dry cough and breathlessness showing a well defined round heterogeneously enhancing mass (*) in the right paravertebral region. (**b**) Axial and (**c**) Sagittal post contrast sequences on MRI showing mass arising from the right T1 nerve root with corresponding neural foramen (arrow). *Histopathology confirmed Schwannoma*

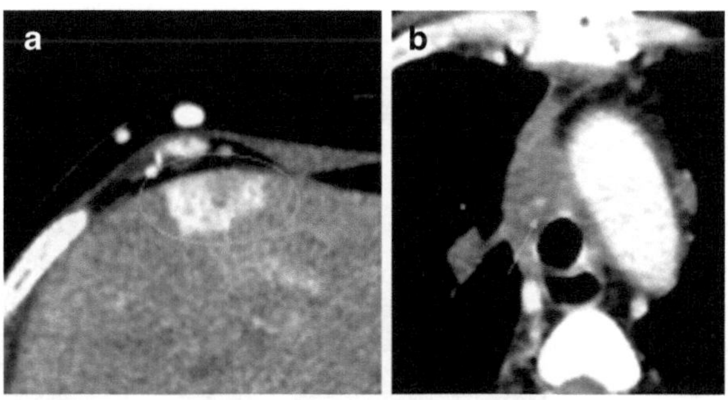

Fig. 15.9 (**a**) Axial CECT abdominal scan in a 38 year old female with complains of cough and pain in right side of neck and chest demonstrating homogenous hyperenhancement seen in segment IV (circle) with subcutaneous venous collateral in the anterior chest wall. (**b**) Anterior mediastinal soft tissue lesion is seen completely encasing the SVC (arrow) in same patient. *The abdominal imaging features are suggestive of Hot quadrate sign and not a metastatic lesion. SVC obstruction causing shunting between SVC and left portal vein via paraumbilical veins along the ligamentum teres*

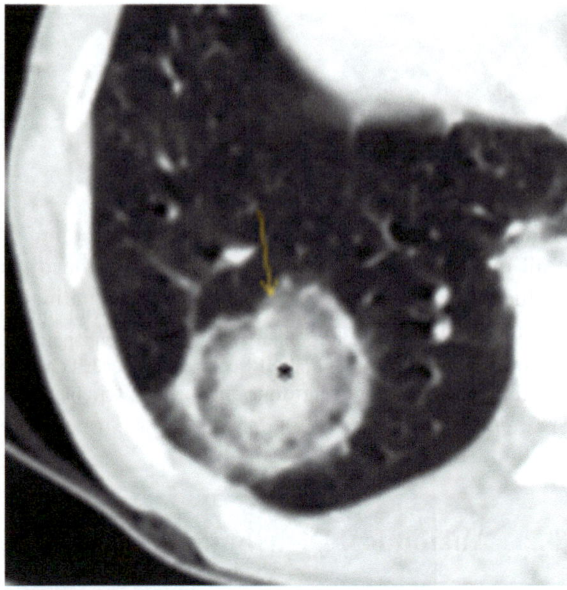

Fig. 15.10 Axial CT lung window in a 56 year old male patient with hemoptysis and shortness of breath since 3 months revealing a central area of ground glass opacity (*) with surrounding incomplete ring of consolidation (arrow) in the right lower lobe lung. *These imaging features are characteristically called as Atoll sign or reverse hallow sign*-which is most commonly seen in *cryptogenic organizing pneumonia*

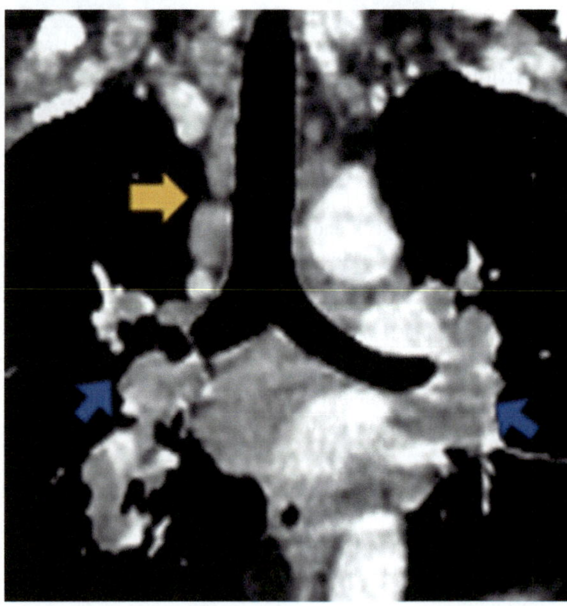

Fig. 15.11 Coronal reformatted CT images in a 48 year female patient undergoing metastatic workup for suspected ca cervix revealing multiple enlarged lymph nodes seen involving the right paratracheal, bilateral hilum and subcarinal region (arrows). *The imaging features and histopathological are suggestive of non-necrotizing granulomatous inflammation -Sarcoidosis*

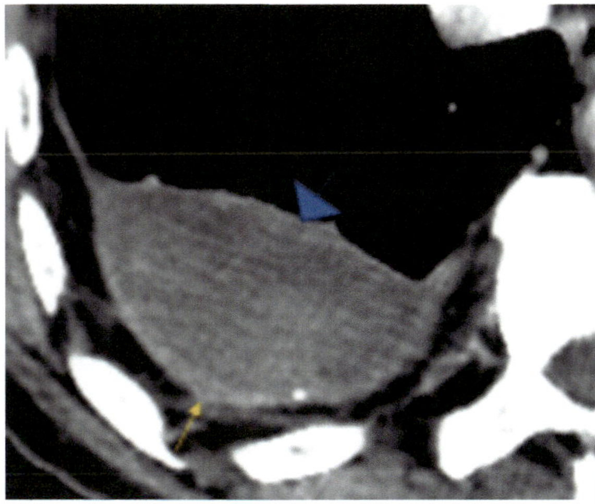

Fig. 15.12 Axial contrast enhanced CT images of lung in a 71 year male patient of carcinoma urinary bladder showing a enhancing parietal (arrow) and visceral pleura (arrow head) with a loculated hyperdense collection within the pleural space. This is a characteristic imaging feature called as *Split pleura sign seen in EMPYEMA*

References

1. Kudzinskas A, Callahan AL. Anatomy, thorax. In: StatPearls [Internet]. Treasure Island: StatPearls Publishing; 2023. [cited 2023 Nov 24]. Available from: http://www.ncbi.nlm.nih.gov/books/NBK557710/.
2. Stoddard N, Heil JR, Lowery DR. Anatomy, thorax, mediastinum. In: StatPearls [Internet]. Treasure Island: StatPearls Publishing; 2023. [cited 2023 Nov 24]. Available from: http://www.ncbi.nlm.nih.gov/books/NBK539819/.
3. Fujimoto K, Hara M, Tomiyama N, Kusumoto M, Sakai F, Fujii Y. Proposal for a new mediastinal compartment classification of transverse plane images according to the Japanese Association for Research on the thymus (JART) general rules for the study of mediastinal tumors. Oncol Rep. 2014;31(2):565–72.
4. Cleveland Clinic [Internet]. [cited 2023 Nov 26]. What are benign lung tumors? Available from: https://my.clevelandclinic.org/health/diseases/15023-benign-lung-tumors.
5. Juanpere S, Cañete N, Ortuño P, Martínez S, Sanchez G, Bernado L. A diagnostic approach to the mediastinal masses. Insights Imaging. 2012;4(1):29–52.
6. Mediastinum Mass - an overview | ScienceDirect Topics [Internet]. [cited 2023 Nov 26]. Available from: https://www.sciencedirect.com/topics/medicine-and-dentistry/mediastinum-mass.
7. Merten DF. Diagnostic imaging of mediastinal masses in children. AJR Am J Roentgenol. 1992;158(4):825–32.
8. Liu H, Chen R, Tong C, Liang XW. MRI versus CT for the detection of pulmonary nodules. Medicine (Baltimore). 2021;100(42):e27270.
9. Suut S, Al-Ani Z, Allen C, Rajiah P, Durr-e-Sabih, AL-Harbi A, et al. Pictorial essay of radiological features of benign intrathoracic masses. Ann Thorac Med. 2015;10(4):231–42.
10. Ananthakrishnan L, Sharma N, Kanne JP. Wegener's granulomatosis in the chest: high-resolution CT findings. AJR Am J Roentgenol. 2009;192(3):676–82.
11. Sykes AMG, Swensen SJ, Tazelaar HD, Jung SH. Computed tomography of benign intrapulmonary lymph nodes: retrospective comparison with sarcoma metastases. Mayo Clin Proc. 2002;77(4):329–33.
12. Gaerte SC, Meyer CA, Winer-Muram HT, Tarver RD, Conces DJ. Fat-containing lesions of the chest. Radiogr Rev Publ Radiol Soc N Am Inc. 2002;22 Spec no:S61–78.
13. Zhang M, Endo M, Adachi S, Kono M. Multilocular thymic cyst: MR findings. AJR Am J Roentgenol. 1994;163(2):479–80.

Chapter 16
Evaluation and Staging of Breast Carcinoma

Satyajit Pradhan, Prashanth Giridhar, Abhishek Chakravarty, and Shreya Shukla

16.1 Introduction and Epidemiology

Breast cancer is the second most common cancer worldwide, with 2.3 million cases (11.5%) diagnosed in women and 670,000 deaths, according to GLOBOCAN 2022 data [1]. Breast cancer is the leading cause of cancer incidence at 23.8% and death at 15.4% among women. Although India's age-standardized rate of female breast cancer is lower than in Western nations, India has a high mortality rate of 14.8%. In very high HDI countries, approximately 1 in 12 women will be diagnosed with breast cancer during their lifetime, compared to 1 in 27 women in low HDI countries [2].

16.2 Risk Factors

Breast cancers are linked to various risk factors; however, most of these factors only slightly to moderately increase the risk.

Female gender is the strongest of all risk factors for breast cancer. A 99% incidence is seen in women, while only 0.5–1% is seen in men [3].

Hormonal factors resulting from longer estrogen exposure are linked to an increased risk of breast carcinoma. Early menarche, later menopause, nulliparity, delayed first childbirth, and lack of breastfeeding all play roles in the development

S. Pradhan (✉) · P. Giridhar · A. Chakravarty
Department of Radiation Oncology, MPMMCC & HBCH Varanasi; Units of Tata Memorial Centre and affliated with Homi Bhabha National Institute, Mumbai, India

S. Shukla
Department of Radio-diagnosis, MPMMCC/HBCH Varanasi, Units of Tata Memorial Centre and affliated with Homi Bhabha National Institute, Mumbai, India

S. Pradhan et al. (eds.), *Evidence Based Handbook on Diagnosis and Staging in Oncology*, https://doi.org/10.1007/978-981-95-9701-7_16

Table 16.1 Risk factors and their associated relative risks for breast cancers

Relative risk <2	Relative risk 2–4	Relative risk >4
Early menarche Late menopause Nulliparity Alcohol use Postmenopausal obesity	One first-degree relative with breast cancer CHEK2 mutation Age older than 35 years for the first birth Proliferative breast disease Mammographic breast density	Mutation BRCA1 or BRCA2 Mutation in PALB2 LCIS Radiation exposure before age 30 years

of breast cancer, with a relative risk (RR) of less than 2. Specifically, delaying the first childbirth past age 30 is associated with a 2–5 times higher risk [4].

A positive family history of BRCA-related cancers, such as breast (in both males and females), ovarian, colorectal, gastric, pancreatic, and prostate cancers in first- and second-degree relatives, is linked to an increased risk of hereditary breast cancer. These cancers tend to occur at a younger age than usual, so screening should begin at least 10 years before the age at diagnosis of the earliest affected family member, or at 25 years old, whichever comes first [5–7].

A notably higher risk has been observed in females with benign proliferative breast diseases. The presence of atypical hyperplasia significantly increases the risk (RR: 4–5). Lobular carcinoma in situ (LCIS), a benign breast lesion, also confers a heightened risk of developing cancer later (RR: 8 to 10) [8, 9].

Postmenopausal women with a body mass index (BMI) of 31.1 or higher are 2.5 times more likely to develop breast cancer than those with a BMI of 22.6 or lower. Obesity is also associated with higher breast cancer mortality rates [10].

Other significant risk factors include older age, previous breast cancer history, early exposure to ionizing radiation (such as mediastinal irradiation for lymphomas), alcohol consumption, and dense breasts seen on mammograms [11] (Table 16.1).

16.3 Clinical Features

Breast cancers usually present as a painless breast lump with progressive increase in size to become noticeable. These lumps commonly drain into the axillary lymph nodes, which may present with axillary swellings or may be found during clinical breast examination. Skin changes like dilated veins and rapidly increasing swelling are usually associated with a malignant phyllodes tumor. Other skin changes like ulceration, bleeding, pus discharge, peau d'orange, and inflammation are suggestive of a locally advanced disease.

Nipple discharge can be associated with both benign and malignant diseases (Table 16.2).

Table 16.2 Types of nipple discharge and their underlying etiology

Color of nipple discharge	Etiology
Milky white (galactorrhoea)	Lactating females, hyperprolactinemia
Greenish	Duct ectasia
Bloody	Intraductal carcinoma, duct papilloma

Patients may also present with swelling of the ipsilateral arm (lymphedema), which may occur due to blockage of draining axillary lymph nodes, preventing the lymphatics from draining from the limb.

Metastatic breast cancers may present with symptoms other than those of local disease. These include the following:

- Cough, shortness of breath, and chest pain (lung metastasis or malignant pleural effusion)
- Vague right-sided rib pain/abdominal pain, jaundice (suggestive of liver metastasis)
- CNS symptoms like headache, nausea, vomiting, blurring of vision, limb weakness (brain metastasis)
- Bony pains, limb weakness, and compressive symptoms—most commonly in the spine and weight-bearing sites (bone metastasis)

16.4 Breast Cancer Screening

The effectiveness of a population-based breast cancer screening program for early detection of breast cancers depends upon the incidence of the disease in the subpopulation and its cost-effectiveness.

The available screening tools include the following:

- Clinical breast examination (CBE)
- Screening mammography ± digital tomosynthesis
- Screening ultrasound
- B/L breast magnetic resonance imaging (MRI)

CBE, performed by trained healthcare practitioners, is a simple and inexpensive method for detecting suspicious breast lumps. It enables early detection and risk assessment during the initial visit, making it a preferred option in healthcare settings with limited resources where mammography screening might not be accessible. The inspection is carried out in both upright and supine positions, with palpation covering all breast areas—including lateral, medial, cephalad, and caudad regions. Additionally, the axilla and supraclavicular fossae are palpated, and findings are documented to compare with imaging results. Mittra et al. conducted a cluster randomized controlled trial in Mumbai, comparing biennial CBE screening with no screening. The results showed a non-significant 15% reduction in breast cancer mortality overall, but a significant 30% reduction was specifically observed in women over 50 years old [12].

Screening mammography is the most crucial screening tool because it uniquely demonstrates a reduction in mortality. It involves taking X-ray images in two views: cranio-caudal (CC) and medio-lateral oblique (MLO). The WHO recommends population-based screening mammography based on resource availability. It is advised only for women aged 50–69 years in well-resourced countries, while it is strongly discouraged in LMICs. A systematic review by USPSTF in 2009 found that annual or biennial screening benefits women aged 39–69, but there is limited data for women older than 69 [13].

The recent USPSTF 2024 update recommends starting screening mammography for women at age 40 and continuing every 2 years until age 74 [14]. A meta-analysis has shown that digital tomosynthesis, when added to screening mammography, offers diagnostic accuracy comparable to standard methods [15].

The presence of dense breast tissue in younger females obscures the detection of cancers by mammography (sensitivity 30–48%) [16]. A screening ultrasound, breast, or contrast-enhanced magnetic resonance imaging (MRI) is being evaluated for its clinical utility. However, recommendations for the use of MRI breast screening pertain to certain high-risk groups.

American Cancer Society guidelines for Annual MRI screening [17]

- BRCA positive
- Li-Fraumeni syndrome and first-degree relatives
- Untested first-degree relative to BRCA carriers
- Women carrying a 20–25% lifetime risk of breast cancer as per family history predictive models
- Radiation to the chest between the ages of 10 and 30 years
- Cowden and Bannayan-Riley-Ruvalcaba syndromes and first-degree relatives

Table 16.3 shows the sensitivity and specificity of breast cancer screening tools.

If a woman shows an abnormal mammogram during screening or has a concerning physical exam finding, further imaging and biopsy might be advised. This additional imaging could include a diagnostic mammogram, a mammogram with supplementary or special views, a targeted breast ultrasound, or a breast MRI. These tests help differentiate whether the lesion is benign or suspicious, guiding the decision on whether a biopsy is necessary [33].

Table 16.3 Sensitivity and specificity of breast cancer screening tools (<2 cm tumor size) [18]

	Sensitivity (%)	Specificity (%)
Clinical breast examination	54	94
Screening mammography	75–85	91
B/L breast MRI	75–100	83–98

16.5 Genetic Testing

Hereditary breast and ovarian cancer syndrome (HBOC) involves BRCA1 and BRCA2 mutations in over 50% of cases. It is characterized by an increased risk of developing breast cancer in both women and men, as well as ovarian cancers (including primary peritoneal cancers), prostate cancer, and pancreatic cancers. The lifetime risk of developing breast cancer for individuals with BRCA 1 mutations is 55–72%, and for BRCA 2 mutations, it is 45–69%.

Individuals who should be offered genetic testing include the following [19]:

- Breast or ovarian cancer diagnosed at or before age 50.
- Family history of male breast cancer.
- Multiple primaries (>1) in one or both breasts.
- Triple negative breast cancers (TNBC).
- History of personal or family cases of prostate and/or pancreatic cancers (metastatic or Gleason Score ≥7), as well as breast and/or ovarian cancers.
- ≥2 relatives diagnosed with breast or ovarian cancers, with at least one on or before 50 years of age.
- ≥3 relatives with breast cancer diagnosed at any age.
- Breast cancer diagnosed at any age in individuals with Ashkenazi Jewish ancestry.
- A family member with a known BRCA1 or BRCA2 pathologic variant.

16.6 Genes Associated with Hereditary Breast and Ovarian Cancers [20]

- ATM—Mutations predispose to breast cancer with high penetrance and may also increase the risk of pancreatic and prostate cancers.
- CDH1—Associated with hereditary diffuse gastric cancer and lobular breast carcinoma, typically presenting before age 40.
- PALB2—Confers elevated risk for breast cancer (up to ~58%), and is linked to ovarian, pancreatic, and male breast cancers.
- PTEN—Germline variants cause PTEN hamartoma tumour syndrome, predisposing to breast, thyroid, renal cell, endometrial, and colorectal cancers, often accompanied by multiple hamartomas, macrocephaly, and characteristic skin lesions.
- STK11 is associated with Peutz–Jeghers syndrome, which features gastrointestinal polyposis, mucocutaneous pigmentation, and an increased risk of cancers in the gastrointestinal tract, pancreas, ovaries (specifically SCTAT), and cervix (notably adenoma malignum).

- TP53—Li-Fraumeni syndrome leads to early-onset breast cancer and various primary tumors, including soft-tissue sarcoma, osteosarcoma, brain tumors, adrenocortical carcinoma, and leukemia.
- BARD1—Variants increase susceptibility to breast cancer.
- BRIP1—Mutations are associated with epithelial ovarian cancer.
- EPCAM, MLH1, MSH2, MSH6, PMS2—Defects in these DNA mismatch-repair genes (Lynch syndrome) predispose to ovarian, colorectal, endometrial, and gastric cancers.
- RAD51C is associated with ovarian cancer and estrogen/progesterone-receptor-negative breast cancer.
- RAD51D—Similar to RAD51C, associated with ovarian and ER/PR-negative breast cancers.
- CHEK2—Variants confer moderate risk for ovarian, endometrial, gastric cancers, and colorectal polyps.

16.7 Histopathology, Immunohistochemistry, and Tumor Markers

Most breast malignancies originate from epithelial cells. They can be invasive or classified as Carcinoma in situ (CIS). CIS is further divided into ductal (ductal carcinoma in situ—DCIS) or lobular (lobular carcinoma in situ and atypical lobular hyperplasia). Lobular neoplasia (LN) refers to a proliferation of small, often loosely cohesive cells in the terminal duct-lobular unit, with or without pagetoid involvement of terminal ducts. It encompasses both LCIS and ALH. LCIS may be multifocal and bilateral, with an associated 1–2% annual risk and a 30–40% lifetime risk of progressing to invasive carcinoma [22]. DCIS is characterized by the proliferation of malignant-appearing mammary ductal epithelial cells without invasion beyond the basement membrane. Most cases present with a non-palpable lump, often discovered incidentally on screening mammography as calcifications. The detection rate of DCIS through screening mammography ranges from 15% to 30%, primarily occurring in individuals aged 49–69 years (Table 16.4).

Table 16.4 Classical morphological patterns of DCIS

Pattern	Description
Comedo	Tumor cells with pleomorphic high-grade nuclei with areas of central necrosis
Cribriform	Tumor cells with "cookie-cutter-like" spaces filled with calcified secretory material
Micropapillary	Complex bulbous protrusions without a fibrovascular core
Papillary	True papillae with fibrovascular core
Solid	Solid sheets of cells within ducts or lobules confined by a basement membrane

Invasive breast carcinomas include various histologic subtypes: infiltrating ductal (76%), invasive lobular (8%), ductal/lobular (7%), mucinous (2.4%), tubular (1.5%), medullary (1.2%), and papillary (1%) [23].

Infiltrating ductal carcinoma is characterized microscopically by cords and nests of tumor cells with varying gland formation. These tumor cells provoke a desmoplastic reaction in the surrounding tissue, which leads to a palpable mass. However, IDC is considered a "diagnosis of exclusion" because it cannot be classified into other specific histologic variants, thus being labeled as infiltrating ductal carcinoma, not otherwise specified (NOS), or infiltrating carcinoma no special type (NST) [21]. Invasive breast carcinomas are further categorized based on nuclear or histological grading. Nuclear grading assesses nuclear atypia relative to normal breast tissue, dividing tumors into well-differentiated, moderately differentiated, and poorly differentiated. Histological grading is performed using the Nottingham grading system [24] (Table 16.5).

The heterogeneous nature of breast cancer can be further explained by conducting immunohistochemistry tests. IHC identifies tumor-associated growth factor receptors like estrogen receptor (ER), progesterone receptor (PR), and HER2. These markers can distinguish breast cancers into 4 subcategories, which hold prognostic as well as predictive importance. These subgroups affect the response to therapy and pattern of failure (Table 16.6).

Serum biomarkers like CA 15–3, CA 27.29, and CEA have been evaluated for surveillance and changing therapy in metastatic breast cancers. Elevated biomarkers have shown variable false positivity and no benefit in clinical outcomes and hence are not routinely recommended in staging workup or decision for changing therapy [26].

Table 16.5 Nottingham grading system

Criteria	Score	Description
Mitotic count	1	Less than 11 mitosis in 10 HPF
	2	Between 11 and 20 mitosis in 10 HPF
	3	Greater than 20 mitosis in 10 HPF
Nuclear atypia	1	Small, regular, uniform nuclei
	2	Moderate increase in size and variability
	3	Marked variation
Tubule formation	1	More than 75% of the tumor forms a gland
	2	10–75% of the tumor forms a gland
	3	Less than 10% of the tumor forms a gland

Score = 3–5 Grade 1 (well differentiated), 6–7 Grade 2 (moderately differentiated), 8–9 Grade 3 (poorly differentiated)

Table 16.6 Luminal subtypes with clinico-pathological features [25]

Intrinsic subtype	Luminal A	Luminal B	HER2 enriched	Basal-like
ER/PR expression	Positive—strong	Positive—variable	Positive or negative	Negative
HER2 amplification	Rare	Rare, though a small percentage is positive	Common	Negative
Grade	Low to intermediate	Intermediate to high	Intermediate to high	High
P53 mutation	Rare	Uncommon	Common	Common
Ki67	Low	Intermediate to high	High	High
mRNA signature expression	High ER cluster, low proliferation	Low ER cluster, low proliferation	High HER2 amplification, high proliferation	Basal signature, high expression

16.8 Diagnostic and Pre-Treatment Workup

All women with a suspicious breast lump should undergo a "*TRIPLE TEST*" which includes the following:

1. Physical examination by an experienced clinician
2. Breast imaging—Bilateral mammogram and or ultrasound or MRI as appropriate
3. Histopathology—FNAC/core biopsy (ideal). Excision biopsy/incision biopsy if indicated

During the examination, the patient's general well-being should be assessed, and performance status should be recorded using the Eastern Cooperative Oncology Group or Karnofsky performance status. Pallor, jaundice, and lymphadenopathy should be noted. Local examination should assess the site, size, skin puckering, skin involvement (peau d'orange, ulceration, skin nodule), changes in skin color, local rise in temperature, and tenderness. Both axillae, the contralateral breast, and the supraclavicular fossae should also be examined. Emphasis should be placed on respiratory (lung metastasis and malignant pleural effusion), abdominal (liver metastasis), and spinal (bone metastasis) examinations during the systemic examination.

Findings on examination can determine the nature of the lump: cystic, solid, or suspicious solid [27].

Cystic lumps should be evaluated by a Breast ultrasound and undergo USG-guided cyst aspiration and sent for histopathology if complex cyst/hemorrhagic with rapid filling, which could be due to any residual disease.

Solid lumps can be both benign or malignant. They should undergo supplemental imaging, and benign appearing lumps should undergo excisional biopsy.

Suspicious solid lumps should be imaged with mammography, and if they continue to appear suspicious, should undergo FNAC/core needle biopsy.

16.9 Breast Imaging

Initial imaging typically involves diagnostic bilateral mammography, with or without ultrasound. The Breast Imaging Reporting and Data System (BI-RADS) is employed to assess the likelihood of malignancy in a breast lump [28] (Figs. 16.1 and 16.2).

Features of a malignant breast lump on mammography
1. Solid mass with spiculated margins
2. Architectural distortion
3. Clustered micro-calcifications
4. Skin thickening
5. Nipple retraction

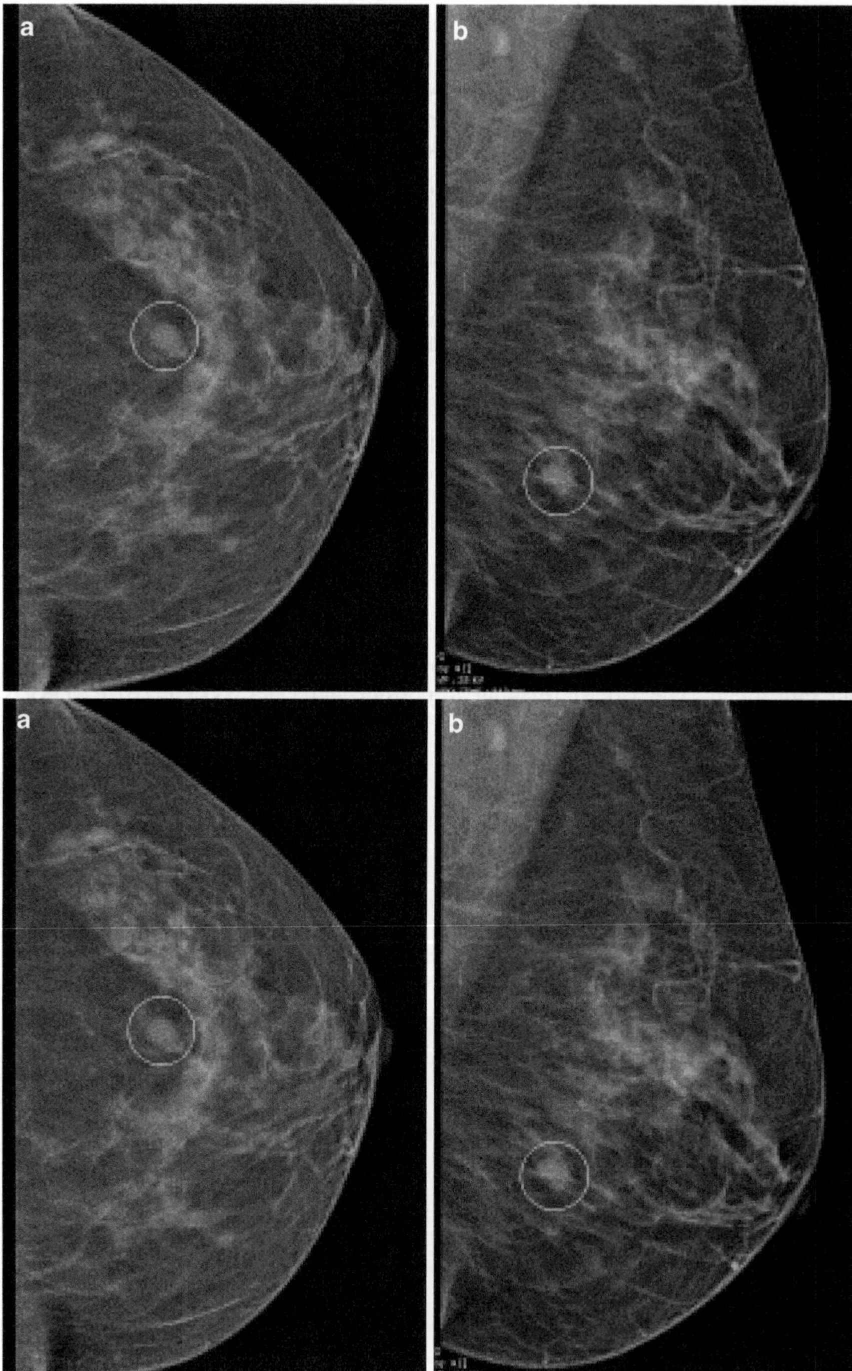

Figs. 16.1 and 16.2 Mammogram showing BIRADS III and BIRADS IV lesions

16.10 MRI Bilateral Breasts

Although not routinely indicated, MRI can be done in special cases, such as

- Occult primary with positive axillary node
- Evaluation in patients with prior breast reconstruction or implants
- In premenopausal females with dense breasts, if an equivocal mammogram is planned for BCT
- Screening in high-risk patients (BRCA carriers) (Fig. 16.3)

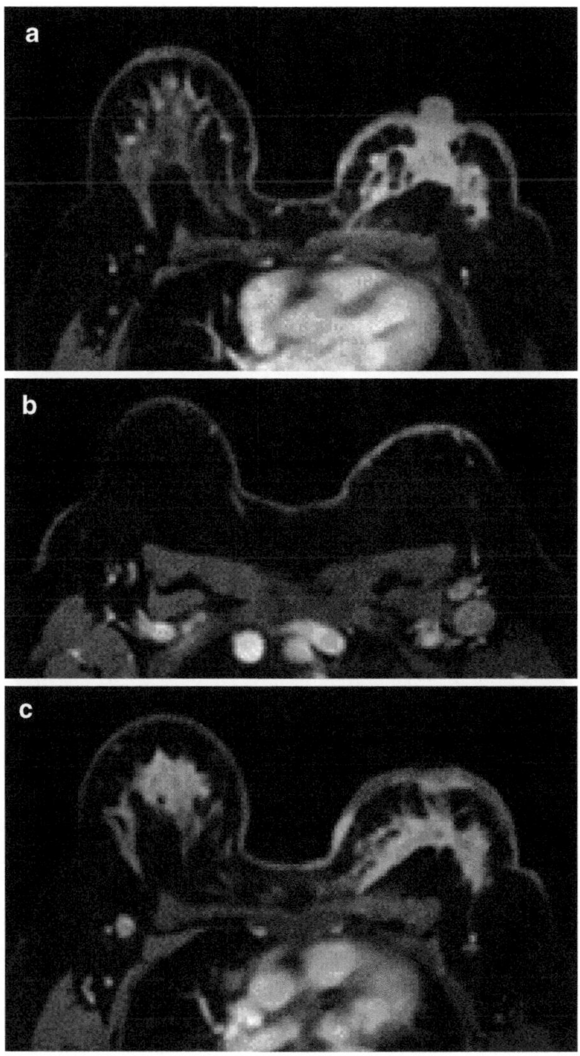

Fig. 16.3 Image of MRI breast with BIRADS 4 and 5 lesions

16.11 Imaging for Metastatic Workup

In T1-T2, N0 or N1, NCCN recommends against imaging for evaluation of distant metastasis [29].

Further investigations may be warranted solely in response to the manifestation of the subsequent signs or symptoms:

- Bone scan indicated if localized bone pain or elevated alkaline phosphatase.
- Contrast-enhanced CT scan of the abdomen and pelvis is indicated if there are elevated alkaline phosphatase levels, abnormal liver function tests, abdominal symptoms, or abnormal physical findings in the abdomen or pelvis.
- Contrast-enhanced CT (if symptomatic for lung metastasis).

For Stage IIIA onwards, metastatic workup with 18-Fluorodeoxyglucose-PET is routinely recommended. A randomised trial including 369 patients with Stage III or IIB showed an absolute difference of 8.2% in upstaging to Stage IV by F-18 PET-CT as compared to CT chest/abdomen/pelvis [30].

Clinical trials are underway to evaluate the clinical utility of fluoroestradiol F-18 PET, which was recently approved by the US Food and Drug Administration for identifying ER-positive breast cancers. This imaging method, when combined with biopsy in cases of recurrent or metastatic breast cancers, seeks to forecast the response to endocrine therapy [31, 32].

16.12 Histopathology

A core needle biopsy is always preferred for tissue diagnosis. The benefit of a core needle biopsy over an FNAC is that it provides information about basement membrane invasion and allows further testing for IHC. Biopsy is preferably performed under USG guidance as it avoids false negative rates. An incisional/excisional biopsy can be performed if repeated biopsies are negative in high clinical and radiological suspicion.

References

1. Cancer (IARC) TIA for R on. Global Cancer Observatory [Internet]. [cited 2024 Jun 9]. Available from: https://gco.iarc.fr/.
2. Global cancer burden growing, amidst mounting need for services [Internet]. [cited 2024 Jun 9]. Available from: https://www.who.int/news/item/01-02-2024-global-cancer-burden-growing%2D%2Damidst-mounting-need-for-services.
3. Breast cancer [Internet]. [cited 2024 Jun 9]. Available from: https://www.who.int/news-room/fact-sheets/detail/breast-cancer.
4. Rosner B, Colditz GA, Willett WC. Reproductive risk factors in a prospective study of breast cancer: the Nurses' Health Study. Am J Epidemiol. 1994;139(8):819–35.

5. Metcalfe KA, Finch A, Poll A, et al. Breast cancer risks in women with a family history of breast or ovarian cancer who have tested negative for a BRCA1 or BRCA2 mutation. Br J Cancer. 2009;100(2):421–5.
6. Narod SA. Modifiers of risk of hereditary breast cancer. Oncogene. 2006;25(43):5832–6.
7. Kurian AW, Gong GD, John EM, et al. Breast cancer risk for noncarriers of family-specific BRCA1 and BRCA2 mutations: findings from the breast cancer family registry. J Clin Oncol. 2011;29(34):4505–9.
8. Fitzgibbons PL, Henson DE, Hutter RV. Benign breast changes and the risk for subsequent breast cancer: an update of the 1985 consensus statement. Cancer Committee of the College of American Pathologists. Arch Pathol Lab Med. 1998;122(12):1053–5.
9. Page DL, Kidd TE, Dupont WD, Simpson JF, Rogers LW. Lobular neoplasia of the breast: higher risk for subsequent invasive cancer predicted by more extensive disease. Hum Pathol. 1991;22(12):1232–9.
10. Chlebowski RT, Hendrix SL, Langer RD, et al. Influence of estrogen plus progestin on breast cancer and mammography in healthy postmenopausal women: the women's health initiative randomized trial. JAMA. 2003;289(24):3243–53.
11. Boyd NF, Guo H, Martin LJ, et al. Mammographic density and the risk and detection of breast cancer. N Engl J Med. 2007;356(3):227–36.
12. Mittra I, Mishra GA, Dikshit RP, et al. Effect of screening by clinical breast examination on breast cancer incidence and mortality after 20 years: prospective, cluster randomised controlled trial in Mumbai. BMJ. 2021;372:n256.
13. Nelson HD, Tyne K, Naik A, Bougatsos C, Chan BK, Humphrey L, U.S. Preventive Services Task Force. Screening for breast cancer: an update for the U.S. preventive services task force. Ann Intern Med. 2009;151(10):727–37, W237–42. https://doi.org/10.7326/0003-4819-151-10-200911170-00009. PMID: 19920273; PMCID: PMC2972726.
14. Pace LE, Keating NL. New recommendations for breast cancer screening—in pursuit of health equity. JAMA Netw Open. 2024;7(4):e2411638.
15. Abdullah P, Alabousi M, Ramadan S, et al. Synthetic 2D mammography versus standard 2D digital mammography: a diagnostic test accuracy systematic review and meta-analysis. Am J Roentgenol. 2021;217(2):314–25.
16. Kolb TM, Lichy J, Newhouse JH. Comparison of the performance of screening mammography, physical examination, and breast US and evaluation of factors that influence them: an analysis of 27,825 patient evaluations. Radiology. 2002;225(1):165–75.
17. Saslow D, Boetes C, Burke W, American Cancer Society breast cancer advisory group, et al. American Cancer Society guidelines for breast screening with MRI as an adjunct to mammography. CA Cancer J Clin. 2007;57(2):75–89. https://doi.org/10.3322/canjclin.57.2.75. Erratum in: CA Cancer J Clin 2007 May–Jun;57(3):185.
18. Mann RM, Kuhl CK, Moy L. Contrast-enhanced MRI for breast cancer screening. J Magn Reson Imaging. 2019;50(2):377–90.
19. Robson ME, Bradbury AR, Arun B, et al. American Society of Clinical Oncology policy statement update: genetic and genomic testing for cancer susceptibility. J Clin Oncol. 2015;33(31):3660–7.
20. Petrucelli N, Daly MB, Pal T. BRCA1- and BRCA2-associated hereditary breast and ovarian cancer. In: Adam MP, Feldman J, Mirzaa GM, Pagon RA, Wallace SE, Bean LJH, Gripp KW, Amemiya A, editors. GeneReviews® [Internet]. Seattle: University of Washington, Seattle; 1998. [Updated 2023 Sep 21]. 1993–2024.
21. Sinn H-P, Kreipe H. A brief overview of the WHO classification of breast tumors, 4th edition, focusing on issues and updates from the 3rd edition. Breast Care (Basel) [Internet]. 2013. [cited 2024 Jun 17];8(2):149–54. Available from: https://doi.org/10.1159/000350774.
22. Andersen J. Lobular carcinoma in situ of the breast: an approach to rational treatment. Cancer. 1977;39(6):2597–604.
23. Li CI, Uribe DJ, Daling JR. Clinical characteristics of different histologic types of breast cancer. Br J Cancer. 2005;93(9):1046–52.

24. Sinn HP, Kreipe H. A brief overview of the WHO classification of breast tumors, 4th edition, focusing on issues and updates from the 3rd edition. Breast Care. 2013;8(2):149–54.
25. Elston CW, Ellis IO. Pathological prognostic factors in breast cancer. I. The value of histological grade in breast cancer: experience from a large study with long-term follow-up. Histopathology. 1991;19(5):403–10.
26. Koboldt DC, Fulton RS, McLellan MD, et al. Comprehensive molecular portraits of human breast tumours. Nature. 2012;490(7418):61–70.
27. Van Poznak C, Somerfield MR, Bast RC, et al. Use of biomarkers to guide decisions on systemic therapy for women with metastatic breast cancer: American Society of Clinical Oncology clinical practice guideline. J Clin Oncol Off J Am Soc Clin Oncol. 2015;33(24):2695–704.
28. Breast_Cancer.pdf [Internet]. [cited 2024 Jun 9]. Available from: https://main.icmr.nic.in/sites/default/files/reports/Breast_Cancer.pdf.
29. Gradishar W, Anderson B, Blair S, Burstein H, Cyr A, Elias A. National comprehensive cancer network breast cancer panel. Breast Cancer. 2014;3:542–90.
30. Dayes IS, Metser U, Hodgson N, et al. Impact of 18F-labeled fluorodeoxyglucose positron emission tomography-computed tomography versus conventional staging in patients with locally advanced breast cancer. J Clin Oncol. 2023;41(23):3909–16.
31. Jones EF, Ray KM, Li W, et al. Initial experience of dedicated breast PET imaging of ER+ breast cancers using [F-18]fluoroestradiol. Npj Breast Cancer. 2019;5(1):1–6.
32. Linden HM, Peterson LM, Fowler AM. Clinical potential of estrogen and progesterone receptor imaging. PET Clin. 2018;13(3):415–22.
33. Nelson HD, Tyne K, Naik A, et al. Screening for breast cancer: an update for the U.S. preventive services task force. Ann Intern Med. 2009;151(10):727–W242. https://doi.org/10.7326/0003-4819-151-10-200911170-00009.

Chapter 17
Evaluation of Non-IDC Breast Cancer

Ankita Rungta Kapoor and Prashanth Giridhar

17.1 Invasive Lobular Carcinoma (ILC) (Table 17.1)

17.1.1 Epidemiology

Invasive lobular carcinoma is the second most prevalent histopathological subtype of breast cancer and constitutes approximately 5–15% of invasive breast malignancies [1]. A notable rise in incidence has been observed over the last two decades, particularly among postmenopausal women. This trend has been linked to exposure to hormone replacement therapy [2].

17.1.2 Pathological Characteristics

From a molecular standpoint, ILC is predominantly classified as a luminal-type tumor, with strong estrogen receptor expression (around 95%) and frequent progesterone receptor positivity (approximately 70%), while HER2 overexpression is uncommon. A hallmark feature of ILC is disruption of E-cadherin–dependent cell adhesion, most often caused by inactivating mutations of the CDH1 gene on chromosome 16q22. Additional recurrent genetic alterations have been described in FOXA1, RUNX1, and TBX3 [3].

A. R. Kapoor · P. Giridhar (✉)
Department of Radiation Oncology, MPMMCC & HBCH, Varanasi, Units of Tata Memorial Centre and affiliated with Homi Bhabha National Institute, Mumbai, India

S. Pradhan et al. (eds.), *Evidence Based Handbook on Diagnosis and Staging in Oncology*, https://doi.org/10.1007/978-981-95-9701-7_17

Table 17.1 Types of non-IDC breast cancer

Invasive lobular carcinoma	Classic lobular carcinoma Solid lobular carcinoma Alveolar lobular carcinoma Pleomorphic lobular carcinoma Tubulo-lobular carcinoma Mixed lobular carcinoma
Tubular carcinoma	
Cribriform carcinoma	
Mucinous carcinoma	Pure type Mixed type
Medullary carcinoma	
Carcinoma with apocrine differentiation	
Carcinoma with signet-ring-cell differentiation	
Invasive micropapillary carcinoma	
Metaplastic carcinoma of no special type	Low-grade adeno-squamous carcinoma Fibromatosis-like metaplastic carcinoma Squamous cell carcinoma Spindle cell carcinoma Metaplastic carcinoma with (a) Mesenchymal differentiation (b) Chondroid differentiation (c) Osseous differentiation (d) Other types of mesenchymal differentiation Mixed metaplastic carcinoma Myoepithelial carcinoma
Epithelial–myoepithelial tumors	
Adenomyoepithelioma with carcinoma	
Adenoid cystic carcinoma	
Carcinoma with neuroendocrine features	
Others	Secretory carcinoma Invasive papillary carcinoma Acinic cell carcinoma Muco-epidermoid carcinoma Polymorphous carcinoma Oncocytic carcinoma Lipid-rich carcinoma Glycogen-rich clear cell carcinoma Sebaceous carcinoma

17.1.3 Clinical Presentation

ILC typically demonstrates an infiltrative growth pattern with ill-defined margins, which contributes to difficulty in detection on clinical examination and imaging. Consequently, lesions are often larger when diagnosed. The disease shows a higher tendency toward bilaterality and multifocality and generally exhibits slow tumor progression. Compared with other invasive breast cancer subtypes, axillary lymph node involvement occurs less frequently. Metastatic dissemination follows a distinct pattern, with increased involvement of gastrointestinal and gynecologic organs in addition to conventional metastatic sites such as bone, liver, and lung [4].

17.1.4 Diagnostic Considerations

Detection of ILC by mammography is challenging, with reported false-negative rates ranging from 19% to 43% [5]. Overall mammographic sensitivity varies between 57 and 81%, while false-positive rates range from 8% to 24% [6]. Ultrasound offers improved detection, with sensitivity reported between 68% and 98%. Typical sonographic findings include an irregular hypoechoic mass with poorly defined margins and posterior acoustic shadowing [7]. Owing to the low cellularity and relatively bland cytological features, ILC may be missed on fine-needle aspiration or core needle biopsy. In addition, ILC demonstrates limited sensitivity to neo-adjuvant chemotherapy, with lower rates of pathological complete response compared with other breast cancer subtypes [8].

17.2 Tubular Carcinoma

17.2.1 Epidemiology

Tubular carcinoma is an uncommon subtype of invasive breast cancer, accounting for approximately 1–2% of cases. Its detection rate is higher in populations undergoing routine screening mammography [9]. Patients most frequently present in the sixth to seventh decades of life.

17.2.2 Pathological Features

Histologically, tubular carcinoma is composed of well-formed tubular structures lined by cuboidal to columnar epithelial cells, often displaying apical cytoplasmic projections, commonly described as “snouts.” There is no universal agreement on the minimum proportion of tubular architecture required for diagnosis, with reported thresholds ranging from 75% to complete tubular differentiation. These tumors are typically positive for estrogen and progesterone receptors and lack HER2/neu overexpression.

17.2.3 Clinical Characteristics

Tubular carcinoma is frequently associated with low-grade ductal carcinoma in situ (DCIS). Compared with invasive ductal carcinoma (IDC), it demonstrates a more favorable clinical course, with a reduced likelihood of axillary lymph node involvement. Distant metastatic spread is uncommon [10].

17.2.4 Diagnosis

On mammography, tubular carcinoma often resembles invasive ductal carcinoma, making histopathological examination essential for definitive diagnosis. Tissue biopsy remains the gold standard for confirmation.

17.2.5 Prognosis

Long-term outcomes are excellent, with pooled disease-free survival rates of approximately 96.4% at 5 years and 91.8% at 10 years [11].

17.3 Mucinous (Colloid) Carcinoma

17.3.1 Epidemiology

Mucinous carcinoma represents around 2% of all breast cancers and is most commonly diagnosed in postmenopausal women. The median age at presentation is approximately 70 years.

17.3.2 Pathological Features

Gross examination typically reveals a soft, gelatinous, and well-circumscribed mass. These tumors are usually positive for estrogen and progesterone receptors, while HER2 amplification is uncommon [12]. Transcriptomic profiling suggests alignment with a luminal A molecular subtype. Among mucin-related genes, MUC2 and MUC6 are predominantly expressed.

17.3.3 *Clinical Characteristics*

Mucinous carcinoma generally exhibits indolent growth. Due to its soft consistency, the lesion may attain a relatively large size before detection.

17.3.4 *Diagnosis*

Mammographic evaluation often shows a well-defined, lobulated breast mass, aiding in differentiation from more aggressive subtypes.

17.4 Medullary Carcinoma

17.4.1 *Epidemiology*

Medullary carcinoma tends to occur in younger women, typically between 45 and 54 years of age. It is more frequently observed in patients carrying germline BRCA1 mutations. Among BRCA1-associated breast cancers, medullary carcinoma accounts for approximately 7.8–19% of cases, while medullary features are present in 35–60%. In contrast, only about 2% of sporadic, non–BRCA-related breast cancers are classified as medullary carcinoma.

17.4.2 *Pathological Features*

Despite an aggressive histological appearance, medullary carcinoma is characterized by distinctive diagnostic criteria, including the following:

- Well-circumscribed tumor margins
- A predominantly syncytial growth pattern involving at least 75% of the tumor
- Intermediate to high nuclear grade
- Prominent diffuse lymphocytic infiltration
- Absence of ductal carcinoma in situ or glandular differentiation

Most medullary carcinomas exhibit a triple-negative immunophenotype.

17.4.3 Clinical Characteristics

Axillary lymph node involvement occurs less frequently compared with other high-grade breast cancers.

17.4.4 Diagnosis

On mammographic imaging, medullary carcinoma typically appears as a non-calcified mass with smooth, well-defined borders [13].

17.4.5 Prognosis

Although medullary carcinoma demonstrates high-grade histopathological features, clinical outcomes are generally more favorable than those observed in invasive ductal carcinoma. The reported 10-year overall survival is approximately 74%, exceeding 90% in patients without lymph node involvement.

17.5 Invasive Micropapillary Carcinoma (IMPC)

17.5.1 Epidemiology

Invasive micropapillary carcinoma is an uncommon variant of breast cancer, accounting for approximately 0.9–2% of all breast malignancies. It is most frequently diagnosed in patients between 50 and 60 years of age.

17.5.2 Pathological Features

IMPC is typically associated with a higher histological grade [14]. A defining immunohistochemical feature is the characteristic reverse (inside-out) staining pattern of MUC1/EMA, a finding shared primarily with mucinous carcinoma. These tumors demonstrate a high frequency of lymphovascular invasion. Most IMPCs express estrogen and progesterone receptors. Based on molecular classification, IMPCs are predominantly luminal in subtype, with luminal A accounting for approximately 75.3% of cases, luminal B for 14.8%, HER2-enriched for 4.7%, and triple-negative disease for 5.2% [15]. HER2 gene amplification is identified in about 20.4% of cases when assessed using fluorescence in situ hybridization (FISH).

17.5.3 Clinical Features

Patients often present with relatively large primary tumors. Compared with invasive ductal carcinoma (IDC), IMPC has a greater propensity for regional lymph node involvement.

17.5.4 Diagnosis

Mammographic findings are generally non-specific. On MRI, IMPC typically appears as an irregular, spiculated mass demonstrating rapid contrast uptake followed by delayed washout, a pattern suggestive of malignancy [16, 17].

17.5.5 Prognosis

Despite its aggressive pathological features, disease-free survival and overall survival rates are comparable to those observed in patients with invasive ductal carcinoma [18].

17.6 Metaplastic Breast Carcinoma (MpBC)

17.6.1 Epidemiology

Metaplastic breast carcinoma is a rare entity, comprising approximately 0.2–5% of all breast cancers.

17.6.2 Pathological Features

MpBC is characterized by the presence of one or more tumor cell populations that have undergone metaplastic transformation, whereby glandular epithelial cells differentiate into non-glandular elements. According to the World Health Organization (WHO), MpBC is classified into several subtypes, including mixed metaplastic carcinoma, low-grade adenosquamous carcinoma, fibromatosis-like carcinoma, squamous cell carcinoma, spindle cell carcinoma, and metaplastic carcinoma with mesenchymal differentiation. Although most MpBCs are triple-negative, their genomic, transcriptomic, and proteomic profiles differ significantly from conventional triple-negative breast cancers (TNBC) [19].

17.6.3 Prognosis

Most subtypes of MpBC exhibit aggressive biological behavior with a high metastatic potential. Exceptions include fibromatosis-like carcinoma and low-grade adenosquamous carcinoma, which generally follow a more indolent course. Overall, MpBC is associated with poorer outcomes, including approximately double the risk of recurrence and reduced survival, when compared with non-metaplastic TNBC.

17.7 Adenoid Cystic Carcinoma

17.7.1 Epidemiology

Adenoid cystic carcinoma of the breast is exceedingly rare, representing less than 0.1% of primary breast malignancies [20]. The typical age at presentation is around 60 years. Axillary lymph node metastasis is uncommon, with reported rates below 5%.

17.7.2 Pathological Features

This tumor displays a distinctive biphasic histological architecture, consisting of both epithelial and myoepithelial components. Although most cases exhibit a triple-negative, basal-like immunophenotype, they are generally low-grade and demonstrate indolent clinical behavior. A characteristic chromosomal translocation, t(6;9), results in the formation of a MYB–NFIB fusion gene.

17.7.3 Prognosis

Adenoid cystic carcinoma is associated with an excellent prognosis, even in cases with relatively large tumor size.

17.7.3.1 Secretory Carcinoma

Secretory carcinoma of the breast is an exceptionally rare malignancy and is the most likely diagnosis in pediatric breast cancer cases. Histologically, it closely resembles secretory carcinoma of the salivary glands. This tumor shares a distinctive molecular hallmark—a chromosomal translocation t(12;15)(p13;q25) leading to the ETV6–NTRK3 fusion gene [21, 22]. Despite frequently exhibiting a triple-negative immune phenotype, secretory carcinoma typically follows an indolent course, with excellent long-term outcomes. Distant metastasis is exceedingly rare.

References

1. Li CI, Anderson BO, Daling JO, Moe RE. Trends in incidence rates of invasive lobular and ductal breast carcinoma. JAMA. 2003;289(11):1421–4.
2. Daling JR, Malone KE, Doody DR, Voigt LF, Bernstein L, Coates RJ, et al. Relation of regimens of combined hormone replacement therapy to lobular, ductal, and other histological types of breast carcinoma. Cancer. 2002;95(12):2455–64.
3. Sledge GW, Chagpar A, Perou C. Collective wisdom: lobular carcinoma of the breast. Am Soc Clin Oncol. 2016;35:18–21.
4. McCart Reed AE, Kalinowski L, Simpson PT, Lakhani SR. Invasive lobular carcinoma of the breast: the increasing importance of this special subtype. Breast Cancer Res. 2021;23(1):6.
5. Johnson K, Sarma D, Hwang ES. Lobular breast cancer series: imaging. Breast Cancer Res. 2015;17:94.
6. Biglia N, Mariani L, Srgo L, Mininanni P, Moggio G, Sismondi P. Increased incidence of lobular breast cancer in women treated with hormone replacement therapy: implications for diagnosis, surgical and medical treatment. Endocr Relat Cancer. 2007;14:549–67.
7. Johnson K, Sarma D, Shelley HE. Lobular breast cancer series: imaging. Breast Cancer Res. 2015;17:94.
8. Katz A, Saad ED, Porter P, Pusztai L. Primary systemic chemotherapy of invasive lobular carcinoma of the breast. Lancet Oncol. 2007;8:55–62.
9. Sullivan T, Raad RA, Goldberg S, Assaad SI, Gadd M, Smith BL, Powell SN, Taghian AG. Tubular carcinoma of the breast: a retrospective analysis and review of the literature. Breast Cancer Res Treat. 2005;93(3):199–205.
10. Jorns JM, Thomas DG, Healy PN, Daignault S, Vickery TL, Snider JE, Mardis ER, Davies SR, Ellis MJ, Visscher DW. Estrogen receptor expression is high but is of lower intensity in tubular carcinoma than in well-differentiated invasive ductal carcinoma. Arch Pathol Lab Med. 2014;138(11):1507–13.
11. Metovic J, Bragoni A, Osella-Abate S, et al. Clinical relevance of tubular breast carcinoma: large retrospective study and meta-analysis. Front Oncol. 2021;11:65338.
12. Barkley CR, Ligibel JA, Wong JS, Lipsitz S, Smith BL, Golshan M. Mucinous breast carcinoma: a large contemporary series. Am J Surg. 2008;196(4):549–51.
13. Meyer JE, Amin E, Lindfors KK, Lipman JC, Stomper PC, Genest D. Medullary carcinoma of the breast: mammographic and US appearance. Radiology. 1989;170(1 Pt 1):79–82.
14. Verras GI, Tchabashvili L, Mulita F, Grypari IM, Sourouni S, Panagodimou E, Argentou MI. Micropapillary breast carcinoma: from molecular pathogenesis to prognosis. Breast Cancer (Dove Med Press). 2022;14:41–61.
15. Lewis GD, Xing Y, Haque W, et al. The impact of molecular status on survival outcomes for invasive micropapillary carcinoma of the breast. Breast J. 2019;25:1171–6.
16. Adrada B, Arribas E, Gilcrease M, Yang WT. Invasive micropapillary carcinoma of the breast: mammographic, sonographic, and MRI features. Am J Roentgenol. 2009;193:58–63.
17. Wu SG, Zhang WW, Sun JY, Li FY, Chen YX, Zhen-Yu ZY. Postoperative radiotherapy for invasive micropapillary carcinoma of the breast: an analysis of surveillance, epidemiology, and end results database. Cancer Manag Res. 2017;9:453–9.
18. Invasive micropapillary carcinoma of the breast had no difference in prognosis compared with invasive ductal carcinoma: a propensity-matched analysis. Sci Rep. 2019;9:1–8.

19. Aydiner A, Sen F, Tambas M, Ciftci R, Eralp Y, Saip P, Karanlik H, Fayda M, Kucucuk S, Onder S, et al. Metaplastic breast carcinoma versus triple-negative breast cancer: survival and response to treatment. Medicine (Baltimore). 2015;94(52):e2341.
20. Lakhani SR, Ellis LO, Schnitt SJ, Tan PH, van de Vijver MJ. World Health Organization classification of tumours of the breast. 4th ed. Lyon: IARC Press; 2012.
21. Skálová A, Vanecek T, Sima R, et al. Mammary analogue secretory carcinoma of salivary glands, containing the ETV6-NTRK3 fusion gene: a hitherto undescribed salivary gland tumor entity. Am J Surg Pathol. 2010;34:599.
22. Tognon C, Knezevich SR, Huntsman D, et al. Expression of the ETV6-NTRK3 gene fusion as a primary event in human secretory breast carcinoma. Cancer Cell. 2002;2:367.

Chapter 18
Presentation and Evaluation of Esophageal Carcinoma

Sambit Swarup Nanda and Tanvee Singla

18.1 Introduction and Epidemiology

Esophageal carcinoma is a malignant tumor of the digestive tract and the leading cause of cancer-related mortality due to poor prognosis. There has been a rapid rise in the number of new cases as well as the number of deaths due to esophageal cancer in the last few decades, making it the eighth most commonly diagnosed cancer and the sixth leading cause of death worldwide [1]. As per GLOBOCAN 2020, more than 0.6 million new cases of esophageal cancer and 0.54 million deaths have been found. The age-standardized rate of esophageal cancer is 6.3 per 100,000 population. There is a large predominance of esophageal malignancy in males as compared to females, accounting for approximately 70% of newly diagnosed cases occurring in men. The incidence is highest in Asia and Europe followed by Africa and North America [2]. Countries with a low human development index, like India, have a higher incidence of SCC. In India, the age-standardized rate is 6.5 per 100,000 population for males and 4.2 per 100,000 for females, making it approx. 47,000 new cases each year and 42,000 deaths [3].

The esophagus is a hollow tube of length 25 cm extending from the cricopharyngeus muscle superiorly to the GEJ inferiorly and corresponds to the vertebral level from C6-T10.

S. S. Nanda (✉) · T. Singla
Department of Radiation Oncology, MPMMCC & HBCH Varanasi, Units of Tata Memorial Centre and affliated with Homi Bhabha National Institute, Mumbai, India

S. Pradhan et al. (eds.), *Evidence Based Handbook on Diagnosis and Staging in Oncology*, https://doi.org/10.1007/978-981-95-9701-7_18

The esophagus is divided into three main parts: cervical, thoracic, and abdominal.

Parts of the esophagus	Extension	Distance from incisors
Cervical	UES to the thoracic inlet	15–20 cm
Upper thoracic	Sternal notch to the azygous vein	20–25 cm
Middle thoracic	The azygos vein to the inferior pulmonary vein	25–30 cm
Lower thoracic	Inferior pulmonary vein to GEJ	30–40 cm
Abdominal	GEJ to 5 cm below GEJ	40–45 cm

Based on the etiology and site of malignancy, esophageal carcinoma is divided into two types: squamous cell carcinoma (SCC) and adenocarcinoma. In high-risk countries like Asia and Africa, SCC is most commonly found, accounting for approx. 80–90% of new cases, whereas adenocarcinoma is most commonly seen in high-income Western countries like the US, UK, and France, representing two-thirds of cases [4, 5]. The incidence of SCC has steadily declined in the Western world, whereas adenocarcinoma incidence has increased over the last few decades. Various Indian series have reported 6–54% contribution of adenocarcinoma in the overall incidence of esophageal cancers [6, 7].

18.2 Risk Factors

The risk factors are different for both histologies and are listed below:

Squamous carcinoma Smoking and alcohol Dietary factors Achalasia Age (50–70) *H. pylori* infection	*Adenocarcinoma* Barrett's esophagus GERD Obesity Smoking and alcohol

Smoking and drinking alcohol act synergistically for SCC of the esophagus. Smoking increases the risk of SCC by 3–7 times and alcohol by 3–5 times [5]. The carcinogenic effect of smoke is due to polycyclic aromatic hydrocarbons and nitrosamines and the generation of reactive oxygen species. The metabolite of alcohol, acetyl aldehyde, is thought to cause cellular damage and carcinogenesis. Consumption of nutrition-deficient food and drinking beverages at high temperatures, causing thermal injury to the mucosa, is also associated with ESCC. *H. Pylori* infection is associated with SCC of esophageal cancers. *H. pylori* causes gastric atrophy and promotes bacterial growth f/b increase in the production of nitrosamines, which are risk factors for SCC. Other risk factors deemed potential contributory factors for esophageal carcinoma include low intake of fresh fruit and vegetables, drinking hot tea, and consuming red meat [8, 9].

The major risk factor for adenocarcinoma of the esophagus is gastroesophageal reflux, which causes inflammation of the lower esophagus, converting squamous epithelium into columnar epithelium, known as Barrett's esophagus. Abdominal obesity increases the risk of GERD, further causing adenocarcinoma. The risk of adenocarcinoma is increased three times with a BMI >30 [10]. Smoking and alcohol are also causative agents of adenocarcinoma of the esophagus.

18.3 Clinical Presentation

The onset of symptoms in esophageal carcinoma is usually gradual and is dependent upon the site of malignancy. The most common complaint is dysphagia, which is progressive and starts with a solid diet followed by a liquid diet. Dysphagia is seen in almost >90% of patients [11]. Dysphagia and resultant decreased food intake and malignancy-related cytokines further lead to weight loss and cachexia. As per the American Cancer Society, an unexplained weight loss of 10 pounds has been attributed to malignancies like esophageal and pancreatic cancer. Thus, rapid weight loss coupled with dysphagia is one of the most common symptoms associated with carcinoma of the esophagus. Other infrequent presentations include hoarseness of voice, chest pain, and bone pain. Hoarseness of voice can be due to left recurrent laryngeal nerve involvement by primary tumor or by nodal metastatic lesion. The symptomatic presentation may vary among patients depending on the extent of the disease. Hematemesis, melena, and hemoptysis can be present in the case of tracheoesophageal or bronchoesophageal fistula.

Symptoms	Percentage of patients (%)
Dysphagia	90
Odynophagia	50
Weight loss	40–70

Differential diagnosis of dysphagia: Dysphagia can be due to oropharyngeal and esophageal disease.

Structural	Propulsive
Zenker's diverticulum Corrosive injury Cervical web Infection	Myasthenia gravis GBS Parkinson's disease

18.3.1 Oropharyngeal Causes

Structural	Propulsive
Schatzki ring Stricture Hernia Congenital stenosis	GERD Achalasia cardia Diffuse esophageal spasm

18.3.2 Esophageal Causes

Diagnosis A detailed clinical history and proper physical examination should be done.

- Documentation of the general condition of the patient as per Eastern Cooperative Oncology Group or Karnofsky performance status has to be noted.
- General physical examination includes documentation of pallor, icterus, cyanosis, clubbing, and any edema/lymphadenopathy.
- Neck examination, including supraclavicular examination to rule out lymphadenopathy.
- Routine blood tests like complete blood count, coagulation profile, viral markers, liver and kidney function tests need to be done before any invasive procedure to establish the baseline fitness and feasibility for biopsy and rule out any infection.
- Proper diagnosis using various investigations has to be done. The list of investigations to be done is explained below:

Upper GI Endoscopy It is one of the principal investigations done for the diagnosis of esophageal carcinoma. It is both diagnostic and therapeutic. All patients presenting with dysphagia, upper GI bleed, and a history of weight loss should undergo upper GI endoscopy. The role of endoscopy is to visualize the mucosa of the esophagus and esophagus-gastric junction, as well as the stomach, and if any suspicious lesion is seen, explain the extent of the disease and biopsy from that suspicious lesion. Approx three-fourths of all esophageal adenocarcinomas are located in the distal one-third of the esophagus, and SCCs are located in the proximal-middle one-third of the esophagus [12]. The extent of the lesion is explained by the upper incisors and EGJ, the length of the tumor, and the circumferential extent to rule out any obstruction. Biopsies are to be taken from suspicious lesions, and at least 6–8 biopsies are to be taken to get sufficient tissue for histologic and molecular interpretation [13]. The early stage of malignancy may appear as ulceration or small nodules on endoscopy, whereas the advanced stage may look like a friable mass or stricture. In the past years, there has been revolutionary development in the techniques of endoscopy, as listed below.

Chromoendoscopy: It helps in better visualization of mucosal lesions using some dyes. The most commonly used dyes are methylene blue, toluidine blue, Lugol's iodine, and indigo carmine. Although it is not 100% sensitive and specific and requires clinical correlation. The limitation of chromoendoscopy is the long duration of the procedure and steep learning curve, but it can be used by experienced hands and provide us with relevant clinical information [14].

Narrow-Band Imaging: It gives 1000 times magnification as compared to conventional endoscopes. In this NBI, light of a small wavelength is used, i.e., blue and green, which gives better information regarding the superficial pattern of lesions, vascular architecture, and contrast enhancement. The sensitivity of NBI to diagnose neoplastic lesions is 100%, and the specificity is 75% [15].

Disadvantages of UGIE—It does not give information about the depth of the lesion and about the involvement of adjacent structures.

Endoscopic Ultrasonography It helps in the delineation of layers of the esophagus by using high-frequency sound waves and also helps in evaluating the primary tumor as well as nodal status. The Radial echo-endoscope uses 7.5–12Mhz with a depth resolution of approx. 3–5 cm, and it gives a 360-degree visualization of the esophageal wall and adjacent structures [16]. The mucosal layer of the esophagus appears hyperechoic, and the muscular layer appears hypoechoic on EUS.

EUS helps in assessing the depth of invasion by the lesion, the extent of the lesion, and nodal status. The overall accuracy for T&N staging is approx. 90% [17] and that for nodal staging it is >70% [18]. In a meta-analysis of 49 studies involving 2558 patients, Puli et al. demonstrated that EUS had excellent sensitivity and specificity in the staging of esophageal cancers. Further, they demonstrated EUS had better-pooled sensitivity in T4 vis-à-vis T1 (sensitivity 92% vs. 82% and specificity 97% vs. 99%, respectively [19]. The interoperator variability, suboptimal staging evaluation in large stenosed tumors, and perforation risk limit its wider applicability. A further limitation of EUS includes its lack of usefulness in restaging post-neoadjuvant therapy, as it is not able to differentiate between fibrosis and residual disease.

Contrast-Enhanced Computed Tomography Thorax, Abdomen, and Pelvis (CECT TAP) The primary role of CECT is to diagnose distant metastasis in the body, particularly hepatic and thoracic. It also has a role in the staging of esophageal cancer with an accuracy of 43–92% in T-staging [20]. It is difficult to differentiate T1 and T2 lesions (for that, EUS is preferred) on CECT, so it mostly helps in the advanced stage, i.e., T3 and T4 [21]. For nodal staging, the accuracy of CECT is 27–86% for nodes >10 mm with a sensitivity of 30–60% and specificity of 60–80% [22]. The meta-analysis by Van Vliet et al. showed that the pooled sensitivity and specificity of CT scans for the detection of regional lymph nodes is 50% (41–60%) and 83% (77–89%). For the detection of distant metastasis, the sensitivity of the CT scan is 52% (33–71%), and the specificity is 91% (86–96%) [23].

Disadvantages of CECT:

- Ionizing radiation exposure
- The extent of the disease is not very clear
- Sensitivity to determine nodal status is low

Magnetic Resonance Imaging (MRI) A T2-weighted MRI sequence is used for T-staging with an accuracy of 81%. It gives better information regarding the extent of the disease. T2WI combined with DW-MRI gives a detection rate of 33% for T1, 58% for T2, 96%, and 100% for T3 and T4, respectively [24]. Conventional MRI has poor sensitivity in nodal detection, but can be improved with contrast-enhanced 1.5 T MRI with a sensitivity of up to 100% and specificity of 78% [25].

Positron Emission Tomography (PET-CT) It has a limited role in the T staging of disease, but can assess the length of the tumor in patients for whom EUS cannot be done. A meta-analysis by Shi et al. showed a sensitivity of 62% and specificity of 96% for nodal detection [26]. PETCT is the imaging of choice for the detection of distant metastasis with a sensitivity of 71% and specificity of 93% [27]. In a study by Duong et al., PET-CT changed the clinical management from either curative to palliative or vice versa in 40% of patients [28].

Further utility of PET CT in detecting nodal metastasis in carcinoma esophagus has been evaluated by Jiang et al. This meta-analysis involving 19 studies with 1089 patients showed per-nodal station basis the pooled sensitivity and specificity of 18F-FDG PET/CT for detecting regional lymph node metastasis were 66% (51–78%) and 96% (92–98%), respectively [29]. Overall nodal detection sensitivity of PET CT remains low, but specificity remains very high. Further utility of PET CT in detecting small (5–1 cm) nodal metastasis remains limited due to the inherent limitation of resolution. Further, due to high cost, infrequent availability, and high false positive rates because of tuberculosis in our country, it is still not used regularly.

18.4 Role of Biomarker Testing in Esophageal Cancer

Her2 Testing It is done in patients who are inoperable, recurrent, and metastatic adenocarcinoma in whom one can target Her2 receptors. Her2 assessment is done using IHC or FISH. Next-generation sequencing (NGS) can also be considered when limited diagnostic tissue is available.

Scoring for Her2 expression:

Scores	IHC pattern	Her2 expression assessment
0	No reactivity or membranous reactivity in <10% of cancer cells.	Negative
1	>10% cells are reactive but only in the membrane part	Negative
2	Weak–moderate reactivity in >10% of cells	Equivocal
3	Strong complete reactivity in >10% of cells	Positive

PDL1 Testing Can be considered for advanced, metastatic, and recurrent cases of esophageal cancer that are candidates for PD-L1 inhibitors. The combined positive score is calculated for the expression of PD-L1. CPS is defined as the number of PD-L1 staining cells divided by the total number of viable tumor cells, multiplied by 100.

Role of Screening in Esophageal Cancer There is no recommendation for routine screening in esophageal carcinoma, but in some premalignant lesions, like Barrett's esophagus, screening to rule out esophageal adenocarcinoma can be done because the risk of death is ten times higher in Barrett's esophagus [30].

Endoscopic surveillance is done in a patient aged >50 years and complaining of GERD symptoms to rule out Barrett's esophagus. The guidelines recommend endoscopic surveillance intervals of 3–5 years for patients without dysplasia, 6–12 months for low-grade dysplasia, and every 3 months for High-grade dysplasia [31]. Mapping biopsies are done at 2-cm intervals from each quadrant in case of non-suspicious segments during surveillance, and for dysplastic segments, biopsies should be taken at 1-cm intervals as per the Seattle protocol. For adequate histological confirmation, a minimum of eight biopsies is recommended [32].

Advanced techniques like chromoendoscopy, narrow-band imaging, and autofluorescence imaging can be used for screening for esophageal adenocarcinoma.

Summary for Diagnosis of Esophageal Cancer

- Baseline workup- complete blood count, LFT and RFT, coagulation profile
- Upper GI endoscopy
- Endoscopic USG
- CECT TAP
- +/– PETCT/MRI
- Fiber-optic bronchoscopy

For Functional Evaluation

- 2D ECHO and PFT + DLCO for cardiac and pulmonary function.
- Nutritional assessment of the patient
- Pulmonary rehabilitation
- Oral hygiene
- Pure tone audiometry

Esophageal cancer is staged as per AJCC staging system

References

1. Lagergren J, Smyth E, Cunningham D, Lagergren P. Oesophageal cancer. Lancet. 2017;390(10110):2383–96. https://doi.org/10.1016/S0140-6736(17)31462-9.
2. Abnet CC, Arnold M, Wei WQ. Epidemiology of esophageal squamous cell carcinoma. Gastroenterology. 2018;154(2):360–73.
3. Globocan. 2008. Accessed online at http://globocan.iarc.fr/factsheet.asp on 9 Dec 2012.
4. Asombang AW, Chishinga N, Nkhoma A, Chipaila J, Nsokolo B, Manda-Mapalo M, et al. Systematic review and meta-analysis of esophageal cancer in Africa: epidemiology, risk factors, management and outcomes. World J Gastroenterol. 2019;25(31):4512–33. https://doi.org/10.3748/wjg.v25.i31.4512.
5. Blot WJ. Esophageal cancer. In: Thun M, Linet MS, Cerhan JR, Haiman CA, Schottenfeld D, editors. Cancer epidemiology and prevention. 4th ed. Oxford University Press; 2018. p. 579–93. https://doi.org/10.1093/ije/dyy166.
6. Tony J, Kumar SK, Thomas V. Time trends and pathological profile of carcinoma lower oesophagus and gastro-esophageal junction over the last 20 years—an experience from South India. Trop Gastroenterol. 2007;28:113–6.

7. Gupta NM, Jindal R, Prakash O, Gupta R, Bhasin DK. Comparison of the clinical profile and outcome for squamous cell carcinoma and adenocarcinoma of the distal esophagus and cardia in India. Surg Today. 2001;31:400–4.
8. Sewram V, Sitas F, O'Connell D, Myers J. Diet and esophageal cancer risk in the Eastern Cape Province of South Africa. Nutr Cancer. 2014;66:791–9.
9. Middleton DR, Menya D, Kigen N, Oduor M, Maina SK, Some F, Chumba D, Ayuo P, Osano O, Schüz J, McCormack V. Hot beverages and oesophageal cancer risk in western Kenya: findings from the ESCCAPE case-control study. Int J Cancer. 2019;144:2669–76.
10. Freedman ND, Abnet CC, Leitzmann MF, Mouw T, et al. A prospective study of tobacco, alcohol, and the risk of esophageal and gastric cancer subtypes. Am J Epidemiol. 2007;165:1424–33.
11. Percik R, Stumvoll M. Obesity and cancer. Exp Clin Endocrinol Diabetes. 2009;117:563–6.
12. Rustgi AK, El-Serag HB. Esophageal carcinoma. N Engl J Med. 2014;371(26):2499–509.
13. Harrison R, Perry I, Haddadin W, McDonald S, Bryan R, Abrams K, Sampliner R, Talley NJ, Moayyedi P, Jankowski JA. Detection of intestinal metaplasia in Barrett's esophagus: an observational comparator study suggests the need for a minimum of eight biopsies. Am J Gastroenterol. 2007;102(6):1154–61. https://doi.org/10.1111/j.1572-0241.2007.01230.x. Epub 2007 Apr 13.
14. Bartel MJ, Picco MF, Wallace MB. Chromocolonoscopy. Gastrointest Endosc Clin N Am. 2015;25:243–60.
15. Guelrud M, Herrera I, Essenfeld H, Castro J. Enhanced magnification endoscopy: a new technique to identify specialized intestinal metaplasia in Barrett's esophagus. Gastrointest Endosc. 2001;53:559–65.
16. DaVee T, Ajani JA, Lee JH. Is endoscopic ultrasound examination necessary in the management of esophageal cancer? World J Gastroenterol. 2017;23(5):751–62.
17. Lee WC, Lee TH, Jang JY, et al. Staging accuracy of endoscopic ultrasound performed by nonexpert endo sonographers in patients with resectable esophageal squamous cell carcinoma: is it possible? Dis Esophagus. 2015;28(6):574–8.
18. Kalaitzakis E, Meenan J. Controversies in the use of endoscopic ultrasound in esophageal cancer staging. Scand J Gastroenterol. 2009;44(2):133–44.
19. Puli SR, Reddy JB, Bechtold ML, Antillon D, Ibdah JA, Antillon MR. Staging accuracy of esophageal cancer by endoscopic ultrasound: a meta-analysis and systematic review. World J Gastroenterol. 2008;14(10):1479–90. https://doi.org/10.3748/wjg.14.1479.
20. Ba-Ssalamah A, Matzek W, Baroud S, et al. Accuracy of hydro-multidetector row CT in the local T staging of oesophageal cancer compared to postoperative histopathological results. Eur Radiol. 2011;21:2326–35. https://doi.org/10.1007/s00330-011-2187-2.
21. Tirumani H, Rosenthal MH, Tirumani SH, et al. Esophageal carcinoma: current concepts in the role of imaging in staging and management. Can Assoc Radiol J. 2015;66:130–9. https://doi.org/10.1016/j.carj.2014.08.006.
22. Liu J, Wang Z, Shao H, et al. Improving CT detection sensitivity for nodal metastases in oesophageal cancer with a combination of smaller size and lymph node axial ratio. Eur Radiol. 2018;28:188–95. https://doi.org/10.1007/s00330-017-4935-4.
23. van Vliet EP, Heijenbrok-Kal MH, Hunink MG, Kuipers EJ, Siersema PD. Staging investigations for oesophageal cancer: a meta-analysis. Br J Cancer. 2008;98(3):547–57.
24. van Rossum PS, van Lier AL, Lips IM, et al. Imaging of oesophageal cancer with FDG-PET/CT and MRI. Clin Radiol. 2015;70:81–95. https://doi.org/10.1016/j.crad.2014.07.017.
25. Zhu Y, Fu L, Jing W, et al. The value of magnetic resonance imaging in esophageal carcinoma: tool or toy? Asia Pac J Clin Oncol. 2019;15:101–7. https://doi.org/10.1111/ajco.13112.
26. Shi W, Wang W, Wang J, et al. Meta-analysis of 18FDG PET-CT for nodal staging in patients with esophageal cancer. Surg Oncol. 2013;22:112–6. https://doi.org/10.1016/j.suronc.2013.02.003.

27. Bunting D, Bracey T, Fox B, et al. Loco-regional staging accuracy in oesophageal cancer-how good are we in the modern era? Eur J Radiol. 2017;97:71–5. https://doi.org/10.1016/j.ejrad.2017.10.015.
28. Duong CP, Demitriou H, Weih L, Thompson A, Williams D, Thomas RJ, et al. Significant clinical impact and prognostic stratification provided by FDG-PET in the staging of oesophageal cancer. Eur J Nucl Med Mol Imaging. 2006;33:759–69.
29. Jiang C, Chen Y, Zhu Y, Xu Y. Systematic review and meta-analysis of the accuracy of 18F-FDG PET/CT for detection of regional lymph node metastasis in esophageal squamous cell carcinoma. J Thorac Dis. 2018;10(11):6066–76. https://doi.org/10.21037/jtd.2018.10.57.
30. Desai TK, Krishnan K, Samala N, et al. The incidence of oesophageal adenocarcinoma in non-dysplastic Barrett's oesophagus: a meta-analysis. Gut. 2012;61:970–6.
31. Wang KK, Sampliner RE. Updated guidelines 2008 for the diagnosis, surveillance and therapy of Barrett's esophagus. Am J Gastroenterol. 2008;103:788–97.
32. Harrison R, Perry I, Haddadin W, et al. Detection of intestinal metaplasia in Barrett's esophagus: an observational comparator study suggests the need for a minimum of eight biopsies. Am J Gastroenterol. 2007;102:1154–61.

Chapter 19
Presentation and Evaluation of Gastric Carcinoma

Prashanth Giridhar and Rahul Sisodiya

19.1 Introduction and Epidemiology

Gastric cancer is ranked the fifth most common cancer and composes 4.9% of all newly diagnosed cases as per the GLOBOCAN 2022 statistics [1] published by the International Agency for Research on Cancer. Gastric cancer is also ranked fifth in terms of cancer deaths, constituting 6.8% of all cancer deaths. Incidence rates are highest in Eastern Asia (with Mongolia having the highest incidence rates in both sexes) alongside Eastern Europe, with rates lowest across the African continent [1]. Gastric cancer is the fifth most commonly detected cancer in Indian males (*but not so common in females or all genders combined*) [2]. Table 19.1 shows the crude number of incidence and deaths attributable to stomach cancer. There is also a significant variation in incidence across different states of India [3]. From the reports available to date, the North Eastern part of India, the district of Aizawl in the state of Mizoram, has recorded the highest incidence in the country, as per NCRP 2013 (64.2/100,000 population), followed by Tamil Nadu, where the incidence is 12.2/100,000 population in men. The lowest incidence in the entire country is in the state of Gujarat, 1.1/100,000 population in men and up to 0.5/100,000 population in women from certain communities [3].

Table 19.1 Incidence and death rates of gastric cancer worldwide (GLOBOCAN 2022)

Data source	Incidence	Deaths
GLOBOCAN		
1. All cancers	19.9 million	9.7 million
2. Stomach cancer	0.96 million	0.65 million (6.8%)

P. Giridhar (✉) · R. Sisodiya
Department of Radiation Oncology, MPMMCC & HBCH, Varanasi, Units of Tata Memorial Centre and affliated with Homi Bhabha National Institute, Mumbai, India

S. Pradhan et al. (eds.), *Evidence Based Handbook on Diagnosis and Staging in Oncology*, https://doi.org/10.1007/978-981-95-9701-7_19

Table 19.2 Risk factors for gastric cancer

Cardia	Non cardia
Age	Age
Male sex	Male sex
Tobacco smoking	Tobacco smoking
Race	Race
Family history	Family history
Physical activity	Physical activity
Fiber intake	Fiber intake
Obesity	*H. pylori*
GERD	High intake of salty and smoked food
	Low consumption of fruits and vegetables

19.2 Risk Factors

Gastric cancer is a multifactorial disease, and both environmental and genetic factors have a role in its etiology. Risk factors for cancers arising from cardia and noncardia regions of the stomach may be different (Table 19.2) [4].

Certain risk factors for gastric cancer, such as age, sex, race/ethnicity, and genetics, are non-modifiable. Conversely, factors like *Helicobacter pylori* (*H. pylori*) infection, gastrointestinal microbiota, obesity, unhealthy dietary habits, lifestyle choices including tobacco and alcohol consumption, exposure to chemicals, radiation, and viruses may be modified [5].

Chronic infection with *Helicobacter pylori* (*H. pylori*) is a major confirmed cause of gastric cancer implicated in approximately 90% of noncardia gastric cancer. *H. pylori*'s long-term presence in the gastric mucosa contributes to chronic conditions such as inflammation, gastritis, mucosal atrophy, and intestinal metaplasia, facilitated by its virulence factors encoded by various genes. Moreover, chronic *H. pylori* infection induces epigenetic and genetic changes in gastric epithelial cells, suggesting cellular instability. These factors underscore the significant role of *H. pylori* in gastric cancer development, highlighting the importance of understanding and managing this infection to mitigate its oncogenic potential [5]. Around 8%–10% of gastric cancers are associated with Epstein-Barr virus (EBV). EBV-associated gastric cancers have distinct clinicopathologic characteristics like male predominance, proximal location, lymphocytic infiltration, and lower frequency of lymph node involvement.

19.3 Clinical Features

Due to vague, non-specific symptoms that characterize gastric cancer, many patients are diagnosed with advanced-stage disease.

Common symptoms are as follows:

1. *Weight loss (22%–61%)*
2. *Abdominal pain (62%–91%)*

3. *Dysphagia*
4. *Hematemesis*
5. *Anorexia (5%–40%)*
6. *Nausea and vomiting* (6%–40%)
7. *Early satiety*
8. *Dyspepsia*

Other symptoms can be postprandial fullness, heartburn, indigestion, and fatigue. In addition, patients may be asymptomatic (4%–17%).

19.4 Metastatic Signs in Gastric Cancer

- *Abdominal mass*: When palpable indicates advanced disease.
- *Virchow node*: Left supraclavicular adenopathy.
- *Sister Mary Joseph node*: Peri-umbilical nodule.
- *Irish node*: Left axillary node.
- *Krukenberg's tumor*: Ovarian mass from metastasis.
- *Blumer's shelf*: Cul-de-sac mass.
- *Ascites*: Peritoneal carcinomatosis.
- *Hepatomegaly*: Often diffuse disease burden.

19.5 Paraneoplastic Manifestations in Gastric Cancer

- *Dermatological*: Diffuse seborrheic keratosis, acanthosis nigricans.
- *Hematological*: Microangiopathic hemolytic anemia, hypercoagulable state (Trousseau's syndrome).
- *Renal*: Membranous nephropathy.
- *Autoimmune*: Polyarteritis nodosa.

19.6 Histopathology

Approximately 95% of all gastric cancers are adenocarcinoma, and the rest include squamous cell carcinoma, adenoacanthoma (adeno-squamous), neuroendocrine, and gastrointestinal stromal tumor [6]. The most widely used histologic classification is the *Lauren classification*, which divides gastric cancer into intestinal and diffuse types [7].

Intestinal gastric cancer	Diffuse gastric cancer
Environmental	Familial
Gastric atrophy, intestinal metaplasia	Blood group A
More common in males	More common in females
Types-polypoidal, superficial	Linitis plastica
APC gene mutation (p53, p16 inactivation)	Decreased E-cadherin (p53, p16 inactivation)

19.7 Molecular Classification

In the TCGA (The Cancer Genome Atlas) study, gastric adenocarcinoma is subdivided into four groups [8].

1. Genetic stable (20%)—Early age at diagnosis, diffuse-type histology, distal location, CDH1, RHOA, and ARID1A mutations.
2. Chromosomally unstable (50%)—Male preponderance, aneuploidy, gastro-esophageal junction, intestinal-type histology, TP53 mutations, and ERBB2 (HER2) amplification.
3. Microsatellite unstable (22%)—Female preponderances, older age at diagnosis, intestinal-type histology, high mutation rate, and MLH1 silencing.
4. EBV positive (9%)—Male preponderance, frequently located at the fundus and body of the stomach, intestinal-type histology, PD-L1/2 amplifications, and PIK3CA mutations.

19.8 Screening

Screening for the early detection of gastric cancer can be performed either in large populations (mass screening) or in individuals considered to be at high risk. Although the effectiveness of mass screening for gastric cancer remains controversial, such programs have been implemented in countries with a high incidence of the disease, including Japan, Venezuela, and Chile [9]. Screening strategies for gastric cancer include four main modalities: upper gastrointestinal (UGI) series, serum pepsinogen testing, *Helicobacter pylori* serology, and endoscopy.

1. *H. pylori serology*—It has low sensitivity and does not detect pre-malignant lesions. It is not useful as a stand-alone screening test.
2. *Serum PG testing*—Decrease in serum PG I and PG I/II ratio is associated with the extent of gastric atrophy. Serum PG is a useful marker of atrophic gastritis, which is a precursor of intestinal-type adenocarcinoma in the stomach. PG I < 70 ng/L and PG I/II ratio < 3 is associated with an increased risk for gastric cancer [10]. In a pooled meta-analysis study, the sensitivity and specificity of serum PG testing for gastric cancer screening were 77% and 73% [11].

3. *Upper GI series*—The barium meal indirect radiograph was introduced as a mass screening program for gastric cancer in 1960 in Japan [12]. The sensitivity was 60%–80%, and the specificity was 90% [13].
4. *Endoscopy*—It is the only method available for direct visual examination of the gastric mucosa and allows for biopsy.

19.9 Hereditary Syndromes

Among 1%–3% gastric cancers are related to hereditary syndromes [14]. A first-degree relative is associated with an OR of 2–10 for developing gastric cancer.

Hereditary syndromes	Genes	Risk for gastric cancer
Hereditary diffuse gastric cancer	CGH1	>80%
Lynch syndrome	MLH1, MSH2, MSH6, PMS2	6%–13%
Hereditary breast/ovarian cancer syndrome	BRCA1/2	2.6%–5.5%
Li-Fraumeni syndrome	P53	2.8%
Familial adenomatous polyposis syndrome	APC	0.5%–2%
Juvenile polyposis	SMAD4, BMPR1A	21%
Peutz-Jeghers syndrome	STK11	29%

19.9.1 Pretreatment Evaluation

19.9.1.1 Endoscopy

Upper endoscopy is widely used to diagnose gastric cancer. It visualizes the gastric mucosa, and a biopsy can be done for histologic diagnosis.

EUS is a combined technique of endoscopy and high-frequency ultrasound (5–12 Hz) that provides high-resolution images with a limited penetration depth (between 1 and 6 cm). There is no consensus on the normal thickness of the gastric wall, but 2–4 mm should be considered the normal range [15]. The overall accuracy of EUS for T staging ranges from 65% to 92.1%. In particular, the sensitivity and specificity for serosa involvement range from 77.8% to 100% and from 67.9% to 100%, respectively [16]. The overall accuracy of EUS in N staging generally ranges from 66% to 90% [17, 18] with low sensitivity values for stages N2 and N3 [16]. One of the most important advantages of EUS in N staging is the possibility of fine needle aspiration (EUS FNA), which contributes to the improvement of the overall accuracy.

19.9.1.2 Computed Tomography

A CT scan of the thorax, abdomen, and pelvis is recommended for evaluation of gastric cancer.

19.9.1.3 Evaluation of T Stage in GC with CT

For optimal gastric distension, neutral (water or methylcellulose) contrast agents are used to visualize enlargement of each layer of the gastric wall. Intravenous contrast is mandatory for the examination of the gastric walls. CT images should be acquired at least in the unenhanced phase and approximately 70 s after injection. The features to identify different T stages are summarized in Table 19.3:

The diagnostic accuracy for T staging with CT is 77%–89%. The sensitivity and specificity of serosal invasion range from 82.8% to 100% and from 80% to 96.8%, respectively, for CT [19].

19.9.1.4 Evaluation of N Stage in GC with CT

There is no consensus on the threshold size for involved nodes (accepted range is 6–10 mm in the upper abdomen). CT sensitivity and specificity of N staging range from 62.5% to 91.9% and 50.0% to 87.9%, respectively [20].

19.9.1.5 Evaluation of M Stage in GC with CT

A CT scan is standard for metastasis detection. Overall M staging accuracy with CT is 96.6%. Good sensitivity and specificity are seen for metastases of the liver (80% and 99%), and pelvis (100% and 99%) [21]. The sensitivity of CT for peritoneal

Table 19.3 CT features to identify T stages [17, 18]

T stage	Features
T1a	Cannot be identified on CT; endoscopy ± EUS to diagnose
T1b	Focal thickening in the inner and/or middle layer with strong enhancement Enhancement of the stomach walls without thickening Focal thickening with intense enhancement of the inner layer associated with a hypo-attenuating peripheral layer
T2/T3	Thickening of the whole stomach walls with a regular outer surface Normal appearance of peri-gastric fat
T4a	Thickening of the whole stomach walls with homogeneous or inhomogeneous enhancement Irregular outer surface Peri-gastric fat stranding Irregular nodules in the peri-gastric fat
T4b	Same as T4a with the absence of fat planes between the primary tumor and adjacent organs or structures

carcinomatosis is low, ranging from 23% to 76% [22]. Therefore, whenever peritoneal involvement is suspected/expected, surgical laparoscopy to assess the peritoneal cancer index is to be performed.

19.9.1.6 FDG PET

FDG-PET is being increasingly applied in the evaluation of gastric cancer. It identifies occult metastatic disease in about 10% patients. International guidelines do not recommend FDG PET as standard imaging for GC as of now. FAPI PET is a new imaging modality found useful in the evaluation of signet ring cell variant with high sensitivity and specificity to identify peritoneal metastases [23].

AJCC Staging system is used for staging of gastric cancer (*VIII edition*).

References

1. Bray F, Laversanne M, Sung H, et al. Global cancer statistics 2022: GLOBOCAN estimates of incidence and mortality worldwide for 36 cancers in 185 countries. CA Cancer J Clin. 2024;74(3):229–63.
2. Sathishkumar K, Chaturvedi M, Das P, Stephen S, Mathur P. Cancer incidence estimates for 2022 & projection for 2025: Result from National Cancer Registry Programme, India. Indian J Med Res. 2022;156(4 & 5):598–607.
3. Servarayan Murugesan C, Manickavasagam K, Chandramohan A, Jebaraj A, Jameel ARA, Jain MS, Venkataraman J. Gastric cancer in India: epidemiology and standard of treatment. Updat Surg. 2018;70(2):233–9.
4. Karimi P, Islami F, Anandasabapathy S, Freedman ND, Kamangar F. Gastric cancer: descriptive epidemiology, risk factors, screening, and prevention. Cancer Epidemiol Biomarkers Prev. 2014;23(5):700–13.
5. Yang WJ, Zhao HP, Yu Y, et al. Updates on global epidemiology, risk, and prognostic factors of gastric cancer. World J Gastroenterol. 2023;29(16):2452–68.
6. Chia NY, Tan P. Molecular classification of gastric cancer. Ann Oncol. 2016;27(5):763–9.
7. Lauren P. The two histological main types of gastric carcinoma: diffuse and so-called intestinal-type carcinoma. An attempt at a histo-clinical classification. Acta Pathol Microbiol Scand. 1965;64:31–49.
8. Zhang W. TCGA divides gastric cancer into four molecular subtypes: implications for individualized therapeutics. Chin J Cancer. 2014;33(10):469–70. https://doi.org/10.5732/cjc.014.10117.
9. Leung WK, Wu M, Kakugawa Y, et al. Screening for gastric cancer in Asia: current evidence and practice. Lancet Oncol. 2008;9:279–87.
10. Borch K, Axelsson CK, Halgreen H, et al. The ratio of pepsinogen A to pepsinogen C: a sensitive test for atrophic gastritis. Scand J Gastroenterol. 1989;24:870–6.
11. Dinis-Ribeiro M, da Costa-Pereira A, Lopes C, et al. Validity of serum pepsinogen I/II ratio for the diagnosis of gastric epithelial dysplasia and intestinal metaplasia during the follow-up of patients at risk for intestinal-type gastric adenocarcinoma. Neoplasia. 2004;6:449–56.
12. Hisamichi S, Sugawara N. Mass screening for gastric cancer by X-ray examination. Jpn J Clin Oncol. 1984;14:211–23.
13. Kato M, Asaka M. Recent development of gastric cancer prevention. Jpn J Clin Oncol. 2012;42:987–94.

14. Lynch HT, Grady W, Suriano G, Huntsman D. Gastric cancer: new genetic developments. J Surg Oncol. 2005;90(3):114–33; discussion 133.
15. Ilson DH. Advances in the treatment of gastric cancer: 2019. Curr Opin Gastroenterol. 2019;35:551–4.
16. Fusaroli P, Caletti G. Endoscopic ultrasonography: current clinical role. Eur J Gastroenterol Hepatol. 2005;17:293–301.
17. Hwang SW, Lee DH, Lee SH, et al. Preoperative staging of gastric cancer by endoscopic ultrasonography and multidetector-row computed tomography: preoperative staging of gastric cancer. J Gastroenterol Hepatol. 2010;25:512–8.
18. Habermann CR, Weiss F, Riecken R, et al. Preoperative staging of gastric adenocarcinoma: comparison of helical CT and endoscopic US. Radiology. 2004;230:465–71.
19. Anand D, Barroeta JE, Gupta PK, Kochman M, Baloch ZW. Endoscopic ultrasound guided fine needle aspiration of non-pancreatic lesions: an institutional experience. J Clin Pathol. 2007;60(11):1254–62.
20. Kwee RM, Kwee TC. Imaging in assessing lymph node status in gastric cancer. Gastric Cancer. 2009;12:6–22.
21. Pan Z, Zhang H, Yan C, et al. Determining gastric cancer resectability by dynamic MDCT. Eur Radiol. 2010;20(3):613–20.
22. Jacquet P, Sugarbaker PH. Clinical research methodologies in diagnosis and staging of patients with peritoneal carcinomatosis. In: Peritoneal carcinomatosis: principles of management. Springer; 1996. p. 359–74.
23. Lin R, Lin Z, Chen Z, et al. [^{68}Ga]ga-DOTA-FAPI-04 PET/CT in the evaluation of gastric cancer: comparison with [^{18}F]FDG PET/CT. Eur J Nucl Med Mol Imaging. 2022;49(8):2960–71.

Chapter 20
Presentation and Evaluation of Colorectal Cancer

Abhishek Shinghal and Soham Sanyal

20.1 Introduction and Epidemiology

Colorectal malignancies were ranked the third most common cancer and composed of 10% of all newly diagnosed cases (colon cancers 6% and rectal cancers 3.8%) as per the GLOBOCAN 2020 statistics [1] published by the International Agency for Research on Cancer. Colorectal malignancies ranked second (9.4%) of all cancer deaths (colon cancers 5.8% and rectal cancers 3.4%). Colorectal cancers are four times more common in developed economies than in developing economies. The 2040 projections expect a 47% rise in all cancer cases worldwide [1]. Cancer cases in India would increase to 2.08 million, a rise of 57.5% in 2040 as compared to 2020 [2]. Rectal cancers accounted for the tenth most commonly detected cancer in Indian males (but not so common in females or all genders combined), and colon cancers were uncommon [2]. Table 20.1 shows the crude number of incidence and deaths attributable to colorectal cancers, both worldwide and in India.

A. Shinghal (✉) · S. Sanyal
Department of Radiation Oncology, MPMMCC & HBCH, Varanasi, Units of Tata Memorial Centre and affliated with Homi Bhabha National institute, Mumbai, India

S. Pradhan et al. (eds.), *Evidence Based Handbook on Diagnosis and Staging in Oncology*, https://doi.org/10.1007/978-981-95-9701-7_20

Table 20.1 Incidence and death rates of colorectal malignancies worldwide (GLOBOCAN 2020) and in India (ICMR cancer registry data)

Data source	**Incidence**		**Deaths**	
GLOBOCAN				
1. All cancers	19.3 million		10 million	
2. Colorectal cancers	1.83 million (10%)		0.9 million (9.4%)	
3. Colon cancers	1.1 million (6%)		0.57 million (5.8%)	
4. Rectal cancers	0.73 million (3.8%)		0.33 million (3.4%)	
Data source	**Incidence**		**Deaths**	
ICMR cancer registry data	Age-standardized rate –per 100,000	Cumulative risk	Age-standardized rate	Cumulative risk
1. All cancers	97.5	10.4%	63.2	7%
2. Colon	11.5	1.3%		
3. Rectum	7.7	0.9%		

Table 20.2 Relative risk of different predisposing and protective factors for colorectal malignancies [3]

Factor	Relative risk
Red meat	1.13
Alcohol	1.58
Western diet	1.28
Dietary fibers	0.84
Dietary calcium	0.77
Dairy products	0.83
Whole grains	0.88
Vegetables	0.96
Fruits	0.93

20.2 Risk Factors

The stark difference in epidemiology and distribution of colorectal cancers between developed and developing countries prompted researchers to explore the differences in lifestyle and eating habits among different countries. Sedentary lifestyle, lack of physical activity, high body mass index, along with increased consumption of red meat, alcohol, and cigarette smoking, have been associated with increased risk of colorectal cancers. Consumption of whole grains, a diet rich in fiber, calcium supplements, vegetables, and dairy products lowers the risk. In all, it can be inferred that a "western" diet and lifestyle can increase the risk of developing colorectal cancers. The shift towards opulence in developing countries and the increased prevalence of obesity with the adoption of a Western diet can be a contributing factor towards the increase in the incidence of colorectal cancers. The relative risks of individual factors are shown in Table 20.2 [3, 4].

20.3 Clinical Features

Out of all colorectal cancers, 36% arise in the right-sided colon (24% in the ascending colon, 12% transverse colon), 26% in the left side (3% in the descending colon, 23% in the sigmoid colon), and 37% arise from the rectal mucosa. The symptom presentation depends on the location of the tumor and its extension. Right-sided tumors generally present as sessile polyps which shows occult bleeding leading to anemia. Left-sided lesions are more invasive and typically described as "apple core" in pattern; this results in bowel obstructive features being the most common presentation. Furthermore, the fresh bleeding from left-sided colon and rectal cancers can be visible on passing stool.

The constellation of symptoms that can be found is as follows:

1. Blood in stool and associated iron deficiency anemia and symptoms like fatigue, palpitation, breathlessness
2. Abdominal pain—if crampy, indicative of obstructive symptoms
3. Change in bowel habits—diarrhea, constipation, tenesmus
4. Change in stool—consistency, caliber, frequency
5. Constitutional symptoms—weight loss, lethargy, loss of appetite
6. In locally advanced disease—palpable abdominal lump, obstruction, perforation, fistula with adjacent organs
7. Symptoms pertaining to the organ involved by metastatic lesions: liver—upper abdominal quadrant pain, jaundice, and hypoproteinemia; lung—breathlessness, cough, pleural effusion

The distant spread can be via three routes [5]:

1. Lymphatic—Virchow node (left supraclavicular node)
2. Intraperitoneal (25%)—Sister Mary Joseph node (periumbilical deposit), Krukenberg tumors in the ovary, omental or peritoneal lesions
3. Hematogenous—liver (49%), lung (10%), bone (6%), brain (7%)

Table 20.3 expounds the differential diagnosis of the common presenting symptoms. Table 20.4 shows the percentage of patients with the symptoms at presentation.

Table 20.3 The differential diagnosis for different signs and symptoms pertaining to colorectal malignancies

1. Rectal bleeding (a) Hemorrhoids (b) Ulcerative colitis (c) Chron's disease (d) Diverticulitis (e) Angiodysplasia (f) Ischemic colitis (g) Intussusception (h) Anal fissure	**2. Change in bowel habit** (a) Change in diet (b) Drug-induced (c) Hypothyroidism (d) Hypokalemia (e) Hypocalcemia (f) Depression (g) Cerebral or spinal cord lesion (h) Irritable bowel syndrome
3. Mass in right lower quadrant (a) Appendix mass (b) Chorn's granuloma (c) Volvulus (d) Ileocecal tuberculosis (e) Right ovarian neoplasm	**4. Mass in the left lower quadrant** (a) Diverticular abscess (b) Fecal impaction (c) Ovarian neoplasm

Table 20.4 Percentage of patients with different clinical features in colorectal malignancies

Symptom	Percentage of patients
Rectal bleeding	55%
Abdominal or rectal pain	57%
Any alteration in bowel habit	56%
Diarrhea	31%
Weight loss	28%
Constipation	17%
Fatigue	12%

20.4 Colorectal Cancer Screening

A disease should have a high prevalence, a long asymptomatic period to allow detection, and should be treatable for screening programs to be successful. Colorectal malignancies fulfil these criteria well, and many countries in the West have established regular screening programs. Different types of tests are available for screening, including invasive and non-invasive tests.

Colonoscopy remains the most widely available modality for screening. But the effectiveness depends on the adequacy of bowel preparation. Also associated is a small but significant risk of complications (prevalence for perforation was 0.5/1000, post-colonoscopy bleeding 2.6/1000, and mortality 2.9/100,000 colonoscopies) owing to the invasive nature of the procedure [6]. Stool sample-based tests, such as FIT and the guaiac test, are recommended only for average-risk patients for whom repeated colonoscopy is not feasible. But these are not diagnostic and should be followed by a colonoscopy for confirmation after a positive result [8]. CT colonography is equivalent to colonoscopy for lesions >=10 mm. The accuracy for lesions 6–9 mm is acceptable, though less than that of colonoscopy. But for lesions less than 5 mm, CT colonography is not reliable [7].

Table 20.5 Sensitivity, specificity, and recommended frequency of different available screening modalities [11]

Modality of screening	Frequency	Sensitivity	Specificity
Colonoscopy	Every 10 years	89–95% (>=10 mm adenomas)	89% (>=10 mm adenomas)
Flexible sigmoidoscopy	Every 5–10 years	72–86%	92%
CT colonography	Every 5 years	89% (>=10 mm adenomas)	94% (>=10 mm adenomas)
Quantitative FIT (OC light-based)	Every year	74%	94%
High-sensitivity Guaiac-based test	Every year	50–75%	96–98%
Mt-sDNA test	Every 3 years	93%	85%

A systematic review done by Lin et al. [8] for the US Preventive Services Task Force in 2021 compared the many available modalities for screening of colorectal malignancies. These include colonoscopy, flexible sigmoidoscopy, CT colonography, high-sensitivity Guaiac-based tests, quantitative FIT, and mt-sDNA test. The summary of the sensitivity and specificity of the tests assessed is mentioned in Table 20.5.

A population-based screening study by Levin et al. showed that after initiation of an organized screening program, the incidence of colorectal malignancies increased. But in the long term, this led to a decrease in the incidence of 36.2% of advanced stages and 14.5% decrease in early-stage disease incidence. Overall, this led to a decrease of 25.5% in incidence and a 52.4% decrease in colorectal cancer-related mortality [9].

The available tests have sufficient accuracy to be inducted for use in a screening program. The disease burden in Western countries warrants a routine screening program to be implemented. But in countries like India, where the prevalence is low, and they have lower life expectancy as compared to their Western counterparts, screening may not yet be justified.

20.5 Genetic Testing

Elucidation of proper family history is important in colorectal cancers. One third of the cases show clustering in families, and in 5–16% of cases, a pathogenic gene could be identified. It was in colon cancers that, for the first time, the adenoma-carcinoma sequence of tumor progression was described. The associated syndromes are classified according to the histopathology of the polyps that precede these malignancies [10].

Familial adenomatous polyposis, MUTYH-associated polyposis, Polymerase proofreading- associated polyposis, AXIN2-associated polyposis, NTLH1-

associated polyposis, and MSH3-associated polyposis come under the group of Adenomatous polyposis syndromes, where the polyps are adenomas originating from the epithelial tissues of the gastrointestinal tract. Tubular, villous, and tubulo-villous are the subtypes of the polyps [10]. Peutz-Jeghers syndrome, PTEN hamartoma tumor (Cowden) syndrome, juvenile polyposis syndrome, serrated polyposis syndrome, mixed type polyposis syndrome, from the group of hamartomatous polyposis syndrome, where the polyps are composed of normal gastrointestinal tract cells but arranged in a distorted architecture [10]. Non-polyposis syndromes include Lynch syndrome, Turcot syndrome, Muir Torre syndrome, Constitutional Mismatch Repair Deficiency Syndrome, Lynch-like syndrome, Familial Colorectal Cancer Type X syndrome, and Li-Fraumeni syndrome. Polyps are not characteristic of these syndromes [10].

According to the NCCN guidelines, a person diagnosed with colorectal cancer who is less than 50 years of age should be tested for genetic mutations with next-generation sequencing. If older than 50 years, family history and number of members affected should be considered according to the disease-specific criteria mentioned in the guidelines [11]. Table 20.6 summarizes Genes associated with the known risk of colorectal cancers in syndrome complexes.

Table 20.6 Associated genes and the known risk of colorectal cancers in syndrome complexes

Syndrome	Gene involved	Risk of colorectal malignancy
Hereditary non-polyposis colon cancer		
Lynch syndrome [12]	MLH1 MSH2 MSH6 PMS2 EPCAM	46–61% 33–52% 10–44% 8.7–20% 33–52%
Li-Fraumeni syndrome [13]	TP53	20%
Hereditary polyposis colorectal cancer		
Familial adenomatous polyposis [14]	APC	100%
MUTYH-associated polyposis [15]	MUTYH	70–90%
NTLH1-associated polyposis [16]	NTLH1	20%
Polymerase proofreading-associated polyposis [17]	POLE, POLD1	20%
Peutz-Jeghers syndrome [18]	STK11	39%
PTEN hamartoma tumor (Cowden) syndrome [19]	PTEN	11–20%
Juvenile polyposis syndrome [20]	BMPR1A, SMAD4	50%
Mixed type polyposis syndrome [21]	GREM1	11–20%

20.6 Histopathology and Tumor Markers

The majority of colorectal cancers are adenocarcinomas (90%). Rarer entities include neuroendocrine, squamous cell, adenosquamous, spindle cell, and undifferentiated carcinomas. Grading of the tumor is dependent on the percentage of gland formation in the tissue (more than 95% is well differentiated, 50–95% is moderately differentiated, and less than 50% is poorly differentiated). Moderately differentiated accounts for 70% of the cases, followed by poorly differentiated (20%) and well differentiated (10%). Adenocarcinomas can be subdivided into histological variants such as mucinous adenocarcinomas, signet ring cell adenocarcinomas, medullary carcinomas, and other less common variants [22]. Mucinous adenocarcinomas have strips of cancerous cells floating in extracellular lakes of mucin, which comprises at least half of the tumor mass. Whereas signet ring cells have intracellular mucin pushing their nucleus to the side, with more than half of the tumor comprising signet cells. Sometimes they may also show pools of extracellular mucin. Signet ring adenocarcinomas have a poorer prognosis and more commonly present with bowel obstruction and infiltrating borders. Medullary adenocarcinomas have a solid growth pattern with very little mucin production [22].

Common phenotypes for colorectal adenocarcinomas are CK 20 positive and negative for CK7, though 20% cases differ from this classic pattern. CDX2 is positive in 90% of colorectal adenocarcinoma and is indicative of enteric mucosal origin and therefore not specific for colon or rectum. Though medullary carcinomas can be CDX2 negative and CD20 negative. Mucinous and medullary adenocarcinomas are more often associated with high-level MSI (MSI-H) [24]. CEA is a glycoprotein derived from the endoderm of the fetus. It is a non-specific blood tumor marker. Its levels can be elevated in colorectal cancer, medullary thyroid cancer, breast cancer, and mucinous ovarian cancer. The levels can be increased in smokers. For colorectal malignancy, it has a sensitivity of 80% and a specificity of 70%. It also has prognostic significance. Levels more than 5 ng/ml indicate a worse prognosis if compared with lower levels in the same stage of cancer. CEA should be documented before any initiation of treatment. Its levels should fall back to normal limits after 4–6 weeks of R0 resection. It is also a marker that should be tested at regular intervals after completion of treatment to detect recurrence [23].

CA 19-9 is a cell surface glycoprotein and is produced naturally by the ductal cells of the pancreas, biliary system, and mucosa of the stomach, colon, salivary glands, and the uterus. Therefore, the levels can be elevated in a wide range of benign and malignant diseases. It has a much lower sensitivity (26–48%) than CEA for colorectal cancers and therefore may not be suitable to be used independently [24] (Table 20.7).

Table 20.7 Prognostic and predictive markers of colorectal malignancies [25]

Prognostic		Predictive	
CEA	MSI	CEA	KRAS
CA 19-9	18qLOH	CA 19-9	BRAF
VGEF	p53	VGEF	PIK3CA
	KRAS		PTEN
	BRAF		UGT1A1
	DPD		

20.7 Diagnostic Confirmation of Colorectal Malignancy

The clinical examination starts with documenting the general condition of the patient and performance status according to the Eastern Cooperative Oncology Group or Karnofsky performance status. Pallor, icterus, and lymphadenopathy are of particular interest, as well as nutritional build. Abdominal examination should be done to rule out obstructive symptoms.

Digital rectal examination is done to identify the tumor and its extent. Its reach depends on the reach of the examiner's fingers. The details that should be noted are as follows:

1. Size, surface, and location of the lesion
2. Distance of the lesion from the anal verge and the anal sphincter
3. Fixity of underlying structures
4. Circumference of the wall involved
5. Percentage of the lumen free for passage of stool
6. Anal tone and sphincter involvement
7. If the patient is having any features of bowel obstruction

Proctoscopy can be done to visualize the full extent of the rectum and obtain a biopsy. Sigmoidoscopy can be done for left-sided lesions. This should be followed by a full colonoscopy evaluation to rule out synchronous colonic lesions. In 5% of cases, a synchronous malignancy can be detected [26].

If a colonoscopy could not be performed completely, virtual CT colonography should be done for completion of the workup. For the patients who have an obstructing lesion and colonoscopy or CT colonography cannot be performed, a full colonoscopy should be done after 3 to 6 months of the surgical resection of the tumor, as advised by the American Society of Colon and Rectal Surgeons [27].

20.8 Surgical Staging

Trans-coelomic spread and peritoneal metastasis in a patient with colorectal cancer are associated with a poor prognosis. The currently available radiological assessments have poor sensitivity and specificity to detect these small disseminations, thereby subjecting the patients to long and arduous radical treatment without much survival benefit. Autopsy series of patients dying from colorectal cancer have reported peritoneal metastasis in 40–80% cases. Tumors with BRAF mutations and CMS4 molecular subtype have been shown to have increased risk of peritoneal metastasis [28].

Peritoneal cancer index (PCI), as proposed by Sugerbaker et al., is a prognostic tool that predicts complete cytoreduction in patients undergoing cytoreductive surgeries, and the PCI score correlates with survival outcomes. It takes into account the size of peritoneal metastases and their distribution in the defined abdominopelvic regions [29].

Direct visualization of the peritoneum may be the most sensible way to detect peritoneal metastasis and proper staging. An observational review by Saklani et al evaluating staging laparoscopy in rectal adenocarcinomas with obstructive features found that 26% and 8% of locally advanced and potentially resectable metastatic cancers were upstaged and prevented unnecessary laparotomies in 21% of patients. Further studies are needed to identify populations that may be appropriate for staging laparoscopy and pre-treatment surgical staging [30].

20.9 Radiological Assessment

20.9.1 Ultrasonography

Endorectal ultrasonography (ERUS) can very well demonstrate the different layers of the rectum as well as the relation of the tumor to surrounding viscera, like the prostate, seminal vesicle, vagina, and uterus. It can also elicit the anal sphincter and muscles. But like all ultrasonography procedures, it is operator dependent and expertise driven. It can differentiate between T1 and T2 tumors and therefore can influence management decisions. There is 69% correlation between ERUS and histopathology, though 18% tumors are overstaged and 13% of tumors are understaged in ERUS. The ability of ERUS to detect mesorectal lymph nodes is superior to many other modalities, even MRI, as it can detect lymph nodes as small as 3 mm. Its limitations include an inability to visualize the mesorectal fascia, a narrower field of exposure, resulting in a poor chance of detecting internal iliac or superior rectal lymph nodes. It can reliably comment on the circumferential resection margin till the level of the seminal vesicles or uterus, but not beyond. Its sensitivity and specificity for nodal staging were 79% and 80%, respectively, making the accuracy to be 64% [31].

20.9.2 Computed Tomography

CECT is one of the most economical and widely available modalities for staging of colorectal cancers. Multidetector CT can well differentiate early and locally advanced colorectal cancers. It can provide details regarding the presence of lymph nodes, involvement of nearby fat, and organs. It has a fair sensitivity (83–88%) and specificity (92–94%) for T1–T3 tumors and reaches 100% for T4 disease. For N disease, the sensitivity is 43% [32, 33].

20.9.3 Magnetic Resonance Imaging

MRI has emerged as a valuable tool not only for preoperative staging but also for guiding neoadjuvant therapy in colorectal cancers. Its ability to comment upon the estimated circumferential resection margin, extramural venous invasion, and fascia and peritoneal involvement has made it a cornerstone for local imaging. The circumferential resection margin (CRM) correlates with cause-specific survival. CRM of less than or equal to 1mm has a hazard ratio of 1.9 as compared to CRM 1.1 to 2 mm [34]. It has high sensitivity (96%) and specificity (96%) to detect mesorectal fascia involvement. The accuracy for mesorectal lymph node involvement was 74%, and pelvic lymph node involvement was 87% [35]. Table 20.8 highlights features to be noted while interpreting MRI.

20.9.4 PET/CT

FDG PET/CT has a sensitivity of 86% and a PPV of 32% for screening of colorectal cancers. False-positive cases accounted for 5–8%. This may be because of the fact that there is physiological elimination of FDG in the bowel mucosa, and this can be found in 11% of all FGD PET/CT studies. The antidiabetic drug metformin may also increase bowel uptake of FDG. The sensitivity and specificity for T3/T4 lesions is 73% and specificity of 99%. For staging of nodal disease, FDG PET/CT shows sensitivity of 42% (stage III) to 63% (stage IV) and specificity of 36% (stage III) to 60% (stage IV) [36]. FDG PET/CT is superior to CECT for liver mets (accuracy 93% vs. 86%). Though there is some evidence that MRI might be better than FDG PET/CT for detecting smaller liver mets (<2 cm) [32].

Fibroblast activating protein inhibitor (FAPI) is highly expressed in tumors and has a very low distribution in normal tissue. FAPI labelled PET/CT has a high

Table 20.8 Features that should be noted while interpreting MR images

Craniocaudal length, distance from the puborectalis fascia
Safety of surgical plane of total mesorectal excision (radial margin, relation to adjacent organs like prostate, seminal vesicles, uterus, vagina)
Extramural venous invasion
Mesorectal tumor, tumor deposits, or mesorectal nodes
Maximum extramural depth spread
Malignant lymph nodes
Minimum distance from mesorectal fascia (circumferential resection margin)
The final TNM stage

signal-to-background noise ratio. FAPI PET/CT has comparable sensitivity (100%) to FDG PET/CT in terms of the primary lesion but superior sensitivity for Lymph node metastasis, liver metastasis, and peritoneal metastasis (90% vs. 80%, 96% vs. 70%, and 100% vs. 55%, respectively). It is intriguing that the specificity of FAPI PET/CT is in the tune of 100% for primary as well as lymph node and peritoneal metastasis [37].

References

1. Sung H, Ferlay J, Siegel RL, Laversanne M, Soerjomataram I, Jemal A, et al. Global cancer statistics 2020: GLOBOCAN estimates of incidence and mortality worldwide for 36 cancers in 185 countries. CA Cancer J Clin. 2021;71(3):209–49.
2. Sathishkumar K, Chaturvedi M, Das P, Stephen S, Mathur P. Cancer incidence estimates for 2022 & projection for 2025: result from National Cancer Registry Programme, India. Indian J Med Res. 2022;156(4 & 5):598–607.
3. Veettil SK, Wong TY, Loo YS, Playdon MC, Lai NM, Giovannucci EL, et al. Role of diet in colorectal cancer incidence: umbrella review of meta-analyses of prospective observational studies. JAMA Netw Open. 2021;4(2):e2037341.
4. Siegel RL, Miller KD, Goding Sauer A, Fedewa SA, Butterly LF, Anderson JC, et al. Colorectal cancer statistics, 2020. CA Cancer J Clin. 2020;70(3):145–64.
5. Stewart CL, Warner S, Ito K, Raoof M, Wu GX, Kessler J, et al. Cytoreduction for colorectal metastases: liver, lung, peritoneum, lymph nodes, bone, brain. When does it palliate, prolong survival, and potentially cure? Curr Probl Surg. 2018;55(9):330–79.
6. Reumkens A, Rondagh EJA, Bakker MC, Winkens B, Masclee AAM, Sanduleanu S. Post-colonoscopy complications: a systematic review, time trends, and meta-analysis of population-based studies. Off J Am Coll Gastroenterol ACG. 2016;111(8):1092.
7. Scalise P, Mantarro A, Pancrazi F, Neri E. Computed tomography colonography for the practicing radiologist: a review of current recommendations on methodology and clinical indications. World J Radiol. 2016;8(5):472–83.
8. Lin JS, Perdue LA, Henrikson NB, Bean SI, Blasi PR. Screening for colorectal cancer: updated evidence report and systematic review for the US Preventive Services Task Force. JAMA. 2021;325(19):1978–98.
9. Levin TR, Corley DA, Jensen CD, Schottinger JE, Quinn VP, Zauber AG, et al. Effects of organized colorectal cancer screening on cancer incidence and mortality in a large community-based population. Gastroenterology. 2018;155(5):1383–1391.e5.
10. Rebuzzi F, Ulivi P, Tedaldi G. Genetic predisposition to colorectal cancer: how many and which genes to test? Int J Mol Sci. 2023;24(3):2137.
11. NCCN [Internet]. [cited 2023 Nov 20]. Guidelines Detail. Available from: https://www.nccn.org/guidelines/guidelines-detail
12. Idos G, Valle L. Lynch syndrome. In: Adam MP, Feldman J, Mirzaa GM, Pagon RA, Wallace SE, Bean LJ, et al., editors. GeneReviews® [Internet]. Seattle: University of Washington, Seattle; 1993. [cited 2023 Nov 20]. Available from: http://www.ncbi.nlm.nih.gov/books/NBK1211/.
13. Schneider K, Zelley K, Nichols KE, Garber J. Li-Fraumeni syndrome. In: Adam MP, Feldman J, Mirzaa GM, Pagon RA, Wallace SE, Bean LJ, et al., editors. GeneReviews® [Internet]. Seattle: University of Washington, Seattle; 1993. [cited 2023 Nov 20]. Available from: http://www.ncbi.nlm.nih.gov/books/NBK1311.
14. Yen T, Stanich PP, Axell L, Patel SG. APC-associated polyposis conditions. In: Adam MP, Feldman J, Mirzaa GM, Pagon RA, Wallace SE, Bean LJ, et al., editors. GeneReviews®

[Internet]. Seattle: University of Washington, Seattle; 1993. [cited 2023 Nov 20]. Available from: http://www.ncbi.nlm.nih.gov/books/NBK1345/.
15. Nielsen M, Infante E, Brand R. MUTYH polyposis. In: Adam MP, Feldman J, Mirzaa GM, Pagon RA, Wallace SE, Bean LJ, et al., editors. GeneReviews® [Internet]. Seattle: University of Washington, Seattle; 1993. [cited 2023 Nov 20]. Available from: http://www.ncbi.nlm.nih.gov/books/NBK107219/.
16. Kuiper RP, Nielsen M, De Voer RM, Hoogerbrugge N. NTHL1 tumor syndrome. In: Adam MP, Feldman J, Mirzaa GM, Pagon RA, Wallace SE, Bean LJ, et al., editors. GeneReviews® [Internet]. Seattle: University of Washington, Seattle; 1993. [cited 2023 Nov 20]. Available from: http://www.ncbi.nlm.nih.gov/books/NBK555473/.
17. Church JM. Polymerase proofreading-associated polyposis: a new, dominantly inherited syndrome of hereditary colorectal cancer predisposition. Dis Colon Rectum. 2014;57(3):396–7.
18. McGarrity TJ, Amos CI, Baker MJ. Peutz-Jeghers syndrome. In: Adam MP, Feldman J, Mirzaa GM, Pagon RA, Wallace SE, Bean LJ, et al., editors. GeneReviews® [Internet]. Seattle: University of Washington, Seattle; 1993. [cited 2023 Nov 20]. Available from: http://www.ncbi.nlm.nih.gov/books/NBK1266/.
19. Yehia L, Eng C. PTEN Hamartoma tumor syndrome. In: Adam MP, Feldman J, Mirzaa GM, Pagon RA, Wallace SE, Bean LJ, et al., editors. GeneReviews® [Internet]. Seattle: University of Washington, Seattle; 1993. [cited 2023 Nov 20]. Available from: http://www.ncbi.nlm.nih.gov/books/NBK1488/.
20. Larsen Haidle J, MacFarland SP, Howe JR. Juvenile polyposis syndrome. In: Adam MP, Feldman J, Mirzaa GM, Pagon RA, Wallace SE, Bean LJ, et al., editors. GeneReviews® [Internet]. Seattle: University of Washington, Seattle; 1993. [cited 2023 Nov 20]. Available from: http://www.ncbi.nlm.nih.gov/books/NBK1469/.
21. Lieberman S, Walsh T, Schechter M, Adar T, Goldin E, Beeri R, et al. Features of patients with hereditary mixed polyposis syndrome caused by duplication of GREM1 and implications for screening and surveillance. Gastroenterology. 2017;152(8):1876–1880.e1.
22. Fleming M, Ravula S, Tatishchev SF, Wang HL. Colorectal carcinoma: pathologic aspects. J Gastrointest Oncol. 2012;3(3):153–73.
23. Duffy MJ. Carcinoembryonic antigen as a marker for colorectal cancer: is it clinically useful? Clin Chem. 2001;47(4):624–30.
24. Lakemeyer L, Sander S, Wittau M, Henne-Bruns D, Kornmann M, Lemke J. Diagnostic and prognostic value of CEA and CA19-9 in colorectal cancer. Dis Basel Switz. 2021;9(1):21.
25. Lech G, Słotwiński R, Słodkowski M, Krasnodębski IW. Colorectal cancer tumour markers and biomarkers: recent therapeutic advances. World J Gastroenterol. 2016;22(5):1745–55.
26. Mulder SA, Kranse R, Damhuis RA, de Wilt JHW, Ouwendijk RJT, Kuipers EJ, et al. Prevalence and prognosis of synchronous colorectal cancer: a Dutch population-based study. Cancer Epidemiol. 2011;35(5):442–7.
27. Chang GJ, Kaiser AM, Mills S, Rafferty JF, Buie WD. Standards Practice Task Force of the American Society of Colon and Rectal Surgeons. Practice parameters for the management of colon cancer. Dis Colon Rectum. 2012;55(8):831–43.
28. Peritoneal Metastases From Colorectal Cancer: Defining and Addressing the Challenges – PubMed [Internet]. [cited 2023 Dec 3]. Available from: https://pubmed.ncbi.nlm.nih.gov/33816304/
29. Wong JSM, Tan GHC, Cheok SHX, Ong CAJ, Chia CS, Teo MCC. Implications of peritoneal cancer index distribution on patients undergoing cytoreductive surgery and hyperthermic intraperitoneal chemotherapy. Pleura Peritoneum. 2022;7(2):95–102.
30. Saklani A, Sugoor P, Chaturvedi A, Bhamre R, Jatal S, Ostwal V, et al. Clinical utility of staging laparoscopy for advanced obstructing rectal adenocarcinoma: emerging tool. Indian J Surg Oncol. 2018;9(4):488–94.
31. Samdani T, Garcia-Aguilar J. Imaging in rectal cancer: magnetic resonance imaging versus endorectal ultrasonography. Surg Oncol Clin N Am. 2014;23(1):59–77.

32. Singla SC, Kaushal D, Sagoo HS, Calton N. Comparative analysis of colorectal carcinoma staging using operative, histopathology and computed tomography findings. Int J Appl Basic Med Res. 2017;7(1):10–4.
33. Kunawudhi A, Sereeborwornthanasak K, Promteangtrong C, Siripongpreeda B, Vanprom S, Chotipanich C. Value of FDG PET/contrast-enhanced CT in initial staging of colorectal cancer – comparison with contrast-enhanced CT. Asian Pac J Cancer Prev APJCP. 2016;17(8):4071–5.
34. Liu Q, Luo D, Cai S, Li Q, Li X. Circumferential resection margin as a prognostic factor after rectal cancer surgery: a large population-based retrospective study. Cancer Med. 2018;7(8):3673–81.
35. Akasu T, Iinuma G, Takawa M, Yamamoto S, Muramatsu Y, Moriyama N. Accuracy of high-resolution magnetic resonance imaging in preoperative staging of rectal cancer. Ann Surg Oncol. 2009;16(10):2787–94.
36. Maffione AM, Rubello D, Caroli P, Colletti PM, Matteucci F. Is it time to introduce PET/CT in colon cancer guidelines? Clin Nucl Med. 2020;45(7):525–30.
37. Cheng Z, Wang S, Xu S, Du B, Li X, Li Y. FAPI PET/CT in diagnostic and treatment management of colorectal cancer: review of current research status. J Clin Med. 2023;12(2):577.

Chapter 21
Presentation and Evaluation of Hepatobiliary Malignancy

Lincoln Pujari, Zarmina Alam, and Satyendra Narayan Singh

21.1 Introduction

Hepatobiliary tumors comprise a heterogeneous group of malignancies including hepatocellular carcinoma (HCC), gall bladder carcinoma, and cholangiocarcinoma. These tumors are associated with bad prognosis. Other rare cancers of this group include pediatric hepatoblastoma, epithelioid hemangioendothelioma, and angiosarcoma (Fig. 21.1).

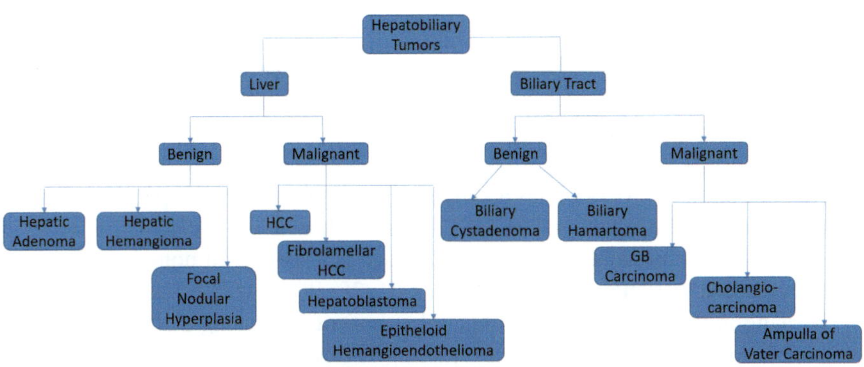

Fig. 21.1 Pictorial representation of hepatobiliary tumors

L. Pujari (✉) · Z. Alam
Department of Radiation Oncology, MPMMCC & HBCH Varanasi, Units of Tata Memorial Centre and also affliated with Homi Bhabha National Institute, Mumbai, India

S. N. Singh
Department of Radio-Diagnosis, MPMMCC and HBCH Varanasi, Units of Tata Memorial Centre and also affliated with Homi Bhabha National Institute, Mumbai, India

S. Pradhan et al. (eds.), *Evidence Based Handbook on Diagnosis and Staging in Oncology*, https://doi.org/10.1007/978-981-95-9701-7_21

21.2 Hepatocellular Carcinoma

21.2.1 Introduction and Epidemiology

Liver cancer is the most frequently diagnosed hepatobiliary malignancy in adults. It accounts for 4.7% of all newly diagnosed cancer cases & ranks as the 6th most common cancer worldwide [1]. HCC constitutes 90% of liver cancer cases [2]. The incidence of HCC increases with age with a peak at 65–70 years. Males are more commonly affected than females. Age-standardized incidence rate of liver cancer is 14.1 in males and 5.2 in females [1]. In terms of mortality, it ranks as the third most common cause of cancer-related deaths after lung and colorectal cancers [1]. In India, liver cancer is reported to be the fourth leading cause of cancer-related deaths in men and ranks eighth in women [3]. Geographically, the incidence of HCC is higher in developing countries of Asia and Africa as compared to developed nations of North America and Europe.

21.2.1.1 Risk Factors

Liver cirrhosis, regardless of etiology, is the most important risk factor for HCC. Around 60–80% of HCCs have been reported in cirrhotic liver [4]. Individuals with cirrhosis have a 2% annual risk of developing HCC [5]. Causative factors for cirrhosis can be:

1. *Viral infections*: Chronic hepatitis B virus (HBV) infection is the leading cause of liver cancer (~60% of cases) in highly prevalent areas like Asia and Africa while hepatitis C virus (HCV) is more prevalent in Europe, North America, and Japan [6].
2. *Alcohol-induced*: Alcohol has a synergistic action with viral hepatitis and other cofactors, increasing the risk of HCC to as much as fivefold [7].
3. *Non-alcoholic steatohepatitis*: NASH, which is a sequela of non-alcoholic fatty liver disease, has an annual risk of around 1–2% [8]. NASH-associated cirrhosis is rising in the Western world, largely because of increasing diabetic and obese population. A subgroup of people with NASH can have HCC even in the absence of cirrhosis.
4. *Environmental toxins*: Aflatoxin B1 is a hepatocarcinogen, produced by *Aspergillus* fungus which is found on crops. Dietary exposure to aflatoxin can induce genetic mutations like TP53.
5. *Inherited disorders*: Inherited metabolic syndromes like Wilsons's disease, hereditary hemochromatosis, and alpha-1 antitrypsin deficiency are also associated with an increased risk for HCC.

21.2.1.2 Surveillance

Various organizations like American Association for the Study of Liver Disease (AASLD), National Comprehensive Cancer Network (NCCN), European Association for the Study of the Liver (EASL), Asian Pacific Association for the Study of the Liver (APASL), and Japanese Society of Hepatology (JSH) have proposed surveillance guidelines for HCC. As per the AASLD recommendations [9]:

At-Risk Population
Table 21.1 showing high-risk population groups for screening of HCC.

Tests for Surveillance
Ultrasound (USG) has a good sensitivity rate of 65–80% for HCC, but it is quite operator dependent. A raised alpha-fetoprotein (AFP) level is often seen in this disease but is not a specific marker for HCC. A meta-analysis conducted by Tzartzeva K et al. defined that the sensitivity of USG alone was 53% (95% CI, 35%–70%), whereas USG plus AFP had a sensitivity of 63% (95% CI, 48%–75%) for early-stage HCC detection [10]. Therefore, as per recent AASLD recommendations, high-risk population for HCC should be screened using both USG and serum AFP [9].

Recommended Interval for Surveillance
Screening is recommended every 6 months for high-risk populations [9].

Table 21.1 Risk stratification showing per year incidence of HCC

Population group	Incidence of HCC
Child-Pugh A–B cirrhosis, any etiology 1. Hepatitis B 2. Hepatitis C 3. Alcohol-associated cirrhosis 4. Nonalcoholic steatohepatitis 5. Others	≥1.0% per year
Child-Pugh C cirrhosis, transplant Candidate	≥1.0% per year
Non-cirrhotic chronic hepatitis B 1. Man from endemic country age >40 years 2. Woman from endemic country age >50 years 3. Person from Africa at earlier age 4. Family history of HCC 5. PAGE-B score ≥10[a]	≥0.2% per year
Hepatitis C and stage 3 fibrosis Non-cirrhotic NAFLD	<0.2% per year

[a]PAGE-B score is an HCC risk stratification model that has been widely validated. It includes factors like sex, age, and platelet counts, with scores ≤9, 10–17, and ≥18 corresponding to low, intermediate, and high-risk groups, respectively

21.3 Clinical Presentation

21.3.1 History

The clinical presentation of HCC can range from no symptoms to symptoms of chronic liver damage and liver cirrhosis. Early-stage patients are usually asymptomatic. Patients with advanced HCC present with non-specific symptoms like jaundice, anorexia, weight loss, fatigue, dyspepsia, fever, and vomiting.

Patients with decompensated cirrhosis may present with abdominal distension, swelling of legs, hematemesis, and encephalopathy.

At-Risk Population

Rarely, HCC may present with paraneoplastic syndromes such as hypercalcemia, hypoglycemia, and watery diarrhea. Some cutaneous features like dermatomyositis, pityriasis and pemphigus can be seen.

Symptoms pertaining to distant metastases to organs like lungs, adrenal gland, bone, and brain (10–15% of total cases) can be shortness of breath, abdominal pain, bone pain, seizures, and headache.

The high rate of late-stage presentations when symptoms actually develop but curative options terminate is largely the reason behind the dismal prognosis of this disease.

21.3.2 Physical Examination

General physical examination may reveal icterus, leg edema, palmar erythema, gynecomastia, and ecchymosis.

In abdominal examination, signs of ascites, hepatomegaly, splenomegaly, dilated abdominal veins, and testicular atrophy can be seen.

21.4 Diagnosis

21.4.1 Imaging

21.4.1.1 Radiological Anatomy of Liver

Liver is traditionally divided into four lobes—right, left, caudate, and quadrate lobes. However, the most followed classification system is Couinaud segmental division according to which liver has eight segments or functional units [11]. The bifurcation of portal vein into right and left divides the liver into cranial segments VII, VIII, IVA, and II and caudal segments VI, V, IVB, and III. The segment I is located on the undersurface of liver. These segments are supplied by individual hepatic arteries, portal veins, and bile ducts (Fig. 21.2).

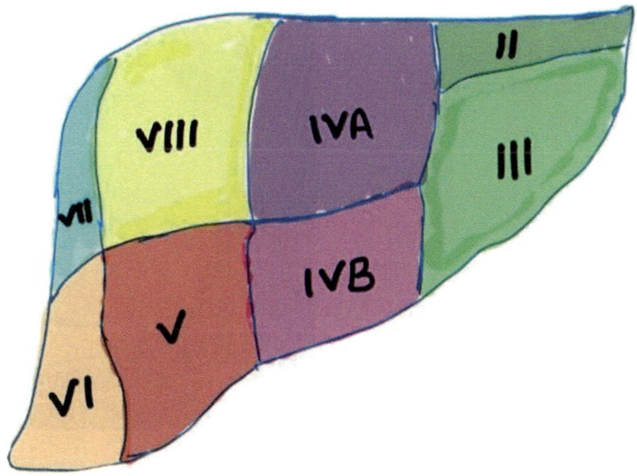

Fig. 21.2 Couinaud classification of hepatic segments

21.4.1.2 Radiological Features in Liver Cirrhosis

USG is the first imaging tool used for any liver pathology (Fig. 21.3). Features suggestive of cirrhosis in USG include the following:

(a) Liver surface nodularity is reported to be ~88% sensitive and 82–95% specific for diagnosing cirrhosis [12].
(b) Coarse and heterogeneous echotexture.
(c) Segmental hypertrophy and atrophy: Hypertrophy of lateral segments of left lobe (segments 2 and 3) and caudate lobe (segment 1) with simultaneous atrophy of posterior segments of right lobe (segments 6 and 7). This is measured by caudate lobe width/right lobe width ratio.
(d) Signs of portal hypertension.

In at-risk patients, HCC can be diagnosed by:

1. Non-invasive (Imaging-Based) Method
   Abdominal contrast-enhanced CT or MRI with four phases (pre-contrast, arterial, portal venous, and delayed) is recommended.

   (a) *Pre-contrast phase*: This phase is required for generation of subtraction images. It helps in identifying fat, calcification, and blood products.
   (b) *Arterial phase (~30–40 s)*: It shows hyper-enhanced aorta and hepatic arteries with no or minimal enhancement of portal vein. This phase is important for arterial anatomy and to delineate lesions receiving blood supply from hepatic arteries.
   (c) *Portal venous phase (~75–90 s)*: This phase is characterized by complete enhancement of portal vein with partial enhancement of hepatic veins. Liver looks brighter in this phase as it receives contrast mixed blood from the portal vein.
   (d) *Delayed phase (~120–180 s)*: In this phase, there is complete enhancement of hepatic veins. This phase helps in identifying hepatic hemangiomas.

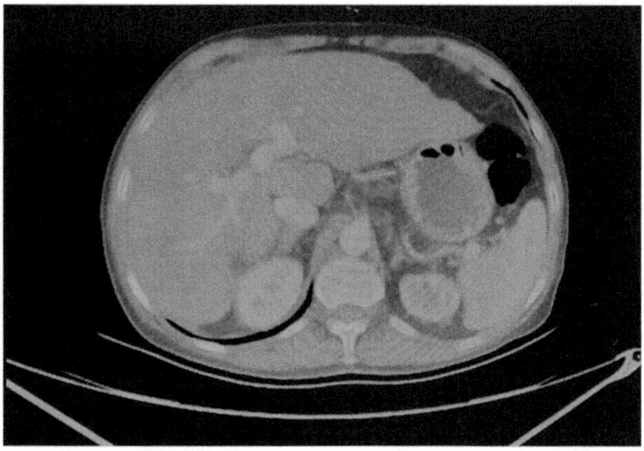

Fig. 21.3 CT showing nodular liver surface with dilated portal vein suggestive of cirrhosis

HCC lesions derive their vascular supply from the hepatic artery, while the normal liver has a dual blood supply, i.e., portal vein (75%) and hepatic artery (25%). This gives rise to a classic feature of arterial phase hyper-enhancement and contrast washout in portal venous or delayed phases for HCC lesions. Another important diagnostic finding is an enhancing capsule which is seen as a thin bright rim around the tumor in portal venous or delayed phases.

These radiological hallmarks have high specificity and positive predictive value in diagnosing HCC for lesions ≥1 cm [13]. A meta-analysis conducted by Roberts LR et al reported that MRI has higher sensitivity (82% vs. 66%), with similar specificity (92% vs. 91%) as compared to CT for diagnosing HCC [14]. As per AASLD, both imaging techniques are equally recommended (Fig. 21.4).

LIRADS Diagnostic Algorithm for HCC

Liver Imaging Reporting and Data System (LIRADS) includes imaging features—tumor size, arterial phase hyper-enhancement, delayed phase washout, and capsule enhancement for diagnosing HCC.

LIRADS score	Risk of cancer
LIRADS 1	Definitely benign
LIRADS 2	Probably benign
LIRADS 3	Intermediate probability of HCC
LIRADS 4	Probably HCC
LIRADS 5	Definitely HCC

Tables 21.2 showing LIRADS algorithm for diagnosis of HCC.

MRI Liver

Sensitivity of MRI for detection of 1–2 cm HCC is around 84%. Liver explant pathology versus prospective MRI staging of HCC demonstrated 97% sensitivity and 100% specificity for the detection of HCC.

The Organ Procurement and Transplantation Network (OPTN) committee recommendations of technical specifications for dynamic contrast-enhanced MRI of the liver

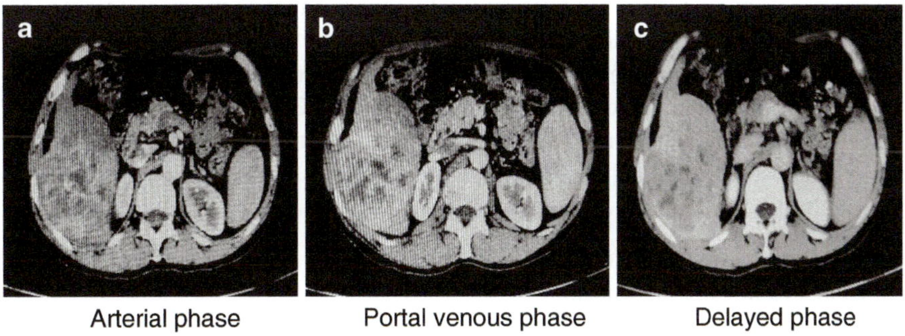

Fig. 21.4 Multiphase CECT showing arterially enhancing HCC lesions in right lobe of liver

Table 21.2 Risk stratification showing per year incidence of HCC

Arterial phase hyper-enhancement (APHE)		Absent		Non-rim APHE		
Lesion size (mm)		<20	≥20	<10	10–19	≥20
Major features: Enhancing capsule Non-peripheral washout Threshold growth	0 features	LR-3	LR-3	LR-3	LR-3	LR-4
	1 feature	LR-3	LR-4	LR-4	LR-4 / LR-5	LR-5
	≥2 features	LR-4	LR-4	LR-4	LR-5	LR-5

Feature	*Specification*
Scanner type	*1.5 Tesla or higher*
Minimum sequences	*Pre-contrast and dynamic post-Gadolinium* *T1-weighted GRE* *T2-weighted (with or without fat saturation)* *T1-weighted in- and out-of-phase imaging*
Contrast injection rate	*2–3 mL/s of gadolinium chelate*
Dynamic phases on CE MRI	*Pre-contrast* *Late arterial* *Portal venous* *Delayed*
Timing of phase	*Bolus tracking preferred*

MRI and HCC—imaging features in a cirrhotic liver

2. Invasive Method (Pathological Diagnosis)

Sequence	*Regenerative nodules*	*Dysplastic nodules*	*HCC*
T1 weighted GRE			
Pre-contrast *Late arterial* *Delayed*	*Hyper or iso* *No* *No*	*Hyper or iso* *Yes* *No*	*Hyper, iso, or hypo* *Yes* *Yes*
T2 weighted	*Iso*	*Iso*	*Hyper or iso*
Gadoxetate disodium	*Iso*	*Iso*	*Hyper or hypo*

Biopsy from HCC lesions is not routinely done because of the risk of tract seeding and the high level of diagnostic accuracy achieved with non-invasive methods. However, a tissue biopsy may be required in patients without cirrhosis or viral hepatitis infection or when the classic imaging finding of HCC is absent. The sensitivity and specificity are superior to any other diagnostic test, and may reach up to 96% and 95%, respectively [15].

Metastatic work-up for extra-hepatic disease:

1. CT thorax: Lung metastasis
2. Bone scan: Bone metastasis

PET Scan

FDG-PET is not a standard investigation for HCC because of its low sensitivity of only 50%–65% [16].

Serum Biomarkers

AFP: Although serum AFP, at a threshold of >400 ng/ml, has long been used in diagnosing HCC, due to lack of sensitivity and specificity, it is no longer recommended as a diagnostic criterion for HCC. In about 30% patients of HCC, serum AFP levels may be normal. Raised AFP levels have been reported in cancers other than HCC like intrahepatic cholangiocarcinoma, stomach cancer, and germ cell tumors [17]. In patients with raised AFP levels, it can be used for post-treatment monitoring.

Laboratory Tests

- HBV and HCV serology
- Liver function test (serum bilirubin, alkaline phosphatase, transaminases)
- Serum albumin, prothrombin time, and activated partial thromboplastin time: for assessment of hepatic functional reserve
- Complete blood count: to rule out hypersplenism and portal hypertension

Child-Pugh Functional Classification [18]

It is used to assess the severity and prognosis of chronic liver disease.

Parameters	Score 1	Score 2	Score 3
Bilirubin (mg/dL)	<2	2–3	>3
Albumin (g/dL)	>3.5	2.8–3.5	<2.8
Prothrombin time (sec)	<4	4–6	>6
Hepatic encephalopathy (grade)	None	1–2	3–4
Ascites	Absent	Moderate	Severe

Score	Class	2-year overall survival
5–6	A	85%
7–9	B	57%
10–15	C	35%

Staging

Various staging systems have been described for HCC like the American Joint Committee on Cancer (AJCC-TNM) staging, Barcelona Clinic Liver Cancer (BCLC) Staging System, Okuda staging system, and Cancer of the Liver Italian Program (CLIP) scoring system.

Commonly, the recent AJCC-TNM staging of 8th edition (2017) is used for staging of HCC [19]:

AJCC prognostic stage groups

- IA: T1a N0 M0
- IB: T1b N0 M0
- II: T2 N0 M0
- IIIA: T3 N0 M0
- IIIB: T4 N0 M0
- IVA: Any T, N1 M0
- IVB: Any T, Any N M1

BCLC staging system for HCC [20]:

BCLC stage	ECOG PS	Tumor characteristics	Child-Pugh class
0	0	Single nodule <2 cm	A
A	0	Single or ≤3 nodules each <3 cm	A–B
B	0	Multinodular	A–B
C	1–2	Portal invasion, N1, M1	A–B
D	3–4	Any tumor burden	C

21.5 Cholangiocarcinoma

21.5.1 Introduction and Epidemiology

Cholangiocarcinomas (CCA) are the biliary tract malignancies that originate from the epithelial lining. ~90% of cholangiocarcinomas are adenocarcinomas [21]. The usual age of presentation is 60–65 years and is slightly more common in men [22]. The incidence of cholangiocarcinoma is low worldwide (0.3–6 cases per 100,000 population per year), but in endemic regions of Thailand, China, and South Korea, incidence >6 per 100,000 population has been reported [23]. Among the biliary tract malignancies, cholangiocarcinoma is the second most common cancer after gall bladder carcinoma [1, 24].

Cholangiocarcinomas are classified as intrahepatic, peri-hilar, and extrahepatic tumors based on their site of origin. Apart from the anatomic location, these subtypes of tumors also differ in their molecular biology, prognosis, and clinical management.

21.5.2 Intrahepatic Cholangiocarcinoma (iCCA)

Cholangiocarcinoma that originates from the intrahepatic portion of biliary tract between the bile ductules and the second-order/segmental bile ducts is iCCA. This is the rarest subtype and accounts for ~10% of cholangiocarcinoma cases [25].

21.5.3 Peri-hilar Cholangiocarcinoma (pCCA)

Cholangiocarcinoma that arises anywhere after the segmental bile ducts till the insertion of cystic duct, i.e., either in the right or left hepatic duct or common hepatic duct, is pCCA. Worldwide, this is the most frequently seen subtype (~50–70%) among all cholangiocarcinoma cases [25].

21.5.4 Distal Cholangiocarcinoma (dCCA)

These are the distal-most cholangiocarcinomas which are located in the common bile duct till its insertion into the ampulla of Vater. These tumors comprise ~30–40% of cholangiocarcinomas [25].

Peri-hilar and distal cholangiocarcinomas are many a times collectively referred to as extrahepatic cholangiocarcinoma (eCCA).

Pathways of Spread

1. Local invasion into the surrounding structures. Cholangiocarcinoma is characterized by early and frequent biliary wall invasion and spread to peri-ductal spaces and portal tracts.
2. Lymphatic spread is via the rich lymphatic network along the submucosa of bile ducts. The commonly involved lymph nodes are peri-choledochal, peri-portal, hepatoduodenal, common hepatic artery, pancreaticoduodenal, celiac axis, and para-aortic nodal groups. The incidence of lymph node metastasis is ~50% [26].
3. Hematogenous spread to distant organs.

Risk Factors

In the majority of patients diagnosed with cholangiocarcinoma, no predisposing factor is usually identified, though evidences are there to support the role of some risk factors in the development of disease (Tables 21.3 and 21.4).

Table 21.3 Risk factors for development of cholangiocarcinoma

Risk factors	OR[a]	
Hepatobiliary conditions	iCCA	eCCA
Choledochal cyst	26.71	34.94
Primary sclerosing cholangitis	22	41
Biliary calculi	10.08	18.58
Cirrhosis	15.32	3.82
Liver flukes	5 (iCCA > eCCA)	
Viral hepatitis	4	2
Extrahepatic conditions		
Nonalcoholic fatty liver disease	2.2	1.5
Diabetes	1.73	1.5
Obesity	1.14	1.2
Lifestyle habits		
Alcohol	3.15	1.75
Cigarette smoking	1.25	1.69
Toxic exposure		
Thorotrast	RR[b] >300	

From Banales et al. [27]
[a]Odds ratio
[b]Relative risk

Table 21.4 Genetic conditions associated with risk of cholangiocarcinoma

Genetic syndromes associated with CCA	Gene involved
Lynch syndrome (HNPCC)	MMR gene
BAP 1 tumor predisposition syndrome	BAP1 gene
Multiple biliary papillomatosis	K-RAS P53 gene
Cystic fibrosis	CFTR gene

21.6 Diagnosis

21.6.1 Clinical Presentation

Early-stage patients are often asymptomatic. Intrahepatic cholangiocarcinoma usually presents late and with nonspecific symptoms like weight loss, fever, anorexia, malaise, fullness, and abdominal pain. Patients with distal or extrahepatic cholangiocarcinoma most of the time present with obstructive biliary symptoms like jaundice, clay-colored stools, dark yellow urine, and pruritus.

21.6.2 Examination

Jaundice is typically accompanied by observable signs of cachexia, and if the obstruction is in the distal common bile duct, a palpable gallbladder may be present, which is known as Courvoisier's sign.

21.6.3 Workup

1. Liver function test
2. Viral hepatitis serology: This testing should be considered in iCCA.
3. Tumor markers
   - Serum carbohydrate antigen 19-9 (CA 19-9) and serum carcinoembryonic antigen (CEA) may be considered for baseline assessment, but they lack specificity for cholangiocarcinoma as elevated levels can be seen in other malignancies as well as in benign conditions. Mild elevation in serum CA 19-9 level may occur due to cholangitis. A serum CA 19-9 level >100 U/mL has been reported to be ~75% sensitive and ~80% specific for cholangiocarcinoma [28]. The sensitivity of serum CEA is low.
   - AFP may be done in iCCA to help rule out HCC.
4. Imaging

   For primary:
   - Ultrasound

     Ultrasonography may be helpful as a first imaging tool to raise the suspicion for CCA. It will reveal a solid mass with variable echogenicity (hypoechoic, hyperechoic or mixed) with possible dilatation of bile ducts.
   - Multiphasic contrast-enhanced delayed CT scan/MRI of the abdomen

     It is the standard imaging test to diagnose cholangiocarcinoma and to assess for tumor resectability. CT/MRI gives information like:

     (a) Primary tumor characteristics
     (b) Relationship with nearby structures like major vessels, liver, and biliary ducts
     (c) Lymph nodal involvement
     (d) Biliary duct dilation
     (e) Presence of satellite lesion
     (f) Distant metastasis, e.g., to liver (Fig. 21.5)

The radiological feature of iCCA in contrast-enhanced CT/MRI is a well-defined mass with peripheral rim enhancement in the arterial phase followed by gradual central enhancement on portovenous and delayed phases [29]. Kim et al. did a retrospective multicenter study to compare CT versus MRI and found MRI to be superior to CT for diagnosing iCCA [30].

For metastases:

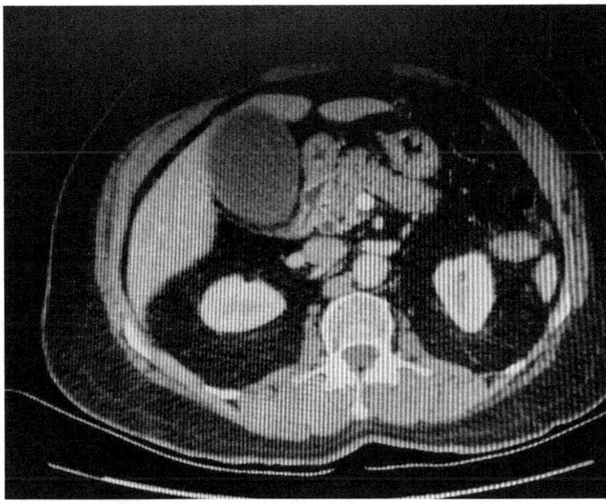

Fig. 21.5 CECT showing enhancing lesion in CBD with overdistended GB

- CT thorax is recommended to rule out distant metastasis to lung.
- PET scan: There is no role of PET in the imaging of primary tumor, but its relevance lies in diagnosing lymph nodal or distant metastasis in patients otherwise considered resectable [31]. Studies have reported PET scan to have a sensitivity of ~56% and specificity of 95% for identifying distant metastases [32].

5. Endoscopic ultrasound (EUS)

   EUS may be helpful in eCCA for diagnosing a mass or abnormal thickening with an additional advantage of directed fine needle aspiration/biopsy.
6. Cholangiography: Patients presenting with obstructive jaundice should be considered for cholangiography.

   - *MR cholangiopancreatography (MRCP)*: It is a non-invasive technique that uses nuclear magnetic resonance principles to delineate the biliary tree. It can generate excellent images of the gall bladder and biliary system that can identify intraductal abnormalities, stricture, and obstruction (Fig. 21.6).
   - *Endoscopic retrograde cholangiopancreatography (ERCP)*:
     It involves the use of a side-viewing endoscope to identify and cannulate the ampulla of Vater. It is an invasive technique in which a water-soluble contrast agent is injected into the bile duct, enabling visualization of the ductal anatomy and identification of obstruction-causing factors, such as calculi or malignant strictures. During the ERCP procedure, bile aspirates can be taken for cytological examination. In addition, it also allows therapeutic interventions like stent placement and removal of stones from the common bile duct.
   - *Percutaneous transhepatic cholangiography (PTC)*:
     Like ERCP, it is also an invasive method in which a needle, such as the Chiba or Okuda needle, is percutaneously introduced into the liver under fluoroscopic control. The bile duct is then cannulated using ultrasound or CT guidance. Injection of a water-soluble contrast medium is done to illustrate the biliary system, and numerous images are captured to demonstrate areas of

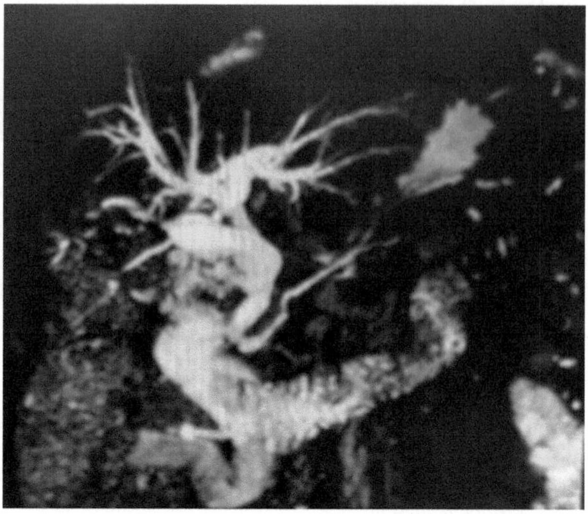

Fig. 21.6 MRCP showing circumferential wall thickening in supra-pancreatic CBD

obstructions or strictures. Additionally, it allows placement of a catheter for external biliary drainage, and bile samples can be obtained for cytological study. PTC is usually done in patients in whom ERCP proves unsuccessful either due to altered biliary tract anatomy or due to proximal biliary obstruction.

7. Staging laparoscopy may be performed before surgery to exclude peritoneal disease/intra-abdominal metastases.
8. Pathological Confirmation

21.6.4 Biopsy

A tissue biopsy is usually not recommended in patients with potentially resectable CCA because of possible complications like tumor dissemination and/or bleeding. However, biopsy has a role in unresectable disease particularly for iCCA which should be distinguished from other liver cancers, e.g., HCC, combined HCC-CCA, and metastatic liver cancers. The biopsy, if done, serves three purposes: (i) pathological confirmation of the diagnosis, (ii) immunohistochemistry (to distinguish iCCA and HCC), and (iii) molecular profiling.

Immunohistochemistry (IHC)

HCC can be distinguished from iCCA by using IHC markers, such as Hep Par 1, arginase 1, and ABCB11, which are specific for hepatocytic component.

21.6.5 Molecular Profiling

Some international guideline organizations like the European Society for Medical Oncology (ESMO) recommend next-generation DNA sequencing (NGS) in patients with CCA, particularly those with advanced or metastatic disease to improve proportion who can receive a targeted therapy. IDH1 mutations, FGFR2 fusions, high microsatellite instability, and NTRK fusions are most frequently targeted mutations in CCA [33].

Bismuth-Corlette Classification of Peri-hilar Cholangiocarcinoma [34]:

A. Type I: Tumors which are distal to the confluence of right and left hepatic ducts.

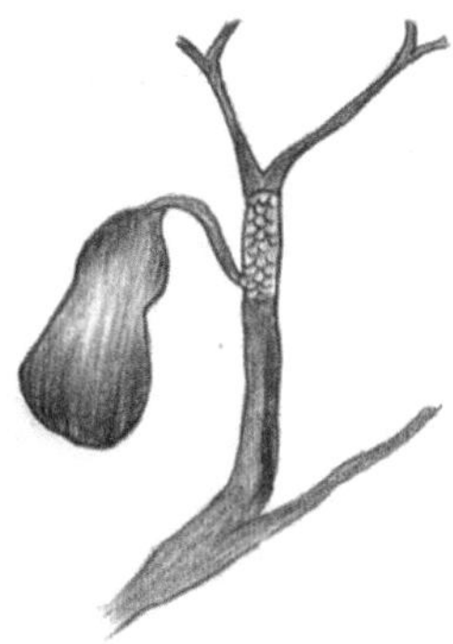

B. Type II: Tumors at the confluence

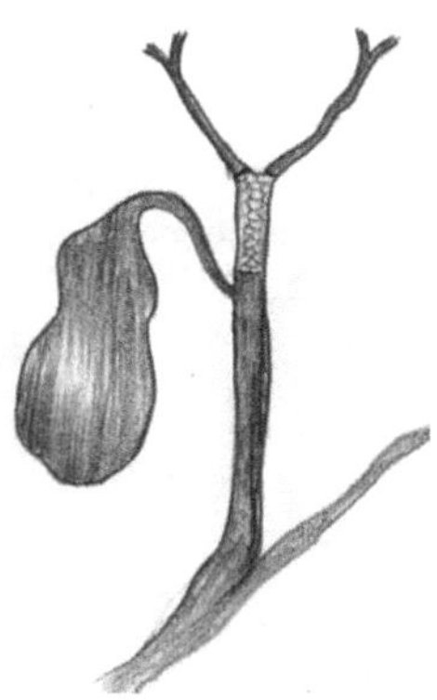

C. Type III (a) Tumors occluding the common and right hepatic ducts

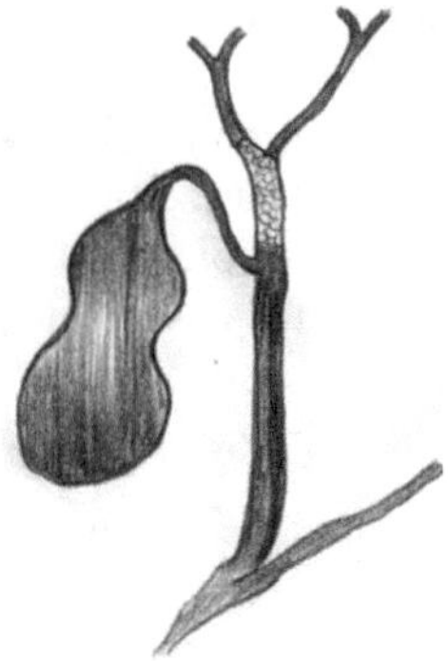

D. Type III (b) Tumors occluding the common and left hepatic ducts.

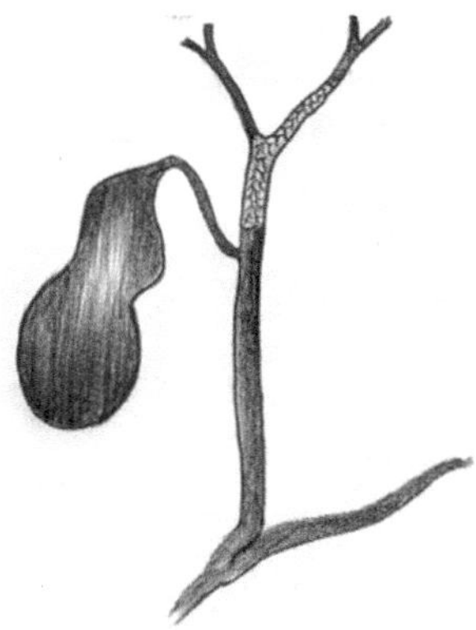

E. Type IV: Tumors involving the confluence and both right and left hepatic ducts.

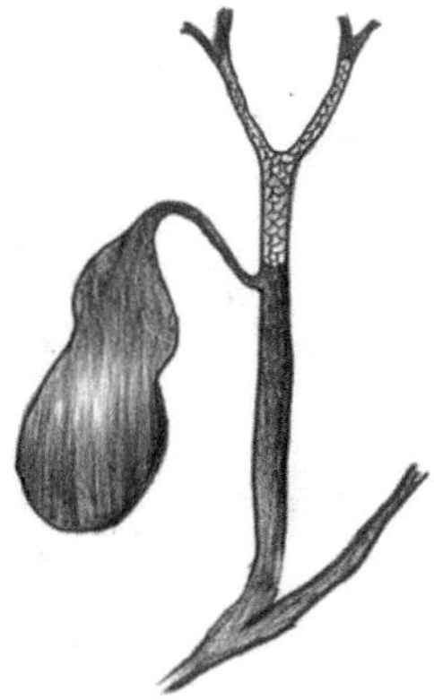

AJCC-TNM staging (2017) is used for intrahepatic cholangiocarcinoma [35]
AJCC prognostic stage groups for intrahepatic cholangiocarcinoma:

- 0: Tis N0 M0
- IA: T1a N0 M0
- IB: T1b N0 M0
- II: T2 N0 M0
- IIIA: T3 N0 M0
- IIIB: T4 N0 M0
- IIIB: Any T, N1 M0
- IV: Any T, Any N M1

AJCC-TNM staging (2017) is used for perihilar cholangiocarcinoma [36]
AJCC prognostic stage groups for perihilar cholangiocarcinoma:

- 0: Tis N0 M0
- I: T1 N0 M0
- II: T2a-b N0 M0
- IIIA: T3 N0 M0
- IIIB: T4 N0 M0
- IIIC: Any T, N1 M0
- IVA: Any T, N2 M0
- IVB: Any T, Any N M1

AJCC-TNM staging (2017) is used for distal cholangiocarcinoma [37]:
AJCC prognostic stage groups for distal cholangiocarcinoma:

- 0: Tis N0 M0
- I: T1 N0 M0
- IIA: T1 N1 M0
- IIIA: T1 N2 M0
- IIA: T2 N0 M0
- IIB: T2 N1 M0
- IIIA: T2 N2 M0
- IIB: T3 N0 M0
- IIB: T3 N1 M0
- IIIA: T3 N2 M0
- IIIB: T4 N0 M0
- IIIB: T4 N1 M0
- IIIB: T4 N2 M0
- IV: Any T, Any N M1

21.7 Gall Bladder Carcinoma

Worldwide gall bladder cancer (GBC) ranks sixth among all GI malignancies and first among biliary tract malignancies, with majority of cases seen in Asian countries [1]. In India, there were 19,570 new cases of gall bladder cancer with 14,736 deaths in the year 2020 [1]. The disease is more prevalent in women and, with a ratio of 2–6 cases for every 1 case in men. Gall bladder cancer was among the leading ten cancers in Indian females as per the National Cancer Registry Programme Report 2020 [38]. The peak age of presentation is fifth to sixth decade of life.

Pathways of Spread

1. Direct invasion: The wall of GB is thin and lacks submucosal layer, thus allowing early direct infiltration of tumor into adjacent structures like liver, CBD, duodenum, pancreas, and porta hepatis.
2. Lymphatic spread: The muscularis propria of GB has a rich lymphatic supply, such that even an early GB cancer can have significant nodal involvement.
3. Peritoneal spread: Peritoneal dissemination is a common occurrence in gallbladder carcinoma, leading to the formation of small deposits on various surfaces, such as the liver, peritoneum, omentum, pelvis, and undersurface of the diaphragm.
4. Hematogenous spread: To distant sites like liver, lung, bone, and brain.

Risk Factors

(a) Cholelithiasis
(b) Gall bladder polyp: >10 mm in diameter
(c) Primary sclerosing cholangitis
(d) Chronic inflammation
(e) Obesity

21.8 Diagnosis

21.8.1 Clinical Presentation

The clinical presentation of GBC can be subgrouped based on the stage of the disease:

A. Early stage

   Gallbladder cancer can remain asymptomatic for an extended period during its early stages. Even when symptoms do manifest, they are nonspecific like dyspepsia or indigestion leading to patients presenting lately when disease advances. Early symptoms in gallbladder cancer can be due to associated gallstone such as biliary colic. These patients, when present to surgeon, get operated for gallstone disease, and GBC is discovered either during surgery or in the gross/histopathological examination of the GB specimen.

B. Locally advanced disease

Symptoms of locally advanced GBC are as follows:

1. Abdominal pain: It is the most common presenting complaint of patients having GBC. In a study reported by Mishra et al. in 2017, pain was present in 89% of total 385 patients [39]. GBC patients may experience colicky pain due to associated gallstones, but as disease advances, the character of pain changes from intermittent biliary colic to continuous, diffuse dull pain in the right upper quadrant or epigastrium (due to local infiltration).
2. Jaundice: Jaundice is the presenting symptom in around one-fourth to one-third of cases and usually results from the direct invasion of biliary tree or compression by an enlarged node.
3. Loss of weight: Weight loss is reported by approximately 63% of GBC patients presenting to a tertiary hospital [39].
4. Anorexia: Loss of appetite is seen in around 60% of patients [39].
5. Gastroparesis: It is an unusual presentation in GBC, prevalent in only 8% of patients [39]. GBC, when infiltrating the first part of duodenum or the antropyloric region of stomach, can cause mechanical gastric outlet obstruction (GOO).

C. Metastatic disease

Symptoms of metastatic disease are pertaining to organs/sites of involvement like:

Chest pain, cough, breathlessness, hemoptysis-> lung metastasis
Right upper abdominal pain, anorexia, indigestion-> liver metastasis
Bone pain, fracture-> bone metastasis
Headache, vomiting, seizures-> brain metastasis

21.8.2 Physical Examination

Examination of a GBC patient may reveal:

1. *Built*: Cachexic and malnourished (due to loss of weight and body fat)
2. *General examination*: Icterus

   Neck node (metastatic supraclavicular node)
   Pruritic scratch marks
   Pedal edema

3. Abdominal examination: Firm to hard non-tender GB lump

   Hepatomegaly
   Ascites
   Periumbilical nodule
   Port-site nodule (GBC-diagnosed post-laparoscopic cholecystectomy)

Differential diagnosis of GBC:

(i) Gallstone disease
(ii) Chronic cholecystitis or xanthogranulomatous cholecystitis
(iii) Mirizzi syndrome
(iv) Other malignancies like cholangiocarcinoma, HCC, and periampullary carcinoma
(v) Tuberculosis of biliary tract

21.8.3 Imaging

1. Ultrasonography
   Transabdominal USG is usually the first-line investigation which raises the suspicion for gall bladder cancer in patients exhibiting symptoms of biliary disease. The following findings in USG may indicate gallbladder cancer:

   (a) Mass replacing the gallbladder and/or infiltrating liver
   (b) Diffuse irregular thickening of the gallbladder wall
   (c) Intraluminal heterogeneous mass with no posterior acoustic shadowing
   However, USG can miss early-stage gallbladder cancer and is highly operator-dependent.

2. Multiphasic contrast-enhanced CT or MRI
   Triphasic, multi-slice, contrast-enhanced helical CT of abdomen and pelvis helps in better assessment of gall bladder mass, its resectability, nodal involvement, and accurate staging of disease. A retrospective study by Tao et al. including 211 patients showed that triple phase dynamic, contrast-enhanced CT has a sensitivity of 86.7%, specificity of 75.2%, and an accuracy of 80.5% in diagnosing malignant gallbladder-occupying lesions [40]. CT can assess local infiltration into the liver, duodenum, and pancreas as well as metastasis to distant sites like liver and ovaries. However, CT has poor sensitivity when it comes to detecting peritoneal and omental metastases (unless they are large) (Fig. 21.7).

MRI reveals the same findings as CT. GBC appears hypointense on T1 and hyperintense on T2 images, with early phase enhancement that persists in the delayed phase (early enhancement followed by washout is visible in benign masses). Diffusion-weighted MRI (DW MRI) has been utilized to differentiate between GBC and benign diseases. Lee et al. did a retrospective study including 126 GBC patients and concluded that T2W MRI combined with DWI has a sensitivity of 97.2%, specificity of 92.2%, PPV of 83.3%, and NPV of 98.8% [41].

3. CECT Thorax: To rule out lung metastasis.
4. 18-Fluorodeoxy-glucose (FDG) positron emission tomography (PET)

It is useful in detecting radiologically occult diseases such as lymph nodes and distant metastasis that may go undetected in CT or MRI scans. In a meta-analysis

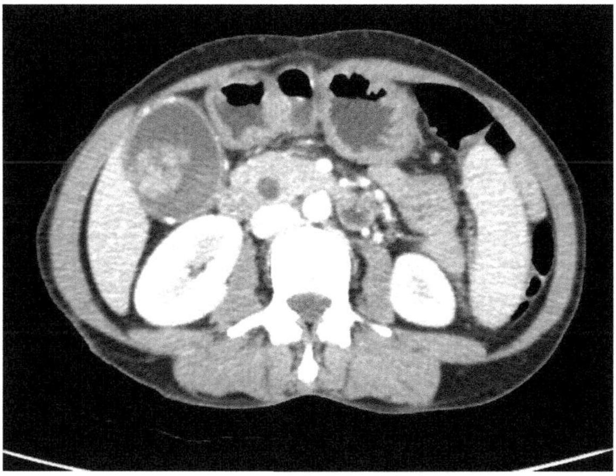

Fig. 21.7 CECT showing distended GB with intraluminal mass

by Annunziata et al., 18-F FDG PET or PET-CT was found to be 87% sensitive and 78% specific in evaluating gall bladder primary tumor [42]. However, PET can yield false-negative result for peritoneal disease which is very small (<0.5 cm).

21.8.4 Cholangiography

Magnetic resonance cholangiography (MRCP) is often the preferred choice as a non-invasive technique for patients with obstructive jaundice to determine the level of biliary obstruction. Invasive cholangiography technique, such as endoscopic retrograde cholangiography (ERCP) or percutaneous transhepatic cholangiography (PTC), is usually done as part of a therapeutic intervention for biliary drainage.

21.8.5 Tissue Diagnosis

Gall bladder mass which is unresectable upfront is subjected to tissue diagnosis for pathologic confirmation of malignancy. Fine needle aspiration cytology (FNAC) or biopsy is usually not recommended in operable lesions to avoid the risk of tumor seeding in the needle track. In a systematic review by Georgios D. et al., the efficacy of FNAC as a diagnostic tool was highlighted with a pooled sensitivity and specificity of 0.85 and 0.94, respectively [43]. However, FNAC can yield false-negative result in certain situations, such as sampling from non-representative areas or presence of necrosis inside tumor [43]. Tissue diagnosis can also be obtained from bile cytology taken during ERCP or PTC. Ascites, if present, should be aspirated for cytological examination to look for malignant cells.

21.8.6 Laboratory Tests

(i) Liver function test: Elevated levels of direct bilirubin and liver enzymes may indicate biliary obstruction. Serum albumin and prothrombin time tests are useful to evaluate functions of liver synthesis.
(ii) Serum markers, carcinoma-embryonic antigen (CEA) and carbohydrate antigen 19.9 (CA 19.9) are non-specific for GBC, but their elevated levels in patients exhibiting clinical symptoms may indicate the possibility of GBC and warrant further investigation. A baseline CA 19.9 level can predict disease burden, determine prognosis, and also monitor the response to neoadjuvant therapy, as per Agrawal et al. [44].

21.8.7 Staging Laparoscopy

All imaging studies, including PET, have poor sensitivity in detecting small peritoneal and omental deposits; therefore, a laparoscopic examination is beneficial in selected cases of surgically resectable GBC to rule out any peritoneal or liver metastasis that would otherwise preclude a surgical resection.

21.8.8 Other Investigations

Upper gastrointestinal endoscopy (UGIE) is recommended in cases where there are symptoms of gastric outlet obstruction (GOO), or if CT scan shows suspicion of duodenal involvement.

Staging
AJCC-TNM staging is the most commonly used staging system for gall bladder carcinoma [45].

AJCC Prognostic Stage groups

- 0: Tis N0 M0
- I: T1 N0 M0
- IIA: T2a N0 M0
- IIB: T2b N0 M0
- IIIA: T3 N0 M0
- IIIB: T1–3 N1 M0
- IVA: T4 N0–1 M0
- IVB: Any T, N2 M0
- IVB: Any T, Any N M1

References

1. Sung H, Ferlay J, Siegel RL, et al. Global cancer statistics 2020: GLOBOCAN estimates of incidence and mortality worldwide for 36 cancers in 185 countries. CA Cancer J Clin. 2021;71(3):209–49.
2. Chatterjee A, Mukhopadhyay S, Ghosh P, et al. Imaging recommendations for diagnosis, staging, and management of hepatic and biliary tract cancer. Ind J Med Paediatr Oncol. 2023;44:241–50.
3. Dikshit R, Gupta PC, Ramasundarahettige C, et al. Cancer mortality in India: a nationally representative survey. Lancet. 2012;379:1807–16.
4. Bartlett DL, Di Bisceglie AM, Dawson LA. Cancer of the liver. In: DeVita VT, Lawrence TS, Rosenberg SA, editors. Cancer: principles and practice of oncology. 8th ed. Philadelphia: Lippincott Williams & Wilkins; 2008. p. 1129–56.
5. Kanwal F, Khaderi S, Singal AG, et al. Risk factors for HCC in contemporary cohorts of patients with cirrhosis. Hepatology. 2023;77:997–1005.
6. Bruix J, Sherman M. Management of hepatocellular carcinoma. Hepatology. 2005;42:1208–36.
7. Rumgay H, Shield K, Charvat H, et al. Global burden of cancer in 2020 attributable to alcohol consumption: a population-based study. Lancet Oncol. 2021;2021:1071–80.
8. Larry Jameson J, Dunlop RG, Loscalzo J, et al. Harrison's principles of internal medicine. New York: McGraw-Hill Education; 2018.
9. Singal AG, Llovet JM, et al. AASLD practice guidance on prevention, diagnosis, and treatment of hepatocellular carcinoma. Hepatology. 2023;78:1922–65.
10. Tzartzeva K, Obi J, Rich NE, et al. Surveillance imaging and alpha fetoprotein for early detection of hepatocellular carcinoma in patients with cirrhosis: a meta-analysis. Gastroenterology. 2018;154(1706–718):e1701.
11. Couinaud C. Le Foie: etudes anatomiques et chirurgicales. Paris: Masson; 1957.
12. Bluth EI, Benson CB, Ralls PW, Siegel MJ. Ultrasound: a practical approach to clinical problems. Thieme; 2008.
13. Bolondi L, Gaiani S, Celli N, et al. Characterization of small nodules in cirrhosis by assessment of vascularity: the problem of hypovascular hepatocellular carcinoma. Hepatology. 2005;42:27–34.
14. Roberts LR, Sirlin CB, Zaiem F, et al. Imaging for the diagnosis of hepatocellular carcinoma: a systematic review and meta-analysis. Hepatology. 2018;67:401–21.
15. Borzio M, Borzio F, Macchi R, Croce AM, Bruno S, Ferrari A. The evaluation of fine-needle procedures for the diagnosis of focal liver lesions in cirrhosis. J Hepatol. 1994;20:117–21.
16. Sacks A, Peller PJ, Surasi DS, Chatburn L, Mercier G, Subramaniam RM. Value of PET/CT in the management of primary hepatobiliary tumors, Part 2. AJR Am J Roentgenol. 2011;197:W260–5.
17. Arif D, Mettler T, Adeyi OA. Mimics of hepatocellular carcinoma: a review and an approach to avoiding histopathological diagnostic missteps. Hum Pathol. 2021;112:116–27.
18. Pugh RN, Murray-Lyon IM, Dawson JL, et al. Transection of the oesophagus for bleeding oesophageal varices. Br J Surg. 1973;60(8):646–9.
19. Amin MB, Edge S, Greene F, et al. AJCC cancer staging manual. New York: Springer; 2017. p. 291.
20. Llovet JM, Bru C, Bruix J. Prognosis of hepatocellular carcinoma: the BCLC staging classification. Semin Liver Dis. 1999;19:329–38.
21. Nakajima T, Kondo Y, Miyazaki M, Okui K. A histopathologic study of 102 cases of intrahepatic cholangiocarcinoma: histologic classification and mode of spreading. Hum Pathol. 1988;19:1228–34.

22. Landis SH, Murray T, Bolden S, et al. Cancer statistics, 1998. CA Cancer J Clin. 1998;48:6–29.
23. Banales JM. Expert consensus document: cholangiocarcinoma: current knowledge and future perspectives consensus statement from the European Network for the Study of Cholangiocarcinoma (ENS-CCA). Nat Rev Gastroenterol Hepatol. 2016;13:261–80.
24. Nakeeb A, Pitt HA, Sohn TA, et al. Cholangiocarcinoma. A spectrum of intrahepatic, perihilar and distal tumors. Ann Surg. 1996;224:463–75.
25. Rizvi S, Gores GJ. Pathogenesis, diagnosis and management of cholangiocarcinoma. Gastroenterology. 2013;145(6):1215–29.
26. Halperin Edward C, Wazer David E, Carlos P, Brady LW. Perez and Brady's principles and practice of radiation oncology. Philadelphia: Wolters Kluwer; 2018.
27. Banales JM, Marin JJG, Lamarca A, et al. Cholangiocarcinoma 2020: the next horizon in mechanisms and management. Nat Rev Gastroenterol Hepatol. 2020;17:557–88.
28. Nakeeb A, Lipsett PA, Lillemoe KD, et al. Biliary carcinoembryonic antigen levels are a marker for cholangiocarcinoma. Am J Surg. 1996;171:147–53.
29. Lim JH. Cholangiocarcinoma: morphologic classification according to growth pattern and imaging findings. AJR Am J Roentgenol. 2003;181(03):819–27.
30. Kim Y, Yeom S, Shin H, et al. Clinical staging of mass-forming intrahepatic cholangiocarcinoma: computed tomography versus magnetic resonance imaging. Hepatol Commun. 2021;5:2009–18.
31. Lamarca A, Barriuso J, Chander A, et al. 18F-fluorodeoxyglucose positron emission tomography (18FDG-PET) for patients with biliary tract cancer: systematic review and meta-analysis. J Hepatol. 2019;71(01):115–29.
32. Huang X, Yang J, Li J, Xiong Y. Comparison of magnetic resonance imaging and 18-fludeoxyglucose positron emission tomography/computed tomography in the diagnostic accuracy of staging in patients with cholangiocarcinoma. Medicine. 2020;99:e20932.
33. Mosele F, Remon J, Mateo J, et al. Recommendations for the use of next-generation sequencing (NGS) for patients with metastatic cancers: a report from the ESMO Precision Medicine Working Group. Ann Oncol. 2020;31:1491–505.
34. Cho E, Kim SH, Choi SJ, et al. Study Group for Biliary Diseases; Korean Pancreatobiliary Association. Diagnosis and treatment of perihilar cholangiocarcinoma: a national survey from the Korean Pancreatobiliary Association. Gut Liver. 2024;18(1):174–83.
35. Lee AJ, Chun YS. Intrahepatic cholangiocarcinoma: the AJCC/UICC 8th edition updates. Chin Clin Oncol. 2018;7(5):52.
36. Gaspersz MP, Buettner S, van Vugt JLA, et al. Evaluation of the New American Joint Committee on Cancer staging manual 8th edition for perihilar cholangiocarcinoma. J Gastrointest Surg. 2020;24(7):1612–8.
37. Bajracharya AD, Shrestha S, Kim HS, Nahm JH, Park K, Park JS. Retrospective analysis of 8th edition American Joint Cancer Classification: distal cholangiocarcinoma. Ann Hepatobiliary Pancreat Surg. 2023;27(3):251–7.
38. Sathishkumar K, Chaturvedi M, Das P, Stephen S, Mathur P. Cancer incidence estimates for 2022 & projection for 2025: result from National Cancer Registry Programme, India. Indian J Med Res. 2022;156(4–5):598–607.
39. Mishra PK, Saluja SS, Prithiviraj N, Varshney V, Goel N, Patil N. Predictors of curative resection and long term survival of gallbladder cancer – a retrospective analysis. Am J Surg. 2017;214(2):278–86.
40. Tao J, Zhang Y, Chen H, Wang S, et al. Triphasic dynamic contrast-enhanced computed tomography predictive model of benign and malignant risk of gallbladder occupying lesions. Medicine. 2020;99:e19539.
41. Lee N, Kim S, Kim T, et al. Diffusion-weighted MRI for differentiation of benign from malignant lesions in the gallbladder. Clin Radiol. 2014;69:e78–85.

42. Annunziata S, Pizzuto DA, Caldarella C, et al. Diagnostic accuracy of fluorine-18-fluorodeoxyglucose positron emission tomography in gallbladder cancer: a meta-analysis. World J Gastroenterol. 2015;21:11481–8.
43. Georgios DK, Christopher GC, Eliot C, et al. The role of fine needle aspiration cytology in the diagnosis of gallbladder cancer: a systematic review. Diagnostics. 2021;11(8):1427.
44. Agrawal S, Lawrence A, Saxena R. Does CA 19-9 have prognostic relevance in gallbladder carcinoma (GBC)? J Gastrointest Cancer. 2018;49(2):144–9.
45. Giannis D, Cerullo M, Moris D, et al. Validation of the 8th Edition American Joint Commission on Cancer (AJCC) gallbladder cancer staging system: prognostic discrimination and identification of key predictive factors. Cancers (Basel). 2021;13(3):547.

Chapter 22
Presentation and Evaluation of Anal Canal Cancer

Ankita Rungta Kapoor and Shamila Alim

22.1 Introduction

The incidence of anal cancer is low in the United States, with less than 1000 new cases diagnosed annually [1], but in India, it is the fourth most common *cancer* among men as per the Global *Cancer* Observatory (*GLOBOCAN*) data 2020. The number of people affected with anal cancer has increased over the last 20 years.

22.2 Clinical Definition of Anal Cancer

An anal cancer is clinically defined as a tumor that develops from any of the three types of mucosae located in the anal region (glandular, transitional, and squamous mucosa), whereas perianal skin cancers are clinically defined as tumors that arise in the hair-bearing skin within a 5 cm radius of the anal verge.

22.3 Lymphatic Spread in Anal Cancers

Tumors originating above the dentate line, like rectal cancers, drain to the mesorectal and internal iliac nodes, whereas tumors arising below the dentate line may also spread to the superficial inguinal and external iliac (deep inguinal) nodes (Table 22.1).

A. R. Kapoor (✉) · S. Alim
Department of Radiation Oncology, MPMMCC/HBCH Varanasi, Unit of Tata Memorial Centre and also affliated with Homio Bhaba National Institue, Mumbai, India

S. Pradhan et al. (eds.), *Evidence Based Handbook on Diagnosis and Staging in Oncology*, https://doi.org/10.1007/978-981-95-9701-7_22

Table 22.1 Disease status at diagnosis with 5-year survival [2]

Disease status at diagnosis	Percentage of patients	5-year survival rate
Localized	50%	80%
Nodal metastases	29%	60%
Distant metastases	12%	30.5%

22.3.1 Pathological Classification

WHO termed all squamous cell carcinoma variants of the anal canal as cloacogenic and identified subtypes as large-cell keratinizing, large-cell non-keratinizing (transitional), or basaloid, in the second edition. Terms cloacogenic, transitional, keratinizing, and basaloid were removed from the third and fourth editions. Now, all these have been included under a common heading of squamous cell carcinoma (SCC). Both cloacogenic (or basaloid) and transitional tumors are now considered to be non-keratinizing tumors.

Both keratinizing and non-keratinizing tumors have been reported to have a similar natural history and prognosis.

WHO 2019 Classification of Malignant Epithelial Tumors of the Anal Canal

Squamous cell carcinoma, NOS Verrucous squamous cell carcinoma
Adenocarcinoma, NOS
Neuroendocrine tumor, NOS
Neuroendocrine carcinoma, NOS
Mixed neuroendocrine–non–neuroendocrine neoplasm (MiNEN)

Other uncommon histology includes

- Small cell (anaplastic) carcinoma
- Undifferentiated cancer
- Melanoma

Risk Factors

- Female gender
- Human papillomavirus (HPV)
- Multiple sexual partners
- Genital warts
- Cigarette smoking
- Receptive anal intercourse
- Human immunodeficiency virus (HIV)

Symptoms at Presentation

- Anorectal bleeding
- Anorectal or perianal pain
- Perianal drainage
- Anal pruritus
- Unintentional weight loss
- Recurring abdominal distention or abdominal pain.
- Prolapsing mass per rectum

22.4 Symptom-Based Differential Diagnosis (Tables 22.2 and 22.3)

Table 22.2 Differential diagnosis for different signs and symptoms pertaining to anal canal malignancies

Peri-anal pain	Generalized—pruritus ani, neoplasm Localized—skin trauma, external hemorrhoids, perianal abscess, neoplasm
Anal canal pain	Anal fissure, anal cancer, anal ulceration due to STDs
Bleeding	Secondary to anal fissures, internal hemorrhoids, Thrombosed external hemorrhoids, or anal neoplasms
Prolapsing tissue	Prolapsing internal hemorrhoids, rectal prolapse
Pruritus	Idiopathic
Perianal drainage	Anal fistula, fecal incontinence, and skin conditions such as pilonidal cyst, perianal hidradenitis, and perianal skin cysts (e.g., sebaceous cyst)

Table 22.3 Percentage of patients with different clinical features in anal canal malignancies [3–5]

Symptom	Percentage of patients
Rectal or anal bleeding	45%
Anorectal pain	30%
Asymptomatic	20%

Table 22.4 Differential diagnosis of painful and painless anal mass

Conditions	Characteristic features
Perianal abscess	Erythematous Fluctuant Indurated Tender pustule-like lesion Occasional purulent drainage
Perianal Crohn's disease	Edematous Skin colored or cyanotic "elephant ear" tags Fissures More common in children
Anal condylomata acuminata	Itchy Perianal grey tan cauliflower-like lesion Pain may be present History of anal intercourse
Thrombosed external hemorrhoids	Acutely painful Swollen Purplish-blue perianal mass No history of anal trauma
Anal cancer	Painless Ulcerating lesion with blood in stool More common in middle-aged adults
Primary rectal SCC	
Colorectal adenocarcinoma	
Other perianal tumors	Cutaneous SCC in situ (Bowen disease) Perianal intraepithelial adenocarcinoma (Paget disease) Melanoma Neuroendocrine tumors
Other conditions	Anal Fistulas and Fissures Chancroid Extra-mammary Paget Disease Pruritus ani Psoriasis

22.5 Differential Diagnoses (Table 22.4)

22.6 Evaluation

Painful anal mass	Painless anal mass
Abscess	External anal tags
Perianal hematoma	Condyloma acuminata
Anal fistula	Venereal warts (Molluscum contangiosum)
Antibioma	Fibrous anal polyp
Thrombosed hemorrhoids	Papilloma
Malignancy of the anal canal	Benign neoplasms like leiomyoma, angiomyxoma

History Must Include

- Patient's bowel habits—average number of bowel movements per day, the need for moderate or severe straining to defecate, the average number of minutes required per defecatory episode, any bowel regimen (laxatives) the patient may use.
- Patients with recurring abdominal pain and/or diarrhea should be asked about a family history of inflammatory bowel disease.
- Presence of risk factors
- Sexual history—number of sexual partners, history of receptive anal intercourse, and prior or current history of sexually transmitted infections, including human papillomavirus (HPV) infection
- Prior or current history of other HPV-associated cancers (e.g., cervical cancer in females, penile cancer in males, head and neck cancer)
- Tobacco use
- Prior human immunodeficiency virus (HIV) infection
- Chronic immunosuppression (e.g., organ transplant recipients, autoimmune disease, chronic corticosteroid use)

Physical Examination

- Positioning—Prone "jack knife" position provides optimal visualization, aligns the laterality of the examiner with the patient.
- If a dedicated examination table is not available, the lateral decubitus position is also acceptable
- Complete anorectal examination includes inspection, digital rectal examination (DRE), anoscopy/proctoscopy, and endoscopy
- Inspection, digital rectal examination (DRE), and anoscopy/proctoscopy can be done on an OPD basis; endoscopy requires additional equipment
- Palpation of bilateral inguinal lymph nodes
- Gynecological examination—for all female patients, to check for vaginal involvement (especially in low-lying tumors)
- Women should be screened for cervical cancer, which is also caused by human papillomavirus (HPV), a risk factor for anal SCC

Inspection

- Gently separate the buttock cheeks to visualize the perianal skin (5 cm perimeter surrounding the anal orifice).
- The examiner should denote any gross lesions concerning anal cancer, perianal abscesses, and/or anal fistulas, or external hemorrhoids.
- Any other discrete skin lesions (e.g., skin excoriation, condyloma) should also be recorded, including their anatomic location and distance to the anal orifice.

DRE

- Adequate lubrication
- Proper communication to optimize patients' comfort
- Evaluate for any mass in the anal canal or lower rectum or a stricture secondary to prior surgeries or Crohn disease

- Anal sphincter tone to be noted
- Neither anoscopy nor proctoscopy can replace a digital anorectal examination, as the distal anal canal is difficult to visualize with an end-viewing endoscope
- If an anal fissure is suspected by inspection or by point tenderness upon insertion of the tip of a gloved finger, DRE should be deferred until healing
- General assessment of pelvic floor and anal sphincter function

Anoscopy/Proctoscopy

- Proper positioning, adequate light source, adequate lubrication
- For evaluating anal condylomata, anal neoplasms, internal hemorrhoids, and anal fissures.
- A rigid proctoscopy is appropriate for identifying the location of rectal neoplasms as well as evaluating for proctitis.
- If an anal fissure is suspected by inspection or attempted digital examination-anoscopy or proctoscopy should be deferred until healing

Endoscopy

- An anorectal examination is not complete without endoscopy
- For complaints of anorectal bleeding or abdominal pain, a colonoscopy is preferred to sigmoidoscopy because diseases such as colorectal polyps and cancers from any portion of the large bowel can cause these symptoms.

Biopsy

- Biopsy of primary
- Biopsy/FNAC of the inguinal lymph node
- Characterization of enlarged inguinal nodes can be done by US-guided FNA when confirmatory features of malignancy are not evident on either MRI or PET-CT (Table 22.5)

Staging System: Changes in the Ninth Version of AJCC

- The ninth version of the joint American Joint Committee on Cancer (AJCC) and the Union for International Cancer Control (UICC) Tumor, Node, Metastasis (TNM) staging system for anal cancers is based on tumor size, invasion of adjacent structures, and presence or absence of nodal and distant metastases
- In the eighth edition, nodal disease was classified as a higher stage than tumor stage
- The term Tis has also been omitted altogether
- Metastases in the inguinal, mesorectal, internal, superior rectal, internal iliac, and/or obturator nodes are classified as N1a nodes (Table 22.6)

Table 22.5 Percentage of patients with early and locally advanced disease at presentation [6, 7]

Early-stage disease without nodal involvement	41%
Regional invasion to loco-regional lymph nodes (inguinal, mesorectal, superior rectal, internal iliac, obturator, external iliac) or adjacent organs	36%
Distant metastatic disease	14%

Table 22.6 Adopted and modified ninth AJCC staging with differences from the eighth AJCC

T category	AJCC 9th edition	AJCC 8th edition
Tx	Primary tumor not assessed	Same as 9th edition
T0	No evidence of primary tumor	
T1	Lesions with a maximum diameter not exceeding 2 cm	
T2	Tumors greater than 2 cm but less than or equal to 5 cm in greatest dimension	
T3	Tumors greater than 5 cm in greatest dimension	
T4	Tumors of any size invading adjacent organ(s)—vagina/urethra/bladder	
N category	**AJCC 9th edition**	**AJCC 8th edition**
Nx	Regional lymph nodes cannot be assessed	Same as 9th edition
N0	No regional lymph node metastasis	
N1a	Tumor involving the inguinal, mesorectal, superior rectal, internal iliac, or obturator lymph node(s)	Tumor involving the inguinal, mesorectal, and internal iliac lymph node(s)
N1b	Tumor involving external iliac lymph node(s)	Same as 9th edition
N1c	Tumor involving N1b with any N1a node(s)	
M category	**AJCC 9th edition**	**AJCC 8th edition**
cM0	No distant metastasis	No distant metastasis
cM1	Distant metastasis	Distant metastasis
pM1	Microscopic confirmation of distant metastasis	No such stage
Stage grouping	**AJCC 9th edition**	**AJCC 8th edition**
Stage I	T1 N0 M0	Same as 9th edition
Stage IIA	T2 N0 M0	
Stage IIB	T1-2 N1 M0	
Stage IIIA	T3 N0-1 M0	
Stage IIIB	T4 N0 M0	
Stage IIIC	T4 N1 M0	
Stage IV	Any T Any N M1	

Pre-treatment Evaluation

- Routine laboratory tests—Baseline complete blood count with differential, a chemistry panel, and liver function testing
- HIV testing (review of HIV serology), cluster of differentiation 4 (CD4) count and percentage; viral load; and screening for co-infections, including viral hepatitis
- Tumor markers—not done routinely; serum carcinoembryonic antigen (CEA) can be found in 20–39% patients with anal SCC [8–10]
- Fertility preservation and reproductive counselling

22.7 Imaging for Anal Canal Tumors

Imaging studies, including endo-anal ultrasound (EAUS), CT scan, MRI, and PET CT, are used for staging of the anal canal tumors. MRI is the best investigation to image anal canal tumors (primary and nodes), and CT of the chest and Abdomen is used to evaluate distant metastasis. The role of PET CT is emerging due to its high sensitivity for nodal metastasis and is also useful in radiation planning. Each of these is discussed below.

22.8 Role of MRI

High-resolution T2-weighted MRI is essential for detailed assessment of local tumor extent. A minimum of 1.5T magnetic field intensity is recommended for optimal results. No specific patient preparation is usually needed, although anal canal distension with jelly can help visualize small lesions [11].

On MRI, tumors appear with relatively high/intermediate signal intensity compared to the low signal intensity of the muscle layers forming the internal and external sphincters and the muscularis propria of the rectal wall. This helps assess tumor infiltration and involvement of the sphincters or inter-sphincteric plane [12, 13].

A standard MRI protocol for anal cancer staging includes T2-weighted turbo spin-echo MR sequences in coronal, transversal, and sagittal planes, along with Diffusion Weighted Imaging (DWI), which shows diffusion restriction in anal cancers [14, 15].

Reports should include the tumor's relationship to the anal margin, extent with quadrant involvement, cranio-caudal length, depth of invasion, and any adjacent organ infiltration (e.g., vagina, prostate, urethra, bladder wall). Additionally, noting the tumor/nodes' relationship to the sacral segment levels aids in radiotherapy planning [16]. Scans should cover both inguinal regions, pelvic sidewall compartments, and the top of the mesorectum to L5 to image the primary tumor and draining nodal disease sites. The lower border of scans should cover the cutaneous anal margin to assess anal margin tumors [17].

Malignant nodes often show mixed signal intensity or breach of the lymph node capsule by tumor signal, best assessed with high-resolution T2-weighted MRI [12]. Short-axis threshold values of 8 mm, 5 mm, and 10 mm are suggested for pelvic, perirectal, and inguinal lymph nodes, respectively. Additional features include loss of normal bean-shaped morphology, fatty hilum, internal T1 and T2 signal heterogeneity with central necrosis, and inhomogeneous enhancement [18, 19].

The dentate line's position corresponds approximately to the upper portion of the external sphincter muscles in MRI. MRI also differentiates anal carcinoma from other causes of local pain and perineal masses, such as pilonidal sinus disease,

Gartner duct or Bartholin gland cysts, tail-gut cyst, uncommon soft-tissue neoplasms, urethral cancer, lymphoma, or metastases [20, 21].

Joint guidelines from the European Society for Medical Oncology, the European Society of Surgical Oncology, and the European Society of Radiotherapy and Oncology (ESMO-ESSO-ESTRO), along with the American Society of Colon and Rectal Surgeons, recommend using MRI of the pelvis and endo-anal ultrasound (EAUS) for the standard management of anal cancer [22, 23]. If MRI is unavailable, EAUS is an alternative, though it should be reserved for small T1 lesions due to its limited field of view, which may restrict identifying regional lymph nodes [24, 25].

The sensitivity of trans-anal ultrasound (TRUS) and MRI for identifying squamous cell carcinoma of the anus (SCCA) approaches 90–100%, with high concordance regarding tumor size [26]. TRUS provides more precise results for smaller, superficial tumors.

22.9 Role of FDG PET-CT

The role of PET CT is evolving in anal cancers. We describe the pros and cons of using PET CT in the initial evaluation of patients.

**PET CT changes stage in a significant number of patients:*

Trautmann et al. reported on 21 patients with anal cancer, finding that PET detected involved pelvic nodes in a quarter of cases that CT missed. However, the group stage changed in only about 10% of cases, possibly duc to the lack of attenuation correction in PET scans, limiting sensitivity for deep pelvic lymph node detection [27]. Cotter et al. (2006) studied 41 patients staged with CT and FDG-PET/CT, finding that PET upstaged inguinal nodes in 17% of cases where both CT and physical examination were negative [28]. FDG-PET changed the tumor stage group in 23% of cases (15% upstaged, 8% downstaged). The staging FDG-PET scan altered management intent in 3% and radiotherapy fields in 13%.

**PET CT has a good positive predictive value in non-enlarged nodes*

In a cohort of 61 patients, PET demonstrated superior sensitivity for regional node staging compared to conventional imaging (CT, MRI, EAUS) alone (89% vs. 62%). For inguinal node metastasis, PET had 100% sensitivity versus 85% for conventional imaging, with histological confirmation in 63% of patients. PET showed 67% sensitivity for peri-rectal nodes. PET is less sensitive for nodes smaller than 8 mm due to partial volume effects, but these nodes are also below the size limits for positive detection on CT and MRI. Therefore, false-negative results on PET are typically also false-negative or equivocal on CT and MRI [29]. The advantage of PET CT lies in its high positive predictive value for significantly increased uptake in non-enlarged nodes.

22.10 Diagnostic Evaluation Flow

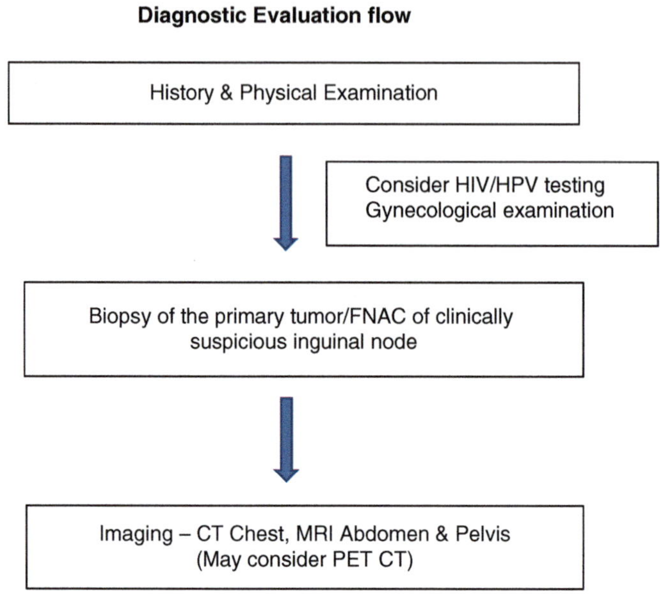

Figure showing steps of workup and clinical staging.

References

1. Welton ML, Steele SR, Goodman KA, et al. Anus. In: Armin MB, editor. AJCC cancer staging manual. 8th ed. Chicago: AJCC; 2017. p. 275.
2. Altekruse SF, Kosary CL, Krapcho M, et al. SEER cancer statistics review, 1975–2007. 2010.
3. Singh R, Nime F, Mittelman A. Malignant epithelial tumors of the anal canal. Cancer. 1981;48:411.
4. Schneider TC, Schulte WJ. Management of carcinoma of anal canal. Surgery. 1981;90:729.
5. Schraut WH, Wang CH, Dawson PJ, Block GE. Depth of invasion, location, and size of cancer of the anus dictate operative treatment. Cancer. 1983;51:1291.
6. James RD, Glynne-Jones R, Meadows HM, et al. Mitomycin or cisplatin chemoradiation with or without maintenance chemotherapy for treatment of squamous-cell carcinoma of the anus (ACT II): a randomised, phase 3, open-label, 2 × 2 factorial trial. Lancet Oncol. 2013;14:516.
7. Gunderson LL, Winter KA, Ajani JA, et al. Long-term update of US GI intergroup RTOG 98-11 phase III trial for anal carcinoma: survival, relapse, and colostomy failure with concurrent chemoradiation involving fluorouracil/mitomycin versus fluorouracil/cisplatin. J Clin Oncol. 2012;30:4344.
8. Raab GT, O'Neil DS, Kiran RP, et al. Elevation of serum CEA in patients with squamous cell carcinoma of the anus. Cancer Invest. 2019;37:288.
9. Tanum G, Stenwig AE, Børmer OP, Tveit KM. Carcinoembryonic antigen in anal carcinoma. Acta Oncol. 1992;31:333.

10. Indinnimeo M, Cicchini C, Izzo P, Stazi A. Anal canal cancer diagnosis: usefulness of serum tumor markers. J Chemother. 1997;9:121.
11. Hemachandran N, et al. Radiology of anal and lower rectal cancers. Clin Radiol. 2021;76(12):871–8.
12. Koh DM, Dzik-Jurasz A, O'Neill B, et al. Pelvic phased-array MR imaging of anal carcinoma before and after chemoradiation. Br J Radiol. 2008;81(962):91–8.
13. Salerno G, Daniels IR, Brown G. Magnetic resonance imaging of the low rectum: defining the radiological anatomy. Colorectal Dis. 2006;8(suppl 3):10–3.
14. Petrillo A, Fusco R, Petrillo M, et al. Standardized Index of Shape (SIS): a quantitative DCE-MRI parameter to discriminate responders by non-responders after neoadjuvant therapy in LARC. Eur Radiol. 2015;25(7):1935–45.
15. Petrillo A, Fusco R, Petrillo M, et al. Value of Time Intensity Curve Visual Inspection to assess neoadjuvant therapy response. J Physiol Health Photon. 2014;110:255–27.
16. Brown G, Rimmer M, Williams S. Colon, rectum and anal canal cancer. In: Nicholson T, editor. Recommendations for cross-sectional imaging in cancer management. 2nd ed. London: The Royal College of Radiologists; 2014. Royal College Recommendations.
17. Glynne-Jones R, et al. Anal cancer: ESMO-ESSO-ESTRO clinical practice guidelines for diagnosis, treatment and follow-up. Radiother Oncol. 2014;111(3):330–9.
18. Parikh J, Shaw A, Grant LA, et al. Anal carcinomas: the role of endoanal ultrasound and magnetic resonance imaging in staging, response evaluation and follow-up. Eur Radiol. 2011;21:776–85.
19. Roach SC, Hulse PA, Moulding FJ, et al. Magnetic resonance imaging of anal cancer. Clin Radiol. 2005;60:1111–9.
20. Tappouni RF, Sarwani NI, Tice JG, et al. Imaging of unusual perineal masses. AJR Am J Roentgenol. 2011;196:W412–20.
21. Hoeffel C, Crema MD, Azizi L, et al. Magnetic resonance imaging of the ischiorectal fossa: spectrum of disease. J Comput Assist Tomogr. 2007;31:251–7.
22. Danti G, Flammia F, Matteuzzi B, Cozzi D, Berti V, Grazzini G, Pradella S, Recchia L, Brunese L, Miele V. Gastrointestinal neuroendocrine neoplasms (GI-NENs): hot topics in morphological, functional, and prognostic imaging. Radiol. Medica. 2021;126:1497–507.
23. Di Serafino M, Vallone G. The role of point of care ultrasound in radiology department: update and prospective. A statement of Italian college ultrasound. Radiol Medica. 2021;126:636–41.
24. Stewart DB, Gaertner WB, Glasgow SC, Herzig DO, Feingold D, Steele SR. Prepared on Behalf of the Clinical Practice Guidelines Committee of the American Society of Colon and Rectal Surgeons. The American society of colon and rectal surgeons clinical practice guidelines for anal squamous cell cancers (Revised 2018). Dis Colon Rectum. 2018;61:755–74.
25. Moureau-Zabotto L, Vendrely V, Abramowitz L, Borg C, Francois E, Goere D, Huguet F, Peiffert D, Siproudhis L, Ducreux M, et al. Anal cancer: French Intergroup Clinical Practice Guidelines for diagnosis, treatment and follow-up (SNFGE, FFCD, GERCOR, UNICANCER, SFCD, SFED, SFRO, SNFCP). Dig. Liver Dis. 2017;49:831–40.
26. Otto SD, Lee L, Buhr HJ, et al. Staging anal cancer: prospective comparison of transanal endoscopic ultrasound and magnetic resonance imaging. J Gastrointest Surg. 2009;13:1292–8.
27. Trautmann T, Zuger J. Positron emission tomography for pre- treatment staging and post-treatment evaluation in cancer of the anal canal. Mol Imaging Biol. 2005;7:309–13.
28. Cotter S, Grigsby P, Siegel B, Dehdashti F, Malyapa R, Fleshman J, Birnbaum E, Wang X, Abbey E, Tan B. FDG-PET/CT in the evaluation of anal carcinoma. Int J Radiat Oncol Biol Phys. 2006;65:720–5.
29. Winton ED, Heriot AG, Ng M, et al. The impact of 18-fluorodeoxyglucose positron emission tomography on the staging, management and outcome of anal cancer. Br J Cancer. 2009;100(5):693–700.

Chapter 23
Presentation and Evaluation of Prostate and Bladder Malignancy

Prashanth Giridhar and Prarabdh Singh

23.1 Introduction

Bladder cancer represents a relatively infrequent malignancy within the Indian population. Data from the GLOBOCAN 2020 database indicate that it is the 17th most common cancer diagnosed in the country [1]. A clear gender disparity is observed, with men being affected far more often than women; most urban population-based cancer registries in India report a male-to-female incidence ratio of nearly 4:1 [2]. The burden of bladder cancer shows notable geographic variation across different regions of India. In men, the highest incidence rates have been documented in Delhi (7.4), followed by Thiruvananthapuram (4.9) and Kolkata (4.0), whereas Dibrugarh reports the lowest incidence (1.1). Among women, Delhi records the highest rate (1.7), with Mumbai and Mizoram both reporting rates of 1.1, while Barshi has the lowest incidence at 0.2 [3]. Tobacco use is recognised as the leading modifiable risk factor for bladder cancer. Individuals who smoke have a three- to fourfold increased risk compared with non-smokers, and tobacco exposure is estimated to contribute to approximately 31% of bladder cancer mortality in men and 16% in women [4, 5]. Additionally, occupational exposure to carcinogenic substances such as aromatic amines and carbon black dust, commonly encountered in the rubber, leather, and dye industries, has been associated with a higher likelihood of developing bladder cancer [6, 7].

P. Giridhar (✉) · P. Singh
Department of Radiation Oncology, MPMMCC & HBCH Varanasi, Units of Tata Memorial Centre and affliated with Homi Bhabha National Institute, Mumbai, India

S. Pradhan et al. (eds.), *Evidence Based Handbook on Diagnosis and Staging in Oncology*, https://doi.org/10.1007/978-981-95-9701-7_23

23.2 Presenting Symptoms and Initial Evaluation

Painless gross haematuria is the most common symptom at presentation in patients with bladder cancer. In a smaller proportion of cases, individuals may also experience irritative lower urinary tract symptoms such as urinary frequency, urgency or pelvic pain.

23.2.1 Clinical Assessment

Patients presenting with these features should undergo a thorough clinical evaluation, including a bimanual examination per rectum and per vagina in the outpatient setting, to assess for possible extension or involvement from a urinary tract malignancy. Based on the clinical findings, further diagnostic investigations should be initiated.

23.2.2 Urine Cytology

Microscopic examination of voided urine for exfoliated malignant cells is particularly sensitive for detecting high-grade tumours and is especially useful in suspected cases of high-grade disease or carcinoma in situ (CIS) [8]. A positive cytology result suggests the presence of malignancy or CIS somewhere within the urinary tract, although it does not provide information regarding the exact site of origin.

23.2.3 Upper Urinary Tract Evaluation

Concomitant upper tract urothelial carcinoma is identified in approximately 2–4% of patients with bladder cancer. Contrast-enhanced CT urography is regarded as the preferred imaging technique for assessment, with MR urography serving as an alternative in patients who cannot undergo CT-based imaging. CT urography demonstrates a sensitivity of around 95% and a specificity approaching 91% and is generally performed after confirmation of positive urine cytology.

23.2.4 Role of Imaging in the Diagnosis and Staging of Bladder Cancer

Assessment of local tumour extent using imaging is advised before undertaking transurethral resection of bladder tumour (TURBT). Both computed tomography (CT) and magnetic resonance imaging (MRI) can be employed for evaluating local invasion; however, MRI provides superior soft-tissue definition when compared with CT. This advantage makes MRI more reliable in differentiating between T1 and T2 stage disease. Evidence from a meta-analysis has shown that 3.0-T MRI combined with diffusion-weighted sequences achieves a sensitivity of 91% and specificity of 96% in distinguishing ≤T1 tumours from ≥T2 tumours prior to surgical intervention [9]. While CT has limited capability in visualising the individual layers of the bladder wall, it remains useful for detecting peri-vesical spread in advanced, high-grade tumours such as T3b and T4 disease [10].

23.2.5 Endoscopic Evaluation and Tissue Diagnosis

Confirmation of bladder cancer requires endoscopic visualisation of the lesion using flexible cystoscopy, followed by biopsy. Transurethral resection of the bladder tumour (TURBT) or biopsy of the bladder mass is essential for histological confirmation and staging, enabling classification into non-muscle invasive bladder cancer (NMIBC) or muscle-invasive bladder cancer (MIBC). During TURBT, maximal tumour removal should be attempted. In patients with NMIBC, a significant proportion may have residual disease or be upstaged at repeat resection, with residual tumour reported in up to 51% of cases [2, 11]. A second TURBT has been shown to improve recurrence-free and progression-free survival [12, 13] and to enhance outcomes following intra-vesical BCG therapy [14].

23.2.6 Assessment for Metastatic Spread

A metastatic work-up is recommended for patients with muscle-invasive bladder cancer identified on imaging or following TURBT. This typically involves contrast-enhanced CT of the chest, abdomen and pelvis. The probability of lymph node metastasis rises with increasing local tumour stage [15, 16], and both MRI and contrast-enhanced CT are useful for detecting enlarged regional lymph nodes, with nodal size being an important indicator of malignant involvement. The lungs and liver represent the most common sites of distant metastatic disease.

Positron emission tomography–CT (PET-CT) is not routinely advised in the evaluation of bladder cancer. Its utility is limited by urinary excretion of 18F-FDG, which accumulates in the bladder and hampers accurate assessment of primary bladder lesions (Tables 23.1, 23.2 and 23.3).

Table 23.1 Adopted and modified from 2017 TNM staging of bladder cancer

	Description	Comments
T stage		
Tx	Primary tumour cannot be assessed	
T0	No evidence of primary tumour	
Ta	Non-invasive papillary carcinoma	Papillary tumour involving mucosa
Tis	Carcinoma in situ: 'flat tumour'	Flat tumour (Usually high grade) non-invasive
T1	Tumour invades subepithelial connective tissue	Papillary tumour involving Lamina propria *Ta, Tis, T1* are *NMIBC*
T2	Tumour invades muscle	
T2a	Tumour invades superficial muscle (inner half)	
T2b	Tumour invades deep muscle (outer half)	
T3	Tumour invades tissue around bladder	
T3a	Extension seen only in microscope	
T3b	Macroscopically (extravesical mass)	
T4	Tumour invades any of the following: prostate stroma, seminal vesicles, uterus, vagina, pelvic wall, abdominal wall	
T4a	Tumour invades prostate stroma, seminal vesicles, uterus or vagina	
T4b	Tumour invades pelvic wall or abdominal wall	
N stage		
N0	No regional lymph node metastasis	
N1	Metastasis in a single lymph node in the true pelvis (hypogastric, obturator, external iliac or presacral)	
N2	Metastasis in multiple regional lymph nodes in the true pelvis (hypogastric, obturator, external iliac or presacral)	
N3	Metastasis in common iliac lymph node(s)	
M stage		
M0	No distant metastasis	
M1a	Non-regional lymph nodes	
M1b	Other distant metastases	

Table 23.2 Grading of bladder cancer (Urothelial carcinoma)

Papillary tumours (WHO classification 2004/2016)
Papillary urothelial neoplasm of low malignant potential (PUNLMP)
Low-grade (LG) papillary urothelial carcinoma
High-grade (HG) papillary urothelial carcinoma
Flat tumours (WHO classification 2004)
Non-malignant lesions Urothelial proliferation of uncertain malignant potential (flat lesion without atypia or papillary aspects) Reactive atypia (flat lesion with atypia) Atypia of unknown significance
Potential pre-malignant lesion Urothelial dysplasia
Malignant lesion Urothelial CIS is always high grade

Table 23.3 Risk category of NMIBC

Risk category	Criterion
Low risk	A primary, single, Ta/T1 LG <3 cm in diameter without CIS in a patient <70 years A primary Ta LG/G1 tumour without CIS with at most ONE of the additional clinical risk factors (Age >70 years, multiple papillary tumours, tumour diameter >3 cm
Intermediate risk	Patients without CIS who are not included in either the low, high or very high-risk groups
High risk	All T1 HG/G3 without CIS, EXCEPT those included in the very high-risk group All CIS patients, EXCEPT those included in the very high-risk group
Very high risk	**Stage, grade with additional clinical risk factors:** Ta HG/G3 and CIS with all 3 risk factors T1 G2 and CIS with at least 2 risk factors T1 HG/G3 and CIS with at least 1 risk factor T1 HG/G3 no CIS with all 3 risk factors

23.2.7 Surveillance After Radical Cystectomy for Bladder Cancer

In patients who have undergone radical cystectomy with curative intent, monitoring of the urethra using urine cytology and/or cystoscopy is advised in selected high-risk groups, such as those with multifocal disease, carcinoma in situ, or involvement of the prostatic urethra. The interval and duration of urethral surveillance should be guided by institutional follow-up protocols. Cross-sectional imaging with CT of the thorax, abdomen and pelvis is recommended every six months for the first three years after surgery, followed by annual imaging thereafter.

23.2.8 Follow-Up After Bladder Preservation Strategies

For patients treated with bladder conservation approaches, including trimodality therapy with curative intent, close surveillance is essential for early detection of disease recurrence. Follow-up evaluations are typically performed every 3–6 months during the initial period after treatment, and after three years, the interval may be extended to six-monthly assessments in most patients. During the first three years, regular cystoscopic examination and urine cytology at 3–6-month intervals are recommended, along with CT imaging of the thorax, abdomen and pelvis every six months. Beyond this period, the frequency of investigations may be gradually reduced based on clinical status and institutional practice.

23.3 Prostate Cancer

23.3.1 Epidemiology and Risk Factors

Prostate cancer is emerging as an increasingly important health concern among men in India, with a consistent rise in incidence over recent years [17]. Data from the National Cancer Database (NCDIR) indicate that prostate cancer ranks among the ten most common malignancies in urban population-based cancer registries, including Bangalore, Delhi, Bhopal and Mumbai [17]. In contrast, its occurrence appears to be relatively lower in rural regions. Over time, prostate cancer has shown a marked upward shift in ranking: from the eighth most common cancer among Indian men in the 1990s to the third most common malignancy in cities such as Delhi and Mumbai by 2014. A similar trend has been observed in Bangalore, where it rose from seventh position in the 1990s to third place.

In absolute numbers, 37,416 prostate cancer cases were reported in India in 2016, increasing to 41,532 cases by 2020, with projections suggesting that the annual burden may exceed 47,000 cases by 2025 [17]. Prostate cancer currently accounts for approximately 3% of all cancers in the country. The average age at diagnosis in India is around 69.7 years [18]. Although metabolic syndrome has been proposed as a potential risk factor, available evidence supporting this association remains limited [19]. Testosterone replacement therapy in hypo-gonadal men has not been shown to increase the risk of developing prostate cancer [20]. At present, no specific lifestyle or dietary interventions are recommended for the prevention of prostate cancer [21].

23.3.2 Screening

Large studies have not demonstrated a clear benefit of routine population-based screening in terms of prostate cancer–specific or overall survival [22]. Given the limited and inconclusive evidence [23], systematic screening using serum prostate-specific antigen (PSA) testing is not recommended, even in individuals with known BRCA2 mutations.

23.3.3 Diagnosis

Men with clinical features suggestive of prostate cancer should undergo estimation of total serum PSA levels.

- If PSA is <4 ng/mL and digital rectal examination (DRE) findings are benign, alternative diagnoses such as benign prostatic hyperplasia or prostatitis should be considered.
- In cases where PSA levels are between 4 and 10 ng/mL with a non-suspicious DRE, a short course of fluoroquinolone antibiotics followed by repeat PSA testing may be considered, although the clinical benefit of this approach remains uncertain [24].
- Patients with PSA levels >10 ng/mL or an abnormal DRE should be evaluated further for prostate cancer.

Ideally, a multi-parametric MRI (mp-MRI) of the prostate should be performed before undertaking a biopsy. When the Prostate Imaging Reporting and Data System (PI-RADS) score is ≥3, targeted biopsies should be obtained in addition to systematic sampling. If mp-MRI is unavailable or if the PI-RADS score is ≤2, systematic biopsy alone is recommended in patients with PSA >10 ng/mL or a suspicious DRE [25, 26].

23.4 Biopsy

1st choice—Systematic 12-core biopsy by trans-perineal route (low infection rates) [27]
2nd choice—Systematic 12-core biopsy by trans-rectal route (Table 23.4)

Once biopsy is performed, imaging is to be recommended for local and distal staging based on risk stratification. If mp-MRI pelvis was done before biopsy, no other local staging is needed. We hereinafter describe the risk stratification followed by recommended staging imaging (Table 23.5).

Table 23.4 Gleason score and grade: International Society of Urologic Pathology grade (group) system

Gleason score	ISUP grade
2–6	1
7 (3 + 4)	2
7 (4 + 3)	3
8 (4 + 4 or 3 + 5 or 5 + 3)	4
9–10	5

Table 23.5 Prostate cancer risk grouping

Definition			
Low-risk	Intermediate-risk	High-risk	
PSA <10 ng/mL	PSA 10–20 ng/mL	PSA >20 ng/mL	Any PSA
and GS <7 (ISUP grade 1)	or GS 7 (ISUP grade 2/3)	or GS >7 (ISUP grade 4/5)	Any GS (any ISUP grade)
and cT1-2a	or cT2b	or cT2c	cT3-4 or cN+
Localised			**Locally advanced**

23.5 Staging Recommendations

Low-risk prostate cancer: mpMRI Pelvis recommended. No other imaging needed
Intermediate risk prostate cancer: PSMA PET/CT, ± mpMRI pelvis (if being planned for radical treatment) **or** CECT TAP (thorax, abdomen, pelvis) ± Bone scan
High risk prostate cancer: PSMA PET/CT ± mpMRI pelvis (if being planned for radical treatment) **or** CECT TAP + Bone scan

23.6 Summary of Evidence for Staging in Prostate Cancer

23.6.1 Initial Staging

The approach to staging prostate cancer is guided by the accessibility of diagnostic techniques and the anticipated therapeutic strategy. With the expanding availability of both conventional and advanced imaging modalities, it is crucial to evaluate the advantages and limitations of each option to ensure selection of the most appropriate staging investigation.

23.7 Local Disease Assessment

23.7.1 Trans-rectal Ultrasound (TRUS)

Although isolated institutional studies have suggested potential utility of three-dimensional TRUS and colour Doppler imaging for local tumour assessment, these findings have not been consistently reproduced in larger, multi-institutional studies [28–30]. As a result, TRUS is not advised for primary tumour (T-stage) evaluation.

23.7.2 Magnetic Resonance Imaging (MRI)

Multi-parametric MRI is currently regarded as the preferred imaging modality for local staging of prostate cancer, with T2-weighted sequences providing the most dependable anatomical detail. In cases of locally advanced (T3) disease, MRI demonstrates high specificity but limited sensitivity for detecting extraprostatic extension and seminal vesicle involvement. The use of higher field strength systems (3T MRI) and the addition of functional imaging techniques may improve detection rates; however, these benefits are tempered by considerable variability in interpretation among readers [31–34].

23.8 Evaluation of Distant Disease

23.8.1 PSMA PET/CT

PSMA PET/CT utilises several radiolabelled tracers, including ^{68}Ga, ^{18}F and ^{64}Cu, as well as Tc-99m–based PSMA SPECT/CT, with ^{68}Ga and ^{18}F tracers being most frequently employed. A recent systematic review and meta-analysis found no meaningful difference in detection performance among commonly used PSMA tracers (^{68}Ga-PSMA-11, ^{18}F-PSMA-1007, and ^{18}F-DCFPyL), while demonstrating superior diagnostic accuracy compared with choline- and fluciclovine-based imaging [35]. Additional meta-analyses have confirmed high sensitivity and specificity of PSMA PET/CT for identifying lymph node and distant metastases, with imaging results influencing treatment decisions in over 10% of patients [36–38].

23.8.2 PSMA PET/MRI

PSMA PET/MRI is an emerging hybrid imaging technique increasingly explored for both staging and follow-up of prostate cancer. A meta-analysis assessing its diagnostic performance reported pooled per-lesion sensitivity and specificity of 61.5% and 90.9%, respectively, for detection of the primary tumour. For lymph node metastases, the corresponding per-lesion sensitivity and specificity were 64.3% and 97.4% [39].

23.9 Assessment of Skeletal Metastases (M Category)

23.9.1 Bone Scintigraphy

Conventional bone scintigraphy remains the most widely used modality for detecting osseous metastases in prostate cancer. Meta-analytic data indicate a pooled sensitivity of 79% (95% CI: 73–83%) and specificity of 82% (95% CI: 78–85%). 18F-NaF PET/CT offers improved sensitivity with comparable specificity for identifying skeletal metastases in newly diagnosed high-risk patients [40, 41]. However, prospective evidence suggests that 18F-NaF PET/CT does not provide additional diagnostic benefit over standard bone scintigraphy in intermediate- or high-risk patients with an initially negative bone scan [42].

23.9.2 Whole-Body MRI (WB-MRI)

Diffusion-weighted whole-body MRI has demonstrated superior sensitivity compared with bone scintigraphy in detecting bone metastases among high-risk prostate cancer patients, as shown in a prospective study involving 100 individuals [43]. WB-MRI has also been shown to outperform combined conventional imaging approaches, including bone scintigraphy, targeted radiographs, and abdominopelvic CT, in both sensitivity and specificity [44]. When compared with choline PET/CT, WB-MRI exhibits higher sensitivity, whereas choline PET/CT demonstrates greater specificity [45].

23.10 Role of Imaging in Recurrent and Metastatic Prostate Cancer

Biochemical recurrence (BCR) following radical prostatectomy (RP) or radiotherapy (RT) typically occurs several years before the development of clinically evident metastatic disease, with an average lead time of approximately 7–8 years. During this asymptomatic phase, particularly at low prostate-specific antigen (PSA) levels, the diagnostic yield of conventional imaging modalities such as bone scintigraphy, CT and MRI is limited. Consequently, in patients experiencing PSA-only recurrence after RP, salvage radiotherapy is often initiated based solely on biochemical criteria, without radiological confirmation of disease recurrence.

Evidence from a meta-analysis indicates that the diagnostic performance of choline PET/CT is highly dependent on PSA values and PSA kinetics [46]. At PSA levels below 1 ng/mL, reported sensitivity is low, ranging from 5% to 24% [47]. In contrast, PSMA PET/CT has demonstrated superior detection rates compared with other imaging techniques, particularly in patients with PSA levels under 1 ng/mL [46]. Reported positivity rates for ^{68}Ga-PSMA PET/CT increase with rising PSA levels, with detection rates of approximately 33% (95% CI: 16–51) for PSA <1 ng/mL, 45% (95% CI: 39–52) for PSA values between 0.2 and 0.49 ng/mL, and 59% (95% CI: 50–68) for PSA levels between 0.5 and 0.99 ng/mL.

In patients who develop biochemical recurrence after definitive radiotherapy, local salvage treatment options are associated with significant morbidity. Therefore, histopathological confirmation of local disease recurrence is recommended prior to initiating salvage therapy [48]. Multi-parametric MRI (mpMRI) has shown high diagnostic accuracy in identifying local tumour recurrence in this setting [48]. While PET imaging offers valuable functional information, its spatial resolution is inferior to that of MRI. As a result, combined PET/MRI may represent a promising approach for evaluating patients with biochemical relapse, warranting further investigation.

Note: Staging of prostate cancer can be done as per updated AJCC TNM Staging

23.11 Follow-Up

Post-definitive or adjuvant treatment patient should get every 3 month PSA for first 2 years and then 6 monthly until 5 years. If the patient is on ADT along with serum PSA, serum calcium, vitamin D and lipid profile must be done. Radiological investigation is needed in case of increasing PSA or if patient is symptomatic.

References

1. https://gco.iarc.fr/today/data/factsheets/populations/356-india-fact-sheets.pdf
2. National Centre for Disease Informatics and Research. Three Year Report of Population Based Cancer Registries 2012–2014. Incidence, Distribution, Trends in Incidence Rates and Projections of Burden of Cancer (Report of 27 PBCRs in India), NCDIR-NCRP ICMR. Bengaluru: National Centre for Disease Informatics and Research; 2016.
3. Mishra V, Balasubramanian G. Urinary bladder cancer and its associated factors – an epidemiological overview. Indian J Med Sci. 2021;73(2):239–48.

4. Bourke L, Bauld L, Bullen C, et al. E-cigarettes and urologic health: a collaborative review of toxicology, epidemiology, and potential risks. Eur Urol. 2017;71:915–23.
5. Wu X, Ros MM, Gu J, Kiemeney L. Epidemiology and genetic susceptibility to bladder cancer. BJUI Int. 2008;102:1207–15.
6. Rushton L, Bagga S, Bevan R, et al. Occupation and cancer in Britain. Br J Cancer. 2010;102:1428–37.
7. Noon AP, Martinsen JI, Catto JW, Pukkala E. Occupation and bladder cancer phenotype: Identification of workplace patterns that increase the risk of advanced disease beyond overall incidence. Eur Urol Focus. 2018;4:725–30.
8. EAU Guidelines. Edn. presented at the EAU Annual Congress Milan 2021. ISBN 978-94-92671-13-4
9. Huang L, Kong Q, Liu Z, Wang J, Kang Z, Zhu Y. The diagnostic value of MR imaging in differentiating t staging of bladder cancer: a meta-analysis. Radiology. 2018;286(2):502–11.
10. Lee CH, Tan CH, de Faria CS, Kundra V. Role of imaging in the local staging of urothelial carcinoma of the bladder. AJR Am J Roentgenol. 2017;208(6):1193–205.
11. Teoh JY, et al. Comparison of detrusor muscle sampling rate in monopolar and bipolar transurethral resection of bladder tumor: a randomized trial. Ann Surg Oncol. 2017;24:1428.
12. Eroglu A, et al. The prognostic value of routine second transurethral resection in patients with newly diagnosed stage pT1 non-muscle-invasive bladder cancer: results from randomized 10-year extension trial. Int J Clin Oncol. 2020;25:698.
13. Gordon PC, et al. Long-term outcomes from re-resection for high-risk non-muscle-invasive bladder cancer: a potential to rationalize use. Eur Urol Focus. 2019;5:650.
14. Hashine K, et al. Results of second transurethral resection for high-grade T1 bladder cancer. Urol Ann. 2016;8:10.
15. Shariat SF, Rink M, Ehdaie B, et al. Pathologic nodal staging score for bladder cancer: a decision tool for adjuvant therapy after radical cystectomy. Eur Urol. 2013;63(2):371–8.
16. Shariat SF, Karakiewicz PI, Palapattu GS, et al. Outcomes of radical cystectomy for transitional cell carcinoma of the bladder: a contemporary series from the Bladder Cancer Research Consortium. J Urol. 2006;176(6 Pt 1):2414–22. discussion 2422
17. https://ncdirindia.org/All_Reports/Report_2020/Factsheet/Fact_Sheet_2020.pdf
18. Hariharan K, Padmanabha V. Demography and disease characteristics of prostate cancer in India. Indian J Urol. 2016;32(2):103–8.
19. Esposito K, et al. Effect of metabolic syndrome and its components on prostate cancer risk: meta-analysis. J Endocrinol Invest. 2013;36:132.
20. Halder, et al. Incidence of prostate cancer in hypogonadal men receiving testosterone therapy; observations from 5 year median follow up of 3 registeries. J Urol. 2015;193:80.
21. Mottet N, van den Bergh RCN, Briers E, et al. EAU-EANM-ESTRO-ESUR-SIOG guidelines on prostate cancer-2020 Update. Part 1: Screening, diagnosis, and local treatment with curative intent. Eur Urol. 2021;79(2):243–62.
22. Ilic D, Neuberger MM, Djulbegovic M, Dahm P. Screening for prostate cancer. Cochrane Database Syst Rev. 2013;1
23. Van Asperen CJ, et al. Cancer risks in BRCA 2 families; estimates for sites other than breast and ovary. J Med Genet. 2005;42:711.
24. Shtricker A, Shefi S, Ringel A, Gillon G. PSA levels of 4.0 – 10 ng/mL and negative digital rectal examination. Antibiotic therapy versus immediate prostate biopsy. Int Braz J Urol. 2009;35(5):551–8.
25. Rouvière O, Puech P, Renard-Penna R, et al. MRI-FIRST Investigators. Use of prostate systematic and targeted biopsy on the basis of multiparametric MRI in biopsy-naive patients (MRI-FIRST): a prospective, multicentre, paired diagnostic study. Lancet Oncol. 2019;20(1):100–9.
26. Kasivisvanathan V, Rannikko AS, Borghi M, et al. PRECISION Study Group Collaborators. MRI-targeted or standard biopsy for prostate-cancer diagnosis. N Engl J Med. 2018;378(19):1767–77.

27. Cerruto MA. Trans rectal versus transperineal 14- core prostate biopsy in detection of prostate cancer: a comparative evaluation at the same institution. Arch Ital Urol Androl. 2014;86:284.
28. Sauvain JL, Palascak P, Bourscheid D, et al. Value of power Doppler and 3D vascular sonography as a method for diagnosis and staging of prostate cancer. Eur Urol. 2003;44(1):21–30. discussion 30–31
29. Mitterberger M, Pinggera G-M, Pallwein L, et al. The value of three-dimensional transrectal ultrasonography in staging prostate cancer. BJU Int. 2007;100(1):47–50.
30. Smith JA, Scardino PT, Resnick MI, Hernandez AD, Rose SC, Egger MJ. Transrectal ultrasound versus digital rectal examination for the staging of carcinoma of the prostate: results of a prospective, multi-institutional trial. J Urol. 1997;157(3):902–6.
31. Fütterer JJ, Engelbrecht MR, Huisman HJ, et al. Staging prostate cancer with dynamic contrast-enhanced endorectal MR imaging prior to radical prostatectomy: experienced versus less experienced readers. Radiology. 2005;237(2):541–9.
32. Wang L, Mullerad M, Chen H-N, et al. Prostate cancer: incremental value of endorectal MR imaging findings for prediction of extracapsular extension. Radiology. 2004;232(1):133–9.
33. D'Amico AV, Whittington R, Malkowicz B, et al. Endorectal magnetic resonance imaging as a predictor of biochemical outcome after radical prostatectomy in men with clinically localized prostate cancer. J Urol. 2000;164(3 Pt 1):759–63.
34. Engelbrecht MR, Jager GJ, Severens JL. Patient selection for magnetic resonance imaging of prostate cancer. Eur Urol. 2001;40(3):300–7.
35. Budiharto T, Joniau S, Lerut E, et al. Prospective evaluation of 11C-choline positron emission tomography/computed tomography and diffusion-weighted magnetic resonance imaging for the nodal staging of prostate cancer with a high risk of lymph node metastases. Eur Urol. 2011;60(1):125–30.
36. Alberts IL, Seide SE, Mingels C, et al. Comparing the diagnostic performance of radiotracers in recurrent prostate cancer: a systematic review and network meta-analysis. Eur J Nucl Med Mol Imaging. 2021;48(9):2978–89.
37. Peng L, Li J, Meng C, et al. Can 68Ga-prostate specific membrane antigen positron emission tomography/computerized tomography provide an accurate lymph node staging for patients with medium/high risk prostate cancer? A diagnostic meta-analysis. Radiat Oncol Lond Engl. 2020;15(1):227.
38. Perera M, Papa N, Roberts M, et al. Gallium-68 prostate-specific membrane antigen positron emission tomography in advanced prostate cancer-updated diagnostic utility, sensitivity, specificity, and distribution of prostate-specific membrane antigen-avid lesions: a systematic review and meta-analysis. Eur Urol. 2020;77(4):403–17.
39. Van Kalmthout LWM, van Melick HHE, Lavalaye J, et al. Prospective validation of gallium-68 prostate specific membrane antigen-positron emission tomography/computerized tomography for primary staging of prostate cancer. J Urol. 2020;203(3):537–45.
40. Evangelista L, Zattoni F, Cassarino G, et al. PET/MRI in prostate cancer: a systematic review and meta-analysis. Eur J Nucl Med Mol Imaging. 2021;48(3):859–73.
41. Ateishi U, Morita S, Taguri M, et al. A meta-analysis of (18)F-Fluoride positron emission tomography for assessment of metastatic bone tumor. Ann Nucl Med. 2010;24(7):523–31.
42. Evangelista L, Bertoldo F, Boccardo F, et al. Diagnostic imaging to detect and evaluate response to therapy in bone metastases from prostate cancer: current modalities and new horizons. Eur J Nucl Med Mol Imaging. 2016;43(8):1546–62.
43. Zacho HD, Jochumsen MR, Langkilde NC, et al. No added value of 18F-Sodium Fluoride PET/CT for the detection of bone metastases in patients with newly diagnosed prostate cancer with normal bone scintigraphy. J Nucl Med Off Publ Soc Nucl Med. 2019;60(12):1713–6.
44. Lecouvet FE, El Mouedden J, Collette L, et al. Can whole-body magnetic resonance imaging with diffusion-weighted imaging replace Tc 99m bone scanning and computed tomography for single-step detection of metastases in patients with high-risk prostate cancer? Eur Urol. 2012;62(1):68–75.

45. One-step TNM staging of high-risk prostate cancer using magnetic resonance imaging (MRI): toward an upfront simplified "all-in-one" imaging approach? – PubMed [Internet]. [cited 2022 Feb 10]. Available from: https://pubmed.ncbi.nlm.nih.gov/24375774
46. Hofman MS, Lawrentschuk N, Francis RJ, et al. Prostate-specific membrane antigen PET-CT in patients with high-risk prostate cancer before curative-intent surgery or radiotherapy (proPSMA): a prospective, randomised, multicentre study. Lancet Lond Engl. 2020;395(10231):1208–16.
47. Prospective Comparison of 18F-Fluoromethylcholine Versus 68Ga-PSMA PET/CT in Prostate Cancer Patients Who Have Rising PSA After Curative Treatment and Are Being Considered for Targeted Therapy | J Nucl Med [Internet]. [cited 2022 Feb 10]. Available from: https://jnm.snmjournals.org/content/56/8/1185
48. Afshar-Oromieh A, Zechmann CM, Malcher A, et al. Comparison of PET imaging with a (68) Ga-labelled PSMA ligand and (18)F-choline-based PET/CT for the diagnosis of recurrent prostate cancer. Eur J Nucl Med Mol Imaging. 2014;41(1):11–20.

Chapter 24
Evaluation and Staging of Testicular Malignancy

Prashanth Giridhar, Abhishek Chakravarty, and Soham Sanyal

24.1 Introduction and Epidemiology

Testis is a heterogeneous organ which consists of all the three layers of origin. However, about 90% of the tumors consist of germ cell tumors which can be broadly classified into seminomatous and non-seminomatous (NSGCT). Testicular cancers are relatively uncommon and are found in less than 1% of male population with median age of presentation between 15 and 35 years. NSGCTs are less common but more aggressive in nature as they arise from multiple cell lines. Germ cell tumors may also present in extra-gonadal sites like retroperitoneum and mediastinum; however, they are managed on similar lines to testicular GCTs.

24.2 Risk Factors

Testicular tumors due to their young age of presentation are generally associated with developmental or familial risk factors. One of such developmental abnormalities during the first decade of life is cryptorchidism (*undescended testis*), which may be associated with approximately 10% of testicular cancers. Orchidopexy, i.e., surgical repositioning of undescended testis, has shown to decrease the risk during the first decade of life [1].

Germ cell neoplasia in situ (GCNIS) is a premalignant condition seen in 90% patients suffering from GCTs. An incidence of 5% is found in cryptorchid testicles [2], prior history of contralateral testicular GCTs [3–5], and in syndromes of abnormal sex differentiation [6].

P. Giridhar (✉) · A. Chakravarty · S. Sanyal
Department of Radiation Oncology, MPMMCC & HBCH Varanasi, Units of Tata Memorial Centre and affliated with Homi Bhabha National Institute, Mumbai, India

S. Pradhan et al. (eds.), *Evidence Based Handbook on Diagnosis and Staging in Oncology*, https://doi.org/10.1007/978-981-95-9701-7_24

Testicular cancer survivors are at an increased risk of a second primary in contralateral testis in up to 2% cases. A population-based study of 29,515 previously treated testicular cancers was evaluated for risk of developing metachronous contralateral testicular cancer. The findings of this study found a cumulative risk of 1.9 % at 15 years. This risk was shown to be lower in non-seminomatous histology and testicular tumors diagnosed at an older age group [7].

Hormonal factors affecting sex differentiation are also associated with increased risk of testicular cancers. Mixed gonadal dysgenesis, males with 45X/46XY karyotype, and malformations of external genitalia carry an increased risk of developing germ cell neoplasia [8]. Klinefelter syndrome has shown a higher incidence of mediastinal germ cell tumors and sarcomas until the age of 30 years [9]. Carney's complex is a syndrome of myxoma, spotty blue nevi pigmentation on face, neck, trunk, and endocrine overactivity (adrenal, pituitary, and thyroid) associated with bilateral sex cord stromal testicular tumors [10].

Family history is also a potential risk factor for developing testicular cancer. A relative risk of 6–10 has been observed in 1st degree relatives with history of testicular cancers [11, 12]. A high percentage, up to 89% of GCTs are characterized by appearance of isochromosome 12p [i(12p)] [13].

Other factors unrelated to developmental and familial causes include testicular microlithiasis and HIV infection. A systematic review of 33 studies was done to evaluate the risk of developing testicular GCT and ITGCN in testicular microlithiasis patients. An overall risk ratio of 8.5% in TGCT and 10.5% in ITGCN was observed in patients with symptomatic testicular microlithiasis [14].

24.3 Clinical Signs and Symptoms

A complaint of painless testicular swelling or nodule, which is usually observed by the patient himself or their partner, is the first presenting complaint. Other symptoms like testicular heaviness, pressure-like sensation, and mild to moderate pain may be present. Testicular pain is not a usual complaint and is seen in only 10% patients. Painful testicular swellings are initially treated on the lines of acute orchitis or epididymitis (suspecting infectious cause) or other causes like testicular torsion. An ultrasound may become necessary to rule out cystic and solid testicular swelling.

About 10% patients present with symptoms related to a metastatic disease like:

- Palpable neck mass (supraclavicular lymph node)
- Cough, dyspnea, hemoptysis (lung metastasis)
- Lower back pain (bulky retroperitoneal lymph nodes with nerve root infiltration)
- Bony pains due to bone metastasis
- Unilateral/bilateral lower limb swelling (to IVC thrombosis)
- Anorexia, melena, vomiting (retroduodenal mass)

Gynecomastia is seen in about 5% males which is associated with production of human chorionic gonadotropin (hCG) by choriocarcinoma or trophoblastic tumors [15].

24.4 Testicular Examination

Testicular examination should begin with bimanual examination of scrotal contents. Examining the normal testis before proceeding to diseased testis is crucial as it gives information about size, contour, and consistency. Any firm or hard fixed area should be considered suspicious until proven otherwise. Cystic swellings can be well differentiated with solid tumors by transillumination test. Inguino-scrotal hernias can be differentiated by checking for reducibility and ring occlusion test, and per abdominal examination may reveal any intra-abdominal mass (possibly due to retroperitoneal lymphadenopathy).

Routine examination of supraclavicular fossa may reveal adenopathy in advanced disease.

Differential diagnosis of testicular mass	
Condition	*Features*
Testicular cancer	Firm, non-tender, non-transilluminable
Inguinal hernia	Cannot get above the swelling, non-transilluminable
Hydrocoele	Non-tender, transilluminable
Epididymal cyst	Non-tender, transilluminable, inferior pole of testis
Testicular torsion	Tender, thickened cord, opposite testis lie horizontal
Hematocele	Tender, history of trauma or surgery
Varicocele	Non-tender, decrease with scrotal elevation, bag of worms
Acute epididymitis	Tender, edema, and redness in scrotum
Acute orchitis	Tender, enlarged testis, fever
Spermatocele	Non-tender, posterior to head of epididymis, may or may not transilluminate

24.5 Histology

Biopsy is of limited value in case of a testicular mass under evaluation as it may lead to upstaging of disease due to scrotal seeding. A radical orchiectomy is usually both diagnostic and therapeutic. Information about histology, pathological staging, and prognosis can be inferred after radical orchiectomy.

Testicular cancers can be broadly classified into seminomatous and non-seminomatous, although non-seminomatous cancers can be of mixed variety and may carry some component of seminoma. Germ cell tumors may contain either single or mixed variety of histology.

24.5.1 Germ Cell Neoplasia In Situ (GCNIS)

All seminomas and post-pubertal NSGCTs develop from GCNIS which are neoplastic gonocyte-like cells with latent totipotent developmental potential, located in the spermatogonial niche of seminiferous tubules [16]. GCNIS can develop into an undifferentiated neoplasm (seminoma) or primitive zygotic neoplasm (embryonal carcinoma) [17]. Further differentiation from embryonal carcinoma results in somatically differentiated tumors (teratoma) or extraembryonal differentiated tumors (yolk sac and choriocarcinoma) [18].

24.5.2 Seminoma

This is the most common type of GCT (~50%) and is commonly seen as a component of mixed GCT. It is derived from transformed gonocytes and commonly presents at 30–49 years of age. Less than 5% patients present with metastatic disease at diagnosis. These tumors are almost always treated with curative intent with a 5-year overall survival of Stage I tumors ranging between 95 and 98%. Poor prognostic factors include age >40 years and advanced stage. Microscopically, seminomas contain sheets of neoplastic cells with abundant cytoplasm and round nuclei with lymphocytic infiltrates, which may be confused with lymphoma. On immunohistochemistry, placental alkaline phosphatase (PLAP) is usually positive and cytokeratin (CK) is weak positive. Negative tests are seen in AFP, CD30, and epithelial membrane antigen (EMA) [19]. Unlike NSGCT, seminomas do not secrete any tumor markers. However, some seminomas may contain syncytiotrophoblastic cells which produce hCG levels up to moderate levels [20].

24.5.3 Embryonal Carcinoma

Embryonal carcinoma is the most undifferentiated variety of GCTs usually presenting 10 years younger as compared to seminomas (25–30 years). Usual site of presentation are testes, anterior mediastinum, and retroperitoneum, and initial presentation could be due to metastatic symptoms such as lower backache, dyspnea, or hemoptysis. They are associated with high risk of metastasis and relapses. Microscopically they appear pleomorphic with scant cytoplasm and usually occur mixed in combination with other types of testicular GCTs (80–90%). IHC is positive for OCT 3/4, PLAP, AFP, hCG, and CD30 and negative for D2-40, CD117, glypican 3. They are mostly marker negative, and elevation of LDH is an important prognostic factor in metastatic embryonal carcinomas. CT abdomen can be used for initial evaluation of retroperitoneal nodes which are seen as heterogeneous and cystic in morphology [21].

24.5.4 Yolk Sac Tumor/Endodermal Sinus Tumor

These tumors are characterized by cells resembling those found in the embryonic or fetal yolk sac, allantois, and extraembryonic mesenchyme. They can be pre-pubertal (GCNIS unrelated) or post-pubertal (GCNIS related and usually seen in mixed GCT). Table 24.1 shows the characteristic features of both entities. Typical histologic appearance of yolk sac tumor is seen as a perivascular arrangement of epithelial cells, which is known as "*glomeruloid or Schillar Duval bodies*." IHC stains diffusely positive for AFP and may also be positive for cytokeratin, SALL4, glipican-3, PLAP, and CD117. These tumors are also associated with high levels of AFP in almost 95–98% cases [22].

24.5.5 Choriocarcinoma

These tumors consist of trophoblastic cells (both cytotrophoblasts and syncytiotrophoblasts) with associated hemorrhage. They strongly express hCG which correlates with burden of disease. The median age of presentation is 20–39 years. About 7–8% of testicular GCT have choriocarcinoma as a component, usually admixed with other GCT types. They spread by hematogenous route to lungs (67%), brain (20%), liver (60%), GIT retroperitoneal nodes, and bones. X-ray chest or CT thorax and abdomen can be used for staging. Metastatic choriocarcinoma creates hemorrhagic masses and presents with a characteristic "cannonball" appearance in the lungs on X-ray and CT scans. Poor prognostic factors include elevated hCG levels >50,000 IU/L (5-year OS—48%) and pure choriocarcinoma histology [23].

Table 24.1 Characteristic features of pre-pubertal and post-pubertal yolk sac tumors

	Pre-pubertal	Post pubertal
Histology	GCNIS unrelated	GCNIS related and mostly seen in mixed GCTs
Age	16–20 months	15–40 years
Risk factors	Unknown	Testicular dysgenesis syndrome; single nucleotide polymorphisms (KITLG, SPRY4, DMRT1)
Disease biology	Less aggressive 80%- Stage I; 6% relapse	More aggressive 40%- Stage I; 33% relapse
Hematogeneous spread	More common	Less common

24.6 Screening for Testicular Tumors

Routine screening is not recommended for testicular neoplasms in asymptomatic male adolescents or adults who do not have any known risk factors due to uncertainty in benefits of screening and relative infrequent incidence of disease. Although screening with clinical or self-examination is not harmful, it may lead to false positive results and anxiety in patients. Tumor markers have insufficient sensitivity and specificity to be used as screening test with no benefit in survival [24].

24.7 Diagnostic and Pre-treatment Workup

Diagnostic evaluation should include imaging (such as scrotal ultrasound), tumor biomarkers, and radical inguinal orchidectomy.

24.7.1 Initial Workup for Suspected Testicular Mass

Patient should be referred for a testicular ultrasound along with color Doppler.

Blood investigations should be sent:

1. Baseline gonadal function: serum levels of Testosterone, FSH and LH
2. Tumor markers: AFP, beta HCG, and LDH
3. Blood investigations as required for surgery in accordance with institutional protocol

If considered suspicious, patient should be prepared for the following:

1. Radical inguinal orchiectomy
2. Sperm banking
3. CECT abdomen and pelvis
4. Inguinal biopsy of contralateral testis, if bilateral testes show abnormalities (to facilitate testes sparing surgery)—inguinal exploration is done with exposure of testes and partial orchiectomy

The staging depends on the histopathological analysis of the surgical specimen, imaging findings, and repeating serum tumor markers after orchiectomy for staging (pre-surgery levels are not taken into consideration for staging purpose) [33].

24.8 Imaging

24.8.1 Testicular Ultrasound

Testicular ultrasound imaging is done through the trans-scrotal approach with linear transducer and is often coupled with color Doppler for better characterization and differentiation between benign and malignant nature of the lesions. It has a high sensitivity (near to 100%) for testicular malignancies and has the advantages of being low-cost, widely available and avoids use of radiation. US elastography can also aid in the diagnosis, as benign lesions are more likely to be "soft" as compared to "hard" malignant masses. About 2-3% of seminomas are bilateral and are often asynchronous. Metastatic lesions in testes can arise from prostate cancer, renal tumors, gastrointestinal carcinoids, and pancreatic tumors.

Scrotal ultrasound is a highly sensitive radiological tool which can differentiate between testicular and extra testicular mass. It can detect intratesticular lesions of size as small as 1-2mm and can simultaneously examine the contralateral testis.

The incidental finding of testicular microlithiasis on ultrasound may also provide evidence of GCNIS in an otherwise healthy man [14]. However, the potential of local staging with ultrasound is poor and unreliable due to difficulty in discerning tunica albuginea on ultrasound [25].

MRI testes: MRI can be considered when the testicular mass is indeterminate on ultrasonography [34].

The imaging characteristics of different conditions are enumerated in the following:

	Ultrasonography		
Condition	Features	Color Doppler	MRI
Seminoma	Homogenous Hypoechoic Solid Sometimes multi-lobulated Fibrinous septae Hemorrhage, necrosis, calcifications uncommon Rarely invade peri-testicular tissue Increased stiffness	Increased vascularity	Homogenous T2 hypo-intense T1 isointense Internal T2 hypo-intense bands On CEMRI Weak progressive wash-in No wash-out
Non-seminomatous germ cell tumors (NSGCTs)	Heterogeneous Ill-defined Infiltrative margins Can contain necrosis, hemorrhage, calcifications, cystic components, or echogenic foci	Increased vascularity	Heterogeneous in both T2 and T1 images T2 hypointense fibrous pseudocapsule

Condition	Ultrasonography		MRI
	Features	Color Doppler	
Embryonal carcinomas	Extensive necrosis and hemorrhage 25% have extra-testicular extension Frequently invades tunica albuginea	Increased vascularity	
Choriocarcinoma	Solitary or multifocal small masses Necrosis and hemorrhage Macroscopic lymphovascular invasion	Increased vascularity	
Yolk sac tumor	Varying proportion of cystic changes, necrosis, and hemorrhage	Increased vascularity	
Teratoma	Predominantly cystic Peripheral solid component Calcifications Echogenic intratumor fat	Increased vascularity	
Spermatocytic tumors	Cannot be differentiated from NSGCTs		
Leydig cell tumor	Round Hypoechoic Lobulated margins Difficult to differentiate from seminomas		T2 hyperintense central scar On CEMRI Rapid wash-in Slow wash-out
Sertoli cell tumors	Multicystic spoke wheel pattern		Homogenous T2 hyperintense Rim enhancement
Hemato-lymphoid testicular tumor	Diffuse or focal Hypoechoic 40% have hydrocele 20–30% bilateral synchronous testes involvement Infiltrate spermatic cord and epididymis	Increased vascularity	
Intratesticular hematoma	Iso-hyperechoic (early) Hypo-anechoic (late)	Avascular	
Intratesticular abscess	Ill-defined Hyperechoic halo	Peripheral hyperemia	
Intratesticular lipoma	Homogenous Hyperechoic	Avascular	Fat signal intensity
Testicular cysts	Thin walled (vs. thick walled in teratoma) Anechoic		

24.8.2 Lymph Node Imaging and Ruling Out Distant Metastasis

The draining lymph nodes of the testes are inter-aortocaval lymph nodes for the right testis and the para-aortic lymph nodes for the left-sided testis. One must be cautious to note the inguinal lymph node involvement if the patient has a history of prior inguinal or scrotal surgeries, breach of the testicular capsule, or involvement of the epididymis in the post-operative histopathology examination. The TNM system of classification considers only the retroperitoneal group of lymph nodes to be draining nodes, and so, all other lymph node involvement is distant metastasis per definition. Also the size of the node has to be mentioned as the sub-classification of stage II changes with increasing size.

While dealing with choriocarcinoma and yolk sac tumors, one needs to be careful to rule out distant mets, as these tumors metastasize commonly to lungs.

24.9 Computed Tomography

CT scan of abdomen, pelvis, and thorax is recommended for staging. CT is the present recommended imaging for retroperitoneal lymph node imaging. However, false negative rates as high as 44% have been described due to occult metastasis in retroperitoneal lymph nodes [26].

The sensitivity and specificity of CT changes with the cut-off considered for size of lymph node. The sensitivity and specificity at different cut-offs are—37% and 100% (10 mm), 70% and 70% (7–8 mm), 90% and 58% (3 mm). Though there is lack of consensus, 8 mm is considered by many to be the suitable cut-off for size of lymph nodes.

CT chest is recommended if retroperitoneal lymph nodes are positive or the histology has a propensity for hematogenous spread like choriocarcinoma or yolk sac tumor.

The advantages of CT are faster acquisition, relatively cheaper, good spatial resolution, and ability to detect necrosis (more in seminomas) or cysts (more in NSGCTs). But the disadvantage is that it is difficult to distinguish between benign and malignant lymph nodes.

24.10 MRI

In comparative studies, it has been found that the sensitivity and specificity for retroperitoneal lymph node detection are similar between CT and MRI. There is some indication that MRI can better predict the histology of cancer by inspecting the nodes, but this ability is hardly essential and mostly would not change management decisions. Taking into consideration the time taken for acquisition, cost, and lesser availability, MRI has not been popular for evaluating lymph node metastasis [35].

24.11 PET/CT

The sensitivity and specificity of PET/CT for lymph node evaluation in seminoma are 92% and 84%, whereas for NSGCTs it is 77% and 95%, respectively. But the role of PET/CT is still not established in the initial evaluation of testicular malignancies. The main role as of now is for the evaluation of residual masses after chemotherapy in seminomas. It can differentiate between fibrosis and true residual disease. It is 100% accurate for lesions more than 3 cm and 95% for lesions less than 3 cm. But the clinical utility for differentiating between fibrosis and residual NSGCT is still not established for PET/CT [27]. Only 56% of viable tumors can be predicted with PET/CT imaging which was not superior to 55% by conventional CT. Some institutes and trials are also exploring the integration of PET/CT as an interim analysis to decrease the cycles of chemotherapy required.

24.12 Immunohistochemistry (IHC)

The International Society of Urological Pathology Consensus Conference has provided recommendations for judicious use of IHC markers for testicular neoplasms [28] (Figs. 24.1 and 24.2).

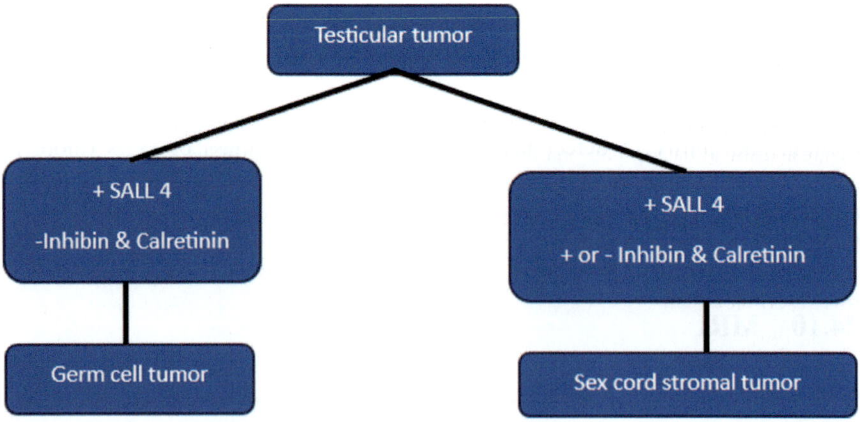

Fig. 24.1 Algorithm to differentiate between Testicular tumors

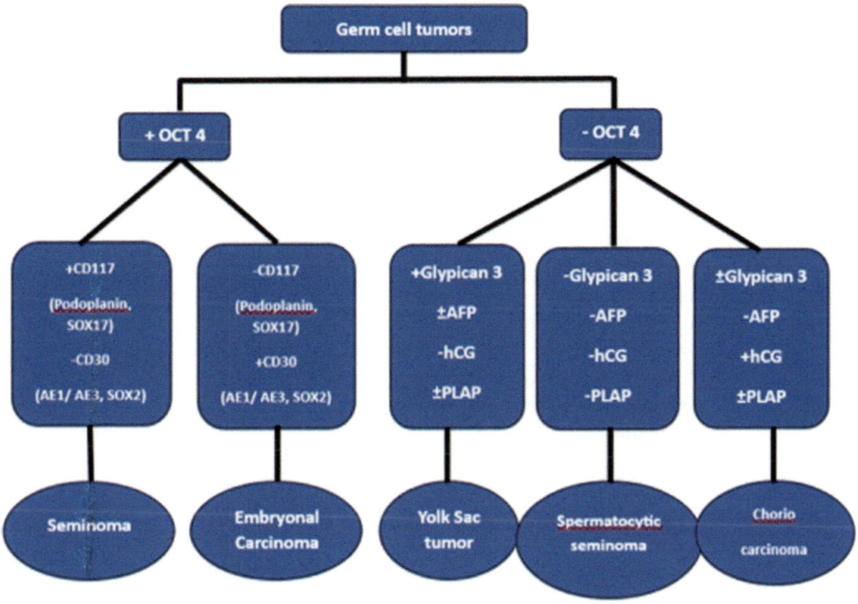

Fig. 24.2 Algorithm to differentiate GCTs on IHC

24.13 Serum Tumor Markers

Serum tumor markers are prognostic factors and important for diagnosis and staging of testicular GCTs. They should be tested before and after orchiectomy. The three classical markers for testicular cancer diagnosis and staging are alpha fetoprotein (AFP), produced in yolk sac tumor, human chorionic gonadotropin (hCG), produced by trophoblasts and lactate dehydrogenase (LDH), less specific marker with its concentration being proportional to tumor volume. They are elevated in 60% testicular cancers, 50–70% being AFP and 40–60% in hCG. Placental alkaline phosphatase (PLAP) is useful marker in monitoring in seminomas but is of limited value in smokers [24].

Utility of serum tumor markers:

- Determine the origin of GCTs, for example, seminomas in orchiectomy specimens showing elevated AFP levels are invariably treated according to NSGCT.
- Pre-orchiectomy and post-orchiectomy tumor marker levels are helpful in staging purposes.
- Response to therapy can be measured with serial monitoring of tumor markers before therapy as increasing concentration may suggest disease progression and need for salvage therapy.
- Rate of decline of tumor markers and their correlation with half-lives may indicate any slow-growing metastatic disease.

Table 24.2 Summary of serum tumor markers used in GCTs [24]

	AFP	HCG	LDH
Normal range	1 mg/L to 10–15 mg/L	1 U/L to 5–10 U/L	Depends on assay method used
Half-life (d)	5–7	1.5–3.0	Not reported
Seminoma	Never	Yes (15–20%)	Yes (40–60%)
NSGCT	Yes (10–20% localized disease; 40–60% advanced disease)	Yes (10–20% localized disease; 40–60% advanced disease)	Yes (40–60%)
Other malignancies	Hepatocellular carcinoma, gastric, lung, colon, pancreas	Neuroendocrine, bladder, kidney, lung, lymphoma, leukemia, GI	Lymphoma, small cell lung, ewings sarcoma, osteogenic sarcoma
Benign conditions	Alcohol abuse, hepatitis, cirrhosis, biliary tract obstruction	Marijuana intake, hypogonadism	Several conditions

Table 24.2 summarizes the key information about traditional serum tumor markers in GCTs.

24.14 Other Serum Biomarkers

A biomarker is defined by the World Health Organization as any measurable substance, structure, or biological process within the body or its products that can influence or predict the development, progression, or outcome of a disease. In the context of testicular cancer, an ideal biomarker would be a readily detectable molecule that is highly specific to germ cell tumors (GCTs).

MicroRNAs (miRNAs) represent a relatively novel class of small, non-coding RNA molecules that play a crucial role in the regulation of gene expression. They are involved not only in normal physiological processes such as cellular differentiation and development, but also in pathological mechanisms including oncogenesis. miRNAs exert their effects by interfering with messenger RNA (mRNA) translation, thereby functioning either as oncogenes or tumor suppressor genes depending on their targets.

Several studies have demonstrated significantly elevated serum levels of miR-371-3 in patients with germ cell tumors compared to healthy individuals. Importantly, these levels show a marked decline following orchiectomy, suggesting a strong association with tumor burden. The rapid postoperative decrease and the correlation between miRNA levels and tumor aggressiveness highlight the potential clinical utility of miR-371-3 as a biomarker. However, this marker is not entirely specific to GCTs, as increased expression has also been reported in other malignancies such as thyroid cancer [29].

In patients with germ cell tumors, circulating levels of miR-367-3p, miR-371a-3p, miR-372-3p, and miR-373-3p have been found to be significantly higher than those observed in healthy controls. Among these, miR-371a-3p has emerged as the most promising candidate, demonstrating a sensitivity of 84.7% and a specificity of 99.0% for the detection of GCTs [30].

Epigenetic alterations, particularly aberrant DNA methylation, have also been implicated in the pathogenesis of testicular cancer. Abnormal methylation patterns have been reported in up to half of affected patients, involving key tumor suppressor genes such as APC, p14 (ARF), p16 (INK4a), PTGS2, and RASSF1A [31]. Despite these observations, the clinical significance of DNA methylation profiles—especially their association with tumor aggressiveness and prognosis—remains uncertain due to limited and heterogeneous available data (Table 24.3).

Newly discovered biomarkers like High Mobility Group A (HMGA), POZ-AT hook-zinc finger protein (PATZ), Aurora-B, Nek-2, Octamer Binding Transcription Factor 3/4 (OCT3/4), c-kit, PLAP, NANOG, SOX2, and CDK10 are being reported to differentiate between histologic subtypes of testicular cancers and appear to be promising. Table 24.4 shows newer biomarkers and their relation with specific GCT.

Table 24.3 Clinical testicular biomarkers [29–31]

Molecular marker	Target	Characteristics	Utility in differentiating between GCT and controls	Correlation with GCT stage
miRNA	miRNA 367-3p, 37—3p, 372-3p, 373-3p	Non-coding RNA; interferes with translation of mRNA	Yes	Yes
mtDNA	mtDNA-79, mtDNA-220	Short length, simple structure	Yes	No
CircDNA	–	Same methylation pattern as tumor cells	Yes	No
CpG island hypermethylation	Gene silencing (APC, GSTP1, p14, p16, PTGS2, RASSF1A)	Easy to detect methylation; techniques already established	Yes	No
CTC	–	Easy to detect; molecular techniques	Yes	Yes

Table 24.4 Newer biomarkers and their relation to specific GCT

Newer biomarkers	Germ cell tumor
HMGA1	Seminoma
HMGA1 and HMGA2	Embryonal carcinoma
PATZ interacting protein RNF4	Role in progression of GCTs like embryonal carcinoma, yolk sac tumors
Aurora-B	Carcinoma in situ, seminoma, embryonal carcinoma; absent in teratoma and yolk sac carcinoma
OCT 3/4	Carcinoma in situ, seminoma, embryonal carcinoma
SOX2	Embryonal carcinoma
SOX17	Differentiated carcinoma in situ, seminoma from embryonal carcinoma

24.15 Staging

Staging Is Done by AJCC TNM Staging of Testicular Tumors

Staging of testicular tumors is pathological. A unique differentiation for germ cell tumors is inclusion of serum tumor markers "S" classifying as S0–S3. Testicular tumors are divided into three stage groupings.

Stage I—disease which is confined to testis

Stage II—confined to retroperitoneal lymph nodes with serum tumor markers in good prognosis range (S0–S1)

Stage III—metastasis beyond retroperitoneum or extra nodal location or tumor markers in poor prognosis range (S2–S3)

24.16 Prognostic Factors

Important prognostic factors include the following:

- Histology: HSGCT versus seminoma
- Lymphovascular invasion (LVI)
- Tumor size >4 cm
- Serum tumor markers (as per IGCCCG risk stratification) [32]
- Presence or absence of non-pulmonary visceral metastasis (NPVM)

References

1. Andreas P, Lorenzo R, Agneta N, Magnus K, Olof A. Age at surgery for undescended testis and risk of testicular cancer. N Engl J Med. 2007;356(18):1835–41.
2. Dieckmann KP, Skakkebaek NE. Carcinoma in situ of the testis: review of biological and clinical features. Int J Cancer. 1999;83(6):815–22.

3. von der Maase H, Rørth M, Walbom-Jørgensen S, et al. Carcinoma in situ of contralateral testis in patients with testicular germ cell cancer: study of 27 cases in 500 patients. Br Med J Clin Res Ed. 1986;293(6559):1398–401.
4. Prevalence of contralateral testicular intraepithelial neoplasia in patients with testicular germ cell neoplasms. | Journal of Clinical Oncology [Abstract]. [cited 2024 Jun 10]. Available from: https://ascopubs.org/doi/10.1200/JCO.1996.14.12.3126
5. Zequi Sde C, da Costa WH, Santana TB, Favaretto RL, Sacomani CA, Guimaraes GC. Bilateral testicular germ cell tumours: a systematic review. BJU Int. 2012;110(8):1102–9.
6. Cassio A, Cacciari E, D'Errico A, et al. Incidence of intratubular germ cell neoplasia in androgen insensitivity syndrome. Acta Endocrinol (Copenh). 1990;123(4):416–22.
7. Fosså SD, Chen J, Schonfeld SJ, et al. Risk of contralateral testicular cancer: a population-based study of 29,515 U.S. men. J Natl Cancer Inst. 2005;97(14):1056–66.
8. Gourlay WA, Johnson HW, Pantzar JT, McGillivray B, Crawford R, Nielsen WR. Gonadal tumors in disorders of sexual differentiation. Urology. 1994;43(4):537–40.
9. Hasle H, Mellemgaard A, Nielsen J, Hansen J. Cancer incidence in men with Klinefelter syndrome. Br J Cancer. 1995;71(2):416–20.
10. Washecka R, Dresner MI, Honda SAA. Testicular tumors in Carney's complex. J Urol. 2002;167(3):1299–302.
11. Han S, Peschel RE. Father-son testicular tumors: evidence for genetic anticipation? A case report and review of the literature. Cancer. 2000;88(10):2319–25.
12. Forman D, Oliver RT, Brett AR, et al. Familial testicular cancer: a report of the UK family register, estimation of risk and an HLA class 1 sib-pair analysis. Br J Cancer. 1992;65(2):255–62.
13. Fichtner A, Richter A, Filmar S, et al. The detection of isochromosome i(12p) in malignant germ cell tumours and tumours with somatic malignant transformation by the use of quantitative real-time polymerase chain reaction. Histopathology. 2021;78(4):593–606.
14. Tan MH, Eng C. Testicular microlithiasis: recent advances in understanding and management. Nat Rev Urol. 2011;8(3):153–63.
15. Tseng A Jr, Horning SJ, Freiha FS, Resser KJ, Hannigan JF Jr, Torti FM. Gynecomastia in testicular cancer patients. Prognostic and therapeutic implications. Cancer. 1985;56(10):2534–8.
16. Pathology Outlines – Germ cell neoplasia in situ [Internet]. [cited 2024 Jun 16]. Available from: https://www.pathologyoutlines.com/topic/testisitgcn.html
17. Almstrup K, Hoei-Hansen CE, Wirkner U, et al. Embryonic stem cell-like features of testicular carcinoma in situ revealed by genome-wide gene expression profiling. Cancer Res. 2004;64(14):4736–43.
18. Houldsworth J, Korkola JE, Bosl GJ, Chaganti RS. Biology and genetics of adult male germ cell tumors. J Clin Oncol. 2006;24(35):5512–8.
19. Chieffi P, Chieffi S, Franco R, Sinisi AA. Recent advances in the biology of germ cell tumors: implications for the diagnosis and treatment. J Endocrinol Invest. 2012;35(11):1015–20.
20. Seminoma [Internet]. [cited 2024 Jun 16]. Available from: http://www.pathologyoutlines.com/topic/testisseminomas.html
21. Embryonal carcinoma [Internet]. [cited 2024 Jun 16]. Available from: http://www.pathologyoutlines.com/topic/testisembryonal.html
22. Yolk sac tumor [Internet]. [cited 2024 Jun 16]. Available from: http://www.pathologyoutlines.com/topic/testisyst.html
23. Choriocarcinoma [Internet]. [cited 2024 Jun 16]. Available from: http://www.pathologyoutlines.com/topic/testischorio.html
24. Mir MC, Pavan N, Gonzalgo ML. Current clinical applications of testicular cancer biomarkers. Urol Clin North Am. 2016;43(1):119–25.
25. Marth D, Scheidegger J, Studer UE. Ultrasonography of testicular tumors. Urol Int. 1990;45(4):237–40.
26. Richie JP, Garnick MB, Finberg H. Computerized tomography: how accurate for abdominal staging of testis tumors? J Urol. 1982;127(4):715–7.

27. de Wit M, Brenner W, Hartmann M, et al. [18F]-FDG-PET in clinical stage I/II non-seminomatous germ cell tumours: results of the German multicentre trial. Ann Oncol. 2008;19(9):1619–23.
28. Ulbright TM, Tickoo SK, Berney DM, Srigley JR, Group M of the II in DUP. Best practices recommendations in the application of immunohistochemistry in testicular tumors: report from the international society of urological pathology consensus conference. Am J Surg Pathol. 2014;38(8):e50.
29. Belge G, Dieckmann KP, Spiekermann M, Balks T, Bullerdiek J. Serum levels of MicroRNAs miR-371-3: a novel class of serum biomarkers for testicular germ cell tumors? Eur Urol. 2012;61(5):1068–9.
30. Syring CI, Bartels J, Holdenrieder S, Kristiansen G, Müller SC, Ellinger J. Circulating serum miRNA (miR-367-3p, miR-371a-3p, miR-372-3p and miR-373-3p) as biomarkers in patients with testicular germ cell cancer. J Urol. 2015;193(1):331–7.
31. Ellinger J, Albers P, Perabo FG, Müller SC, von Ruecker A, Bastian PJ. CpG island hypermethylation of cell-free circulating serum DNA in patients with testicular cancer. J Urol. 2009;182(1):324–9.
32. GSRGT 2020: The International Germ Cell Cancer Collaborative Group (IGCCCG) Update [Internet]. [cited 2024 Jun 17]. Available from: https://www.urotoday.com/conference-highlights/gsrgt-2020/testicular-cancer/126571-gsrgt-2020-clinical-trials-corner-the-international-germ-cell-cancer-collaborative-group-igcccg-update.html
33. Gilligan T, Lin DW, Aggarwal R, et al. Testicular cancer, version 2.2020, NCCN clinical practice guidelines in oncology. J Natl Compr Canc Netw. 2019;17(12):1529–54.
34. Sharbidre KG, Lockhart ME. Imaging of scrotal masses. Abdom Radiol (NY). 2020;45(7):2087–108. https://doi.org/10.1007/s00261-019-02395-4. PMID: 31919649
35. Hale GR, Teplitsky S, Truong H, Gold SA, Bloom JB, Agarwal PK. Lymph node imaging in testicular cancer. Transl Androl Urol. 2018;7(5):864–74.

Chapter 25
Evaluation and Staging of Cervical Cancer

Satyajit Pradhan, Abhishek Shinghal, Shreya Shukla, and Shubham Dokania

Cervical cancer is a major public health problem, ranking as the fourth most common cancer globally among women, with approximately 6.62 lacs new cases and 3.48 lacs deaths in 2022, and age-standardized incidence and mortality rates 14.1 and 7.1 per 1 lac women, respectively [1]. Out of these, 85% new cases and 90% deaths happened in low- and middle-income countries (LMICs). Cervical cancer is the product of poor hygiene, poverty, high parity, and malnutrition. Some factors formerly believed to be associated with risk of cervical cancer are now known to be risk factors for HPV infection. High-risk HPV DNA is found in 99.7% of cervical cancer specimens. This chapter describes the presentation, evaluation, and staging of cervical cancers.

25.1 Epidemiology

Cervical cancer is a major public health problem, ranking as the fourth most common cancer globally among women, with approximately 6.62 lacs new cases and 3.48 lacs deaths in 2022, and age-standardized incidence and mortality rates 14.1 and 7.1 per 1 lac women, respectively [1]. Out of these, 85% new cases and 90% deaths happened in low- and middle-income countries (LMICs), where it is the second most common cancer and the third leading cause of cancer death among women [2, 3]. The highest regional incidence and mortality is in sub-Saharan Africa, Latin America, and the Caribbean, and the lowest in Northern America, Western

S. Pradhan (✉) · A. Shinghal · S. Dokania
Department of Radiation Oncology, MPMMCC & HBCH Varanasi, Units of Tata Memorial Centre and affliated with Homi Bhabha National institute, Mumbai, India

S. Shukla
Department of Radio-diagnosis, MPMMCC/ HBCH Varanasi, Units of Tata Memorial Centre and also affliated with Homi Bhabha National Institute, Mumbai, India

S. Pradhan et al. (eds.), *Evidence Based Handbook on Diagnosis and Staging in Oncology*, https://doi.org/10.1007/978-981-95-9701-7_25

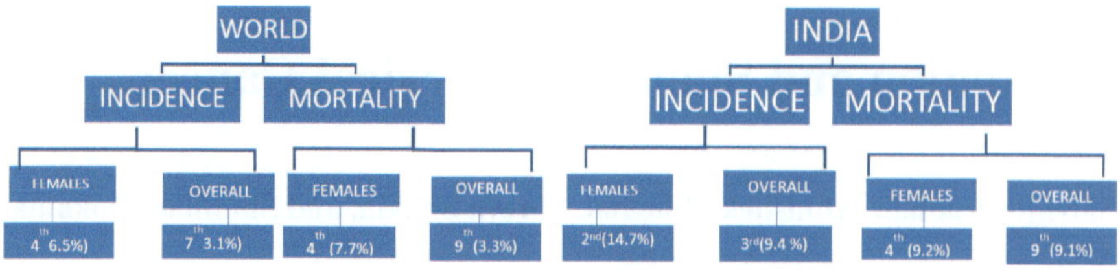

Fig. 25.1 Incidence and mortality of carcinoma cervix (in India and worldwide) [4]

Asia, and Australia/New Zealand [3]. The incidence and mortality data in India and worldwide have been illustrated in Fig. 25.1 [4]. With crude incidence 18.9 per 1 lac women, age-standardized incidence 17.7 per 1 lac women, and 2% cumulative risk of cervical cancer, India had one-fifth of all new cases in the world in 2022 [5, 6]. Rural women are at higher risk of developing cervical cancer as compared to their urban counterparts [7]. Papumpare district, Arunachal Pradesh, India, has the highest incidence rate of cervical cancer (27.7 per 100,000) in Asia [8]. This substantial discrepancy in incidence is explained by the dearth of effective public healthcare screening and facilities for effective treatment globally.

25.2 Risk Factors and Etiopathogenesis

Cervical cancer is the product of poor hygiene, poverty, high parity, and malnutrition. Some factors formerly believed to be associated with risk of cervical cancer are now known to be risk factors for HPV infection. High-risk HPV DNA is found in 99.7% of cervical cancer specimens [9]. Within 12–24 months of exposure to the virus, 90% HPV infections are cleared or become inactive. Infections by the high-risk HPV types (HPV 16 and 18 account for 70%, and HPV 31, 33, 45, 52, and 58 contribute to another 18% of cervical cancer cases worldwide) persist which then increase the risk of progression to cervical cancer [10, 11].

Risk factors with their mechanism of carcinogenesis are as follows:

1. Immunosuppression (e.g., AIDS, organ transplant). *Delays HPV clearance.*
2. Chlamydia infection: *disrupt N-cadherin-dependent cell-cell junctions.*
3. Number of sexual partners *(increased HPV acquisition).*
4. Sexual activity from an early age/giving birth at an age younger than 17 years *(increased HPV acquisition)* [12].
5. Multiple full-term pregnancies: *Increased hormones during pregnancy leading to squamous metaplasia.*
6. Cigarette smoking: *Suppresses immune action against HPV; aberrant DNA methyltransferase functioning, aberrant methylation of TSG p16.*
7. Long-term (> 5 years) use of oral contraceptives (2–four-fold increased risk): *Mechanism NOT clear.*
8. Poverty *(persistent HPV infection, poor immunity, poor genital hygiene).*

25.3 Etiopathogenesis of HPV-Induced Cervical Cancer

HPV infects the stratified epithelia and induces productive replication with differentiation [13]. HPV genome is either integrated host genome or remains into nuclei of infected cells as extrachromosomal plasmids. HPV manages to enter cells in the basal epithelial layer, the sole actively dividing cell layer, which gets exposed through micro-abrasions. HPV genome has 3 genomic regions: (i) 4-kb early (E) region encodes nonstructural proteins, (ii) 3-kb late (L) region encodes capsid proteins, (iii) 1-kb noncoding long control region (LCR) regulates viral replication. The dysplasia lesions as precursors of cervical cancer have characteristic expression of high-risk HPV (HR-HPV) E6/E7 genes, which contribute to genomic stability and malignant progression. HPV-mediated etiopathogenesis of cervical cancer is depicted in Fig. 25.2 [14].

E6 (150-amino acid protein) inactivates TP53 protein through ubiquitination and proteasome-mediated degradation. E7 (100-amino acid protein) alters activity of the cellular transcription factor E2F via its capacity to bind the RB protein. E6/E7 expression also induces telomerase activity and contributes to immortalization of human epithelial cells, thus providing the impetus for human epithelial cell transformation. HR-HPV genomes are integrated into host DNA in the more invasive cancers and cervical intraepithelial neoplasia (CIN) 2/3, while extrachromosomal HPV DNA is found in benign and low-grade lesions. Integration is randomly distributed over the whole host genome, preferably with genomic fragile sites. Loss of fragile Histidine tetrads expression and progression of HPV 16 + ve CIN are shown to be associated. HPV integration disrupts the E2 gene, leading to dysregulated E6/E7 expression. Absent amplification of E2 is a molecular marker of integration or progression in cervical cancer. Another early event in the transformation process is global DNA methylation in cervical tissue, which increases the grade of cervical dysplasia.

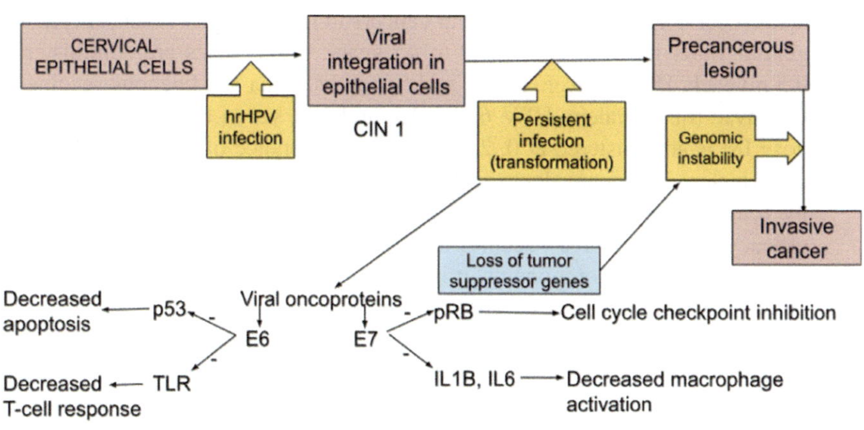

Fig. 25.2 HPV-mediated etiopathogenesis of carcinoma cervix [14]

25.4 Histology

Cervical cancer is classified into two main histological types: squamous cell carcinoma (SCC) and adenocarcinoma. Former is the predominant type, accounting for about 93–95%, while endocervical adenocarcinoma represents 4-6% of the histological types of cervical carcinoma (mainly in FIGO II and III stages) [15]. WHO classifies epithelial tumors of uterine cervix into three groups: SCC, adenocarcinomas, and other epithelial tumors (adenosquamous and undifferentiated carcinoma). Adenocarcinoma and adenosquamous carcinoma have poorer prognosis compared to SCC, specifically in Stage II and III [16].

25.5 Prevention

(i) *Primordial prevention*: Implies the role of administration in decreasing the onset of risk factors, by ensuring better genital hygiene practices (construction of toilets and availability of economical, good-quality sanitary pads), safe sexual practices and better nutritional status of poor females, and spreading awareness pertaining to parity and hygiene.

(ii) *Primary prevention:* This includes vaccines targeting primarily 9–14-year-old females (as per WHO guidelines and 9–26-year-old females as per Indian guidelines) [7, 17, 18], preferably before the onset of sexual activity. Available vaccines include the following: Cervarix, which is active against HPV serotypes 16 and 18. 3 doses, is administered IM, each 0.5 ml at 0, 1, and 6 months. Gardasil is active against HPV serotypes 6, 11, 16, and 18. Three doses are administered IM, each 0.5 ml at 0, 2, and 5 months. Both vaccines were developed using recombinant proteins from L1 (viral capsid)—antibody levels obtained are 100 times than that in natural infections. Gardasil 9 is active against HPV serotypes 6, 11, 16, 18, 31, 33, 45, 52, and 58, and is protective against cervical, vaginal, and vulvar cancers in females, anal canal cancer, and genital warts in the age group 9 to 45 years. Three doses are administered 0.5 ml each, IM are given at 0, 2, and 6 months. India's indigenous vaccine—Cervavac (quadrivalent–HPV 6, 11, 16, and 18), yet to be launched. 0.5 ml dose IM is administered at 0, 2, and 6 months. Choice of vaccine—Bivalent, quadrivalent, and nonavalent vaccines have similar efficacy and immunogenicity for cervical cancer prevention. There is limited data regarding safety or efficacy when the three vaccines are used interchangeably. Due to different characteristics and components, it is better to administer the same vaccine for all doses, unless the prior vaccine is unknown or available [19].

(iii) *Secondary prevention:* This implies identifying disease in the early stage by implementation of population-based screening. Length of survival after a diagnosis of cervical cancer depends on the cancer stage at the time of detection. The survival chance becomes better if detected at the precancerous stage through screening and treated at such a stage [20]. Therefore, it is important for all eligible women to avail cervical cancer screening. Over the past 30 years, cervical cancer incidence and mortality have decreased by more than 50% in high-income countries and by 10–40% in India with maximum attribution to the decrease in unhygienic practices, improved access to screening and early detection, and better treatment facilities [21].

National guidelines for cervical cancer screening recommend screening of females from 30 to 59 years of age at an interval of 3–5 years for VIA and cytology and 5–10 years for HPV testing for screen-negative females.

1. Optimal Resource Setting:

   (a) High-risk HPV (hrHPV) DNA testing: Most sensitive screening test available. It is 97.8% sensitive, 95.3% specific for detecting cervical neoplasm, with a PPV 10.9 and NPV 100% [22]. With such high NPV, screening interval can be prolonged up to 10 years in screen-negative women, minimum of 5 years [23]. As per an Indian trial, 50% reduction in cervical cancer mortality was seen with appropriate treatment of HPV screen-positive women [24]. It can replace cytology as the primary screening tool in optimal resource settings. Cervicovaginal sample is ideally collected by a clinician during a pelvic examination; can also be reliably collected by end users themselves (self-sampling)—acceptable in terms of ease of use, convenience, privacy, and physical and emotional comfort [25]. Most common device used for self-sampling is cervical swab.
   (b) Conventional cytology (Pap smear): Led to major reduction in incidence of cervical cancer over the past 5 decades. It has an advantage of ease of administration, so can be conducted frequently for a large population. But it needs skilled technicians, pathologists, infrastructure, and quality control measures. It is 43.5% sensitive, 98% specific for detecting cervical neoplasm, with a PPV 11.4% and NPV 99.7% [22].
   (c) Co-testing: No longer recommended by European QA guidelines.
   (d) Liquid-based cytology: Uses a brush for sampling instead of spatula used for conventional cytology. It is more expensive with lower false-negative rates and lower rate of unsatisfactory smears [26].

2. Resource-Constrained Setting

Visual inspection with acetic acid (VIA): economical, non-invasive, and real-time test with immediate results, so that management decisions can be taken at the same visit. It can also be performed by trained nurses and health workers. This involves unmagnified visualization of the cervix after application of 5% acetic acid. Aceto-white regions are the abnormal ones. It is 80% sensitive (range 79–82%), 92% specific (range 91–92%), and has PPV of 10% (range 9–10%) and NPV of 99% [27]. It is the best screening tool for resource-constrained settings. Modifications include VIA using magnification (VIAM) 2.5-4x and VILI (visual inspection after Lugol's Iodine) showing suspicious mahogany brown color.

Invasive SCC cervix is the end result of progressive CIN occurring within the metaplastic epithelium of the transformation zone, with the rates of progression varying as per different studies. A grossly abnormal lesion, with a suggestion of malignancy can be biopsied without either colposcopy or VIA; however, it is recommended to identify extent and location of lesions that are not visible. Present screening guidelines clearly define the role of colposcopy and biopsy. Main use of colposcopy in pre-invasive lesions is to determine the best suitable type of treatment—cryotherapy versus loop electrosurgical excision procedures (LEEP). Biopsy is performed with conventional biopsy forceps or with LEEP. The use of ablative and excision techniques in young nulliparous women is of concern as younger women are more likely to spontaneously clear HPV infections [28].

(iv) *Tertiary prevention:* Includes treatment of progressive cervical cancer (surgery, chemotherapy, radiotherapy) and palliative care as per patient's need. This aims to limit the needs augmentation of radiation oncology and gynecological surgery facilities.

WHO has taken an initiative to eliminate cervical cancer and has set various targets to reach by 30 [29]. These include full HPV vaccination of 90% girls by 15 years of age, screening 70% women using a high-performance test by age 35 and again by 45, and ensuring that 90% of women identified with cervical cancer receive adequate treatment.

25.6 Clinical Features

Transvaginal bleeding (constituting post-coital, intermenstrual, and postmenopausal) is the most common symptom. Among these, post-coital is the most specific symptom associated with this pathology. Serosanguinous foul-smelling discharge per vagina can also occur in many patients secondary to either tumor necrosis or secondary bacterial infections. Bleeding and discharge per vagina are more evident early in exophytic tumors; however, the manifestations are subtle in endocervical ones where bulk of disease constitutes the infiltrative component. There may be groin swelling- due to either lower third vaginal involvement or due to non-regional nodal metastasis to inguinal region. Back pain may also occur with involvement of uterosacral ligament or vertebral metastases. Few patients might present with pain per abdomen, which could be due to significant para-aortic lymph node metastases or gross hydroureteronephrosis. In case of advanced disease, bladder or rectal mucosal invasion can lead to hematuria, hematochezia, and/or pelvic pain. Such patients might also present with unilateral gross lower limb edema, probably due to large pelvic nodes causing vascular or lymphatic obstruction.

25.7 Workup

1. *History Taking*

Bleeding per vagina is quantified using the number of pads soaked daily, presence or absence of clots, history of blood transfusion. For per vagina discharge, quantity and history of associated fever should be asked. Onset and duration of bleeding and discharge must be elicited. Abdominal pain, lower back pain, and possible complications (like pedal edema, backache, flank pain radiating to groin, hematuria or bleeding PR, neuropathic pain) should be checked. To exclude causes other than carcinoma cervix, look for any history of hormonal replacement therapy or Tamoxifen use (indicating endometrial cancer), history of chronic pelvic pain with dysmenorrhea (chronic PID, endometriosis), history of mass protruding per vagina (prolapse). History of other STDs, genital warts in the patient or in male partner, multiple sexual partners, age of first intercourse, parity, smoking, any HPV vaccination must be elicited. Patient's socio-economic history including poor nutritional status, poverty, and poor genital hygiene (menstrual or sexual) are significant risk factors. Whether the patient stays in a kutcha house, uses unhygienic clothes during menses, or has a working toilet in her house has a bearing on the risk of cervical cancer. History of comorbidities is important for treatment options.

2. *Local Examination*

Patients must be well counseled before physical examination, with informed verbal and written consent in the presence of a female attendant in a well-lit room. Patients must be asked to void and then lie in lithotomy position before local examination. First a per vagina examination is done to check for any cervical growth—its size, friability, consistency, involvement of anterior/posterior cervical lips, fornices, extent of vaginal involvement, distance from introitus, whether bleeding on touch or any skip lesions in vagina. Per speculum examination is done using well-lubricated Cusco's self-retaining bivalve speculum and lesion checked for friability, size, extent, any bleeding on touch, proliferative/ulcerative/ulceroproliferative, ectocervical/endocervical extension, and vaginal extension (including skip lesions). A clinical drawing of the examination findings should be drawn, both at the time of diagnosis and prior to brachytherapy, to depict the extent of disease, based on IBS-GEC ESTRO-ABS recommendations [30]. The diagram with scaled markings can have erroneous interpretation in some cases as the anatomy is variable; hence, manual marking of tumor dimensions and Near Maximum Distance (NMD) should be done as shown in Fig. 25.3.

Bidigital examination of cervix and vagina involves introducing middle and index fingers of gloved and lubricated hand into the vagina, with the thumb abducted and ring and little fingers flexed into the palm. Bimanual examination is done for palpation of uterus and adnexa. For palpating uterus, vaginal fingers are placed in the posterior fornix to lift the uterus and simultaneously the other hand is placed midway between umbilicus and symphysis pubis and pressed downward toward the

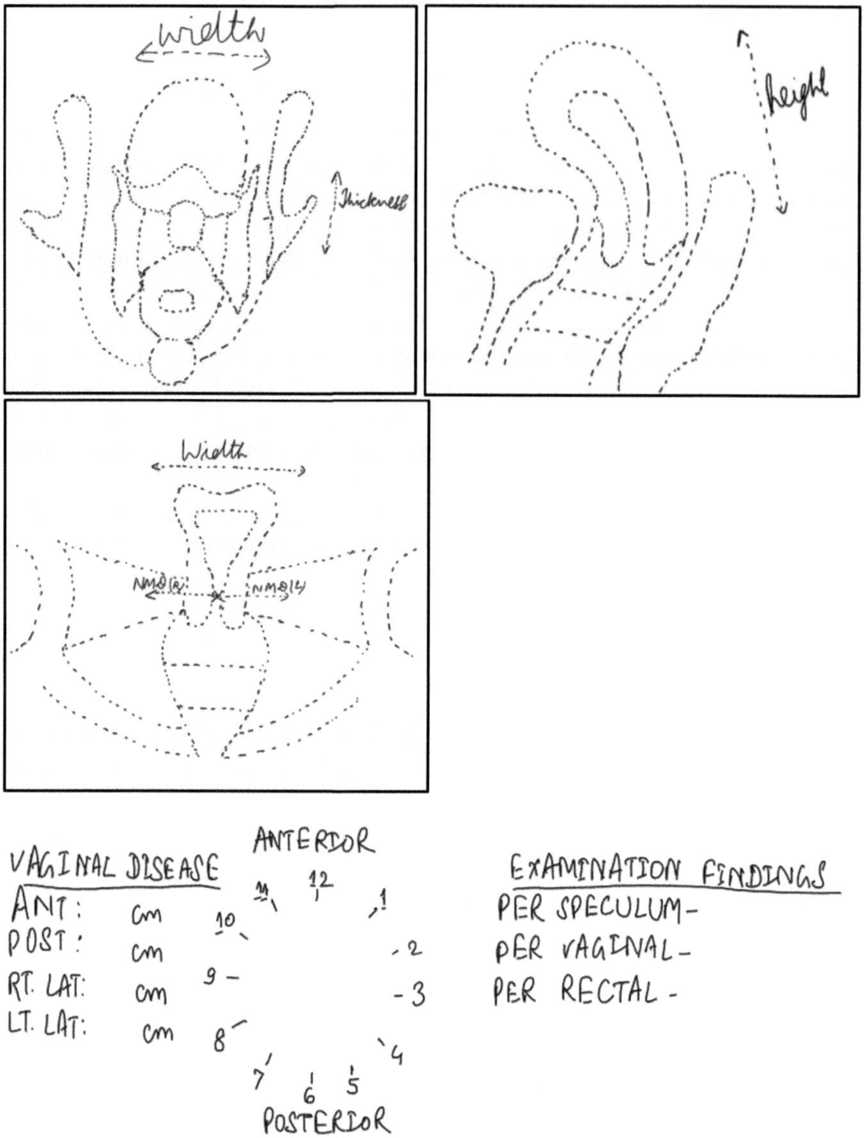

Fig. 25.3 Clinical drawing of examination findings in carcinoma cervix

pelvic hand. For adnexal palpation, vaginal fingers are slid into each lateral fornix and ipsilateral abdominal region, lateral to umbilicus is pressed. Per rectal bidigital examination with one finger in vagina and other in anal canal is done to look for any perineal skin tag, fissure, fistula, or protruding growth; anal tone, smoothness of rectal mucosa; parametrial thickening, nodularity, lateral extent, and fixity to lateral pelvic wall. Inguinal lymph nodes must be examined.

3. *Investigations*:

   (i) *Baseline fitness investigations:* Blood investigations (complete blood count, liver function test, kidney function test, serum electrolytes, coagulation profile) and chest X-ray. Adequate hemoglobin level (preferably above 10 gm/dl) is an important prognostic factor for better local control, and disease-free survival [31].

   (ii) *Investigation for confirmation of diagnosis:* Diagnosis is confirmed using histopathological examination of the biopsied sample. The types of biopsies include punch biopsy (using biopsy forceps), cone biopsy (using laser or scalpel), or endocervical curettage (to scrape endocervical canal). Any palpable ulcero-proliferative growth in cervical region with relevant symptoms can be biopsied while doing per speculum examination achieving adequate hemostasis using a vaginal pack if needed.

   (iii) *Investigations for staging*: Include imaging and endoscopy. Imaging options available include the following:

      1. *Magnetic resonance imaging (MRI):* Advantage of MRI is better soft tissue delineation due to higher soft tissue contrast, so recommended for demonstration of size, location, local extension, stromal ring invasion, involvement of parametrium, and bladder-rectal invasion [32]. It is the standard for local staging of carcinoma cervix and defining local extent of primary disease. Sensitivity and specificity of lymph nodal delineation are similar to CT. Fusion of DWI with T2-weighted images significantly ($p < 0.05$) increases diagnostic accuracy compared to T2-weighted images alone [33]. Vaginal jelly should be used for adequate evaluation of full circumference of vagina and fornices. However, clinical examination cannot be replaced by MRI for accurate assessment of vaginal involvement. Disadvantages of MRI include limited availability, longer duration for scanning, difficulty for claustrophobic patients, and lack of expertise in its interpretation.
      2. *Computed tomography (CT)*: It is widely available imaging modality which provides high spatial resolution images within a shorter period. Cervical lesions are usually hypodense and heterogenous. It has limited value in detection of early parametrial and cervical stromal invasion. In most cases, it overestimates the parametrial and vaginal invasion [34]. It is equally capable than MRI with sensitivity of 31–50%, while specificity of 84–92% in evaluating regional and non-regional lymph node metastases. It is also used as a cheaper modality to rule out distant metastases. It has much lower scan time compared to MRI. The sensitivity, specificity, positive predictive value (PPV), and negative predictive value (NPV) for different parameters individually for CT and MRI are compared in Table 25.1, [32] (Figs. 25.4 and 25.5).

3. *^{11}FDG postitron emission tomography (PET):* Use of whole-body PET CT is on the assent due to its superiority over other imaging in detecting Nodal and distant metastasis. Hence, it is recommended as the investigation of choice to rule out nodal and distant metastasis in locally advanced cervical cancer. Its higher negative predictive value (NPV) than conventional imaging confers advantage in

Table 25.1 Comparison of the available parameters for CT and MRI for locoregional disease

	CT				MRI			
	Sens(%)	Spec(%)	PPV(%)	NPV(%)	Sens(%)	Spec(%)	PPV(%)	NPV(%)
Primary tumor visualization	93	N/A	N/A	N/A	93	N/A	N/A	N/A
Parametrial invasion	43–55	71	53	62	52–80	63–91	55–67	61–95
Bladder invasion	64–100	73–92	40	100	75–100	88–91	7	96–100
Rectal invasion	45–100	88–91	N/A	100	71–100	91	17	96–100
Lymph node metastasis	31–50	84–92	61	64	36–89	78–99	64–68	57

Evaluation [32]

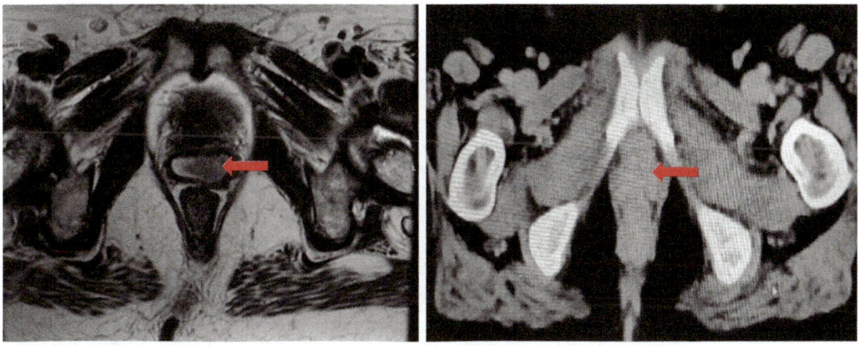

Fig. 25.4 Depicting better visualization of vaginal involvement on MRI than CT

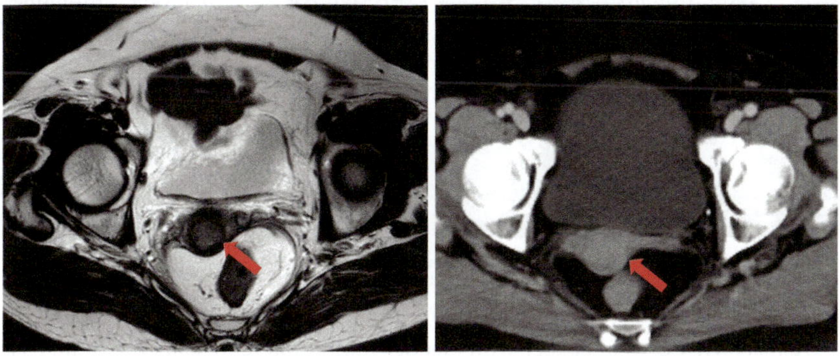

Fig. 25.5 Depicting better visualization of early parametrial involvement on MRI than CT

evaluating recurrent or residual disease. It can also differentiate post radiation fibrosis from residual or recurrence [35].

4. *Ultrasonography (USG):* It is beneficial in resource-constrained settings where CT scan is not available. Transabdominal USG can detect cervical lesion, grossly enlarged pelvic lymph nodes, hydroureteronephrosis, and presence of peritoneal metastasis. Transvaginal USG (TVS), being readily available, is the initial imaging modality for any gynecological disease. It effectively shows presence of hydro/pyometra and extension into the uterine corpus, and for obtaining tissue biopsy samples in case of clinically obscured lesions. Transrectal USG (TRUS) is an alternative in case of excess bleeding per vagina and to assess endophytic components of the cervical mass. It has sensitivity of 87–95% for parametrial invasion detection and 93.6% for tumor detection [36]. TRUS and TVS are very accurate for early-stage tumor classification. Main disadvantage is operator-dependent and limited interpretation value (Fig. 25.6).

The endoscopic investigations for staging include the following:

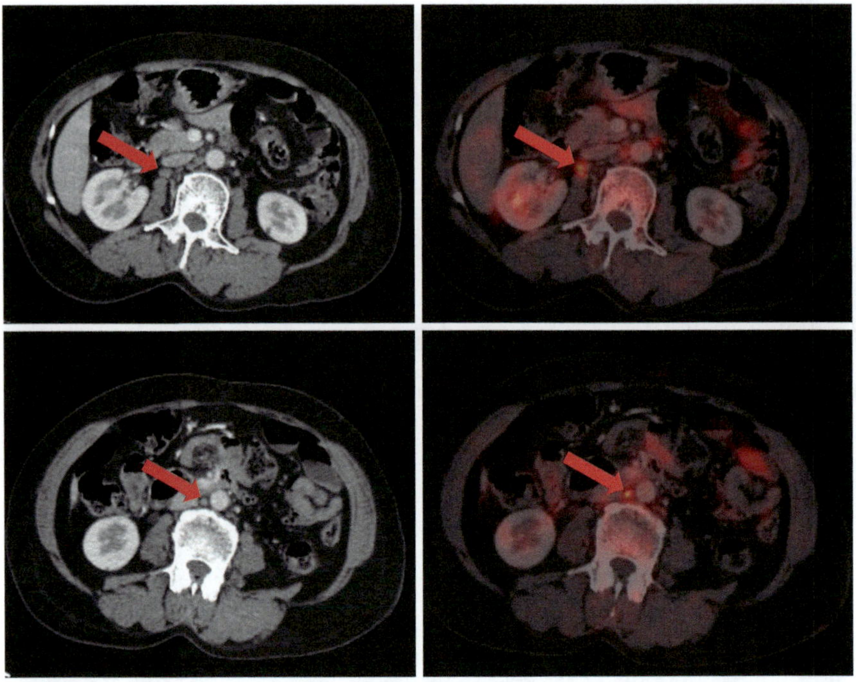

Fig. 25.6 Depicting better visualization of para-aortic LN on PETCT than CT

1. *Cystoscopy:* Cervical cancer with bladder infiltration represents 2% of all cases [37]. In cases with clinically and radiologically suspected bladder infiltration, a cystoscopy should be done to look for mucosal ulcerations or bullous mucosal edema. Bullous edema (caused due to involvement of lymphatics without mucosal involvement) is not considered as bladder infiltration.
2. *Sigmoidoscopy:* In clinically and radiologically suspected rectal infiltration (much less incidence than bladder infiltration), a sigmoidoscopy should be done to confirm the mucosal infiltration.

25.8 FIGO (2018) and TNM Staging

Cervical cancer is staged clinically. Primary tumor and nodal involvement, size, and extent-based staging by FIGO (International Federation of Gynecology and Obstetrics) (2018) and TNM staging by AJCC (American Joint Committee on Cancer) (eighth edition) are used commonly [38].

Figures showing images to identify FIGI stage II, III, and IVA cervical cancer respectively are shown below

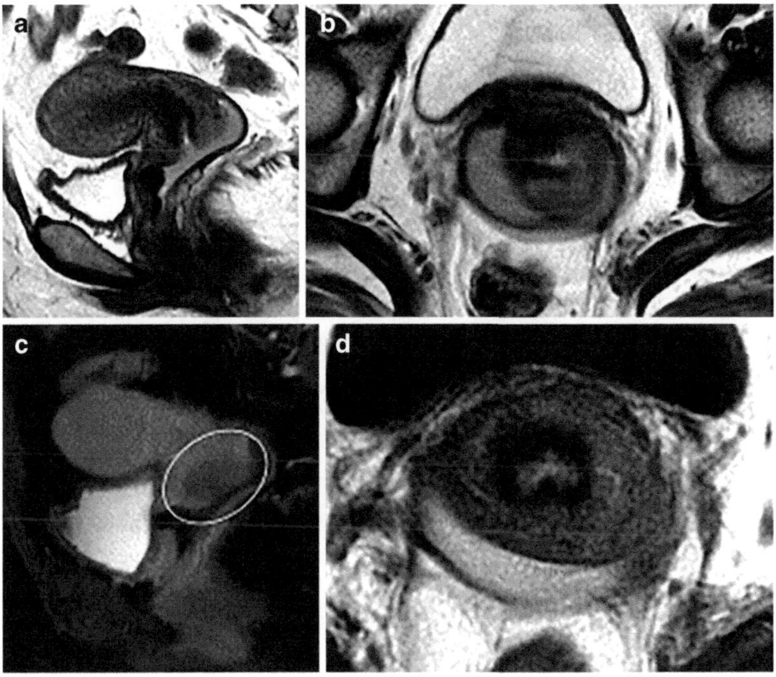
a
b
c
d

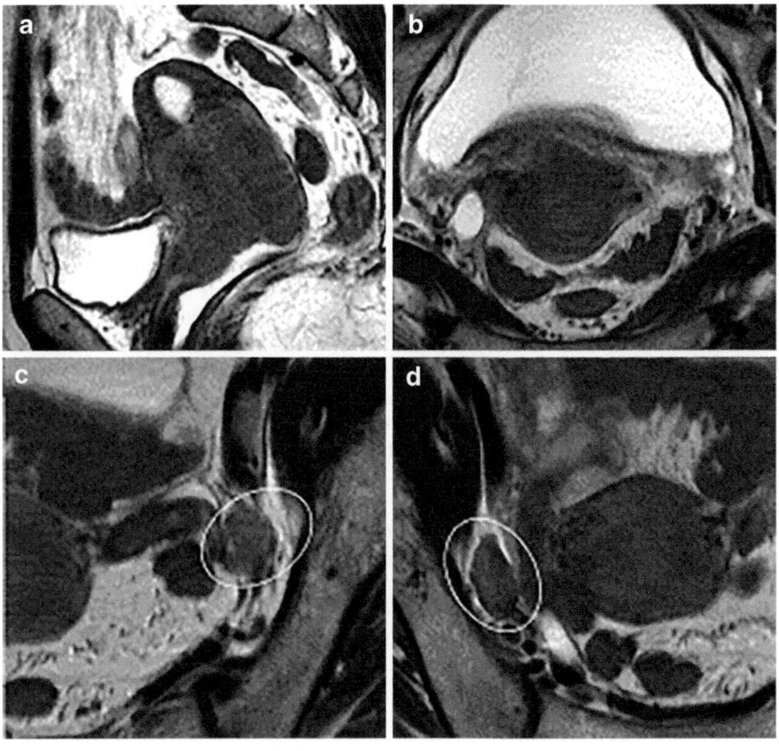
a
b
c
d

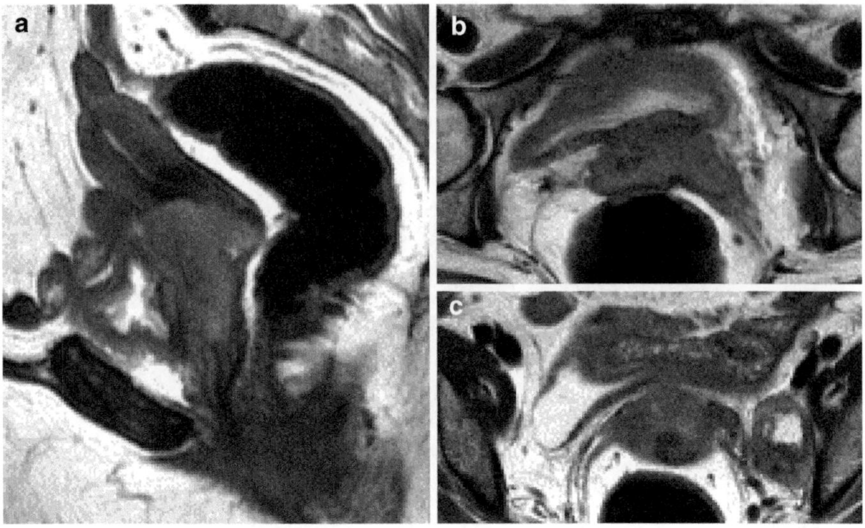

References

1. 23-cervix-uteri-fact-sheet.pdf [Internet]. [cited 2024 May 17]. Available from: https://gco.iarc.who.int/media/globocan/factsheets/cancers/23-cervix-uteri-fact-sheet.pdf
2. WHO fact sheet on cervical cancer [Internet]. Available from: https://www.who.int/news-room/fact-sheets/detail/cervical-cancer#:~:text=Cervical%20cancer%20is%20the%20fourth%20most%20common%20cancer,2020%20occurred%20in%20low-%20and%20middle-income%20countries%20%281%29.
3. Torre LA, Bray F, Siegel RL, Ferlay J, Lortet-Tieulent J, Jemal A. Global cancer statistics, 2012. CA A Cancer J Clin. 2015 Mar;65(2):87–108.
4. Sung H, Ferlay J, Siegel RL, Laversanne M, Soerjomataram I, Jemal A, et al. Global cancer statistics 2020: GLOBOCAN estimates of incidence and mortality worldwide for 36 cancers in 185 countries. CA A Cancer J Clin. 2021;71(3):209–49.
5. Cancer Today [Internet]. [cited 2024 May 16]. Available from: https://gco.iarc.who.int/today/
6. 356-india-fact-sheet.pdf [Internet]. [cited 2024 May 17]. Available from: https://gco.iarc.who.int/media/globocan/factsheets/populations/356-india-fact-sheet.pdf
7. Kaarthigeyan K. Cervical cancer in India and HPV vaccination. Indian J Med Paediatr Oncol. 2012 Jan;33(01):7–12.
8. Report of National Cancer Registry Programme 2012–2016 [Internet]. Available from: http://cancerindia.org.in/wp-content/uploads/2022/08/CancerCervixUteri.pdf
9. Walboomers JMM, Jacobs MV, Manos MM, Bosch FX, Kummer JA, Shah KV, et al. Human papillomavirus is a necessary cause of invasive cervical cancer worldwide. J Pathol. 1999;189(1):12–9.
10. Asiaf A, Ahmad ST, Mohammad SO, Zargar MA. Review of the current knowledge on the epidemiology, pathogenesis, and prevention of human papillomavirus infection. Eur J Cancer Prev. 2014;23(3):206–24.
11. de Sanjose S et al. Human papillomavirus genotype attribution in invas.pdf [Internet]. [cited 2024]. 2010. Available from: https://www.clinicalkey.com/service/content/pdf/watermarked/1-s2.0-S1470204510702308.pdf?locale=en_US&searchIndex=

12. Collins SI, Mazloomzadeh S, Winter H, Rollason TP, Blomfield P, Young LS, et al. Proximity of first intercourse to menarche and the risk of human papillomavirus infection: a longitudinal study. Int J Cancer. 2005;114(3):498–500.
13. Astudillo-de La Vega H, Ruiz-Garcia E, Lopez-Camarillo C, De La Garza-Salazar JG, Meneses-Garcia A, Benitez-Bribiesca L. Malignant transforming mechanisms of human papillomavirus. In: De La Garza-Salazar JG, Morales-Vásquez F, Meneses-Garcia A, editors. Cervical cancer [Internet]. Cham: Springer; 2017. p. 35–56. [cited 2023 Nov 8]/ Available from: http://link.springer.com/10.1007/978-3-319-45231-9_3.
14. Ramachandran D, Dörk T. Genomic risk factors for cervical cancer. Cancer. 2021;13(20):5137.
15. Agarwal S, Malhotra K, Sinha S, Rajaram S. Profile of gynecologic malignancies reported at a tertiary care center in India over the past decade: comparative evaluation with international data. Indian J Cancer. 2012;49(3):298.
16. Meng Y, Chu T, Lin S, Wu P, Zhi W, Peng T, et al. Clinicopathological characteristics and prognosis of cervical cancer with different histological types: a population-based cohort study. Gynecol Oncol. 2021;163(3):545–51.
17. Roy S, Shankar A, Rath GK. HPV vaccination of girl child in India: intervention for primary prevention of cervical cancer. Asian Pac J Cancer Prev. 2018;19(9):2357–8.
18. WHO updates recommendations on HPV vaccination schedule [Internet]. [cited 2023 Nov 9]. Available from: https://www.who.int/news/item/20-12-2022-WHO-updates-recommendations-on-HPV-vaccination-schedule
19. WER9219–241-268.pdf [Internet]. [cited 2023 Nov 8]. Available from: https://iris.who.int/bitstream/handle/10665/255354/WER9219-241-268.pdf?sequence=1
20. 3_ NCG_INDIA_Rev_Preventive Oncology_Primary_Care.pdf [Internet]. [cited 2023 Nov 8]. Available from: https://tmc.gov.in/ncg/docs/PDF/DraftGuidelines/Preventive/3_%20NCG_INDIA_Rev_Preventive%20Oncology_Primary_Care.pdf
21. Singh M, Jha RP, Shri N, Bhattacharyya K, Patel P, Dhamnetiya D. Secular trends in incidence and mortality of cervical cancer in India and its states, 1990–2019: data from the global burden of disease 2019 study. BMC Cancer. 2022 Dec;22(1):149.
22. Petry KU, Menton S, Menton M, Van Loenen-Frosch F, De Carvalho Gomes H, Holz B, et al. Inclusion of HPV testing in routine cervical cancer screening for women above 29 years in Germany: results for 8466 patients. Br J Cancer. 2003;88(10):1570–7.
23. Arbyn M, Anttila A, Jordan J, Ronco G, Schenck U, Segnan N, et al. European guidelines for quality Assurance in Cervical Cancer Screening. Second edition—summary document. Ann Oncol. 2010;21(3):448–58.
24. Sankaranarayanan R, Nene BM, Shastri SS, Jayant K, Muwonge R, Budukh AM, et al. HPV screening for cervical cancer in rural India. N Engl J Med. 2009;360(14):1385–94.
25. Nishimura H, Yeh PT, Oguntade H, Kennedy CE, Narasimhan M. HPV self-sampling for cervical cancer screening: a systematic review of values and preferences. BMJ Glob Health. 2021;6(5):e003743.
26. Pankaj S, Nazneen S, Kumari S, Kumari A, Kumari A, Kumari J, et al. Comparison of conventional pap smear and liquid-based cytology: a study of cervical cancer screening at a tertiary care center in Bihar. Indian J Cancer. 2018;55(1):80.
27. Sauvaget C, Muwonge R, Sankaranarayanan R. Meta-analysis of the effectiveness of cryotherapy in the treatment of cervical intraepithelial neoplasia. Int J Gynecol Obste. 2013;120(3):218–23.
28. Korets S, Cain JM. Diagnosis and therapy of benign and preinvasive disease of the cervix. GLOWM [Internet]. 2015; [cited 2023 Nov 8]; Available from: https://www.glowm.com/section-view/item/20
29. Cervical Cancer Elimination Initiative [Internet]. [cited 2023 Nov 8]. Available from: https://www.who.int/initiatives/cervical-cancer-elimination-initiative
30. Mahantshetty U, Poetter R, Beriwal S, Grover S, Lavanya G, Rai B, et al. IBS-GEC ESTRO-ABS recommendations for CT based contouring in image guided adaptive brachytherapy for cervical cancer. Radiother Oncol. 2021;160:273–84.

31. Thomas G. The effect of hemoglobin level on radiotherapy outcomes: the Canadian experience. Semin Oncol. 2001;28:60–5.
32. Petsuksiri J, Jaishuen A, Pattaranutaporn P, Chansilpa Y. Advanced imaging applications for locally advanced cervical cancer. Asian Pac J Cancer Prev. 2012;13(5):1713–8.
33. Park JJ, Kim CK, Park SY, Park BK. Parametrial invasion in cervical cancer: fused T2-weighted imaging and high- *b* -value diffusion-weighted imaging with background body signal suppression at 3 T. Radiology. 2015;274(3):734–41.
34. Yitta S, Hecht EM, Mausner EV, Bennett GL. Normal or abnormal? Demystifying uterine and cervical contrast enhancement at multidetector CT. Radiographics. 2011;31(3):647–61.
35. Grant P, Sakellis C, Jacene HA. Gynecologic oncologic imaging with PET/CT. Semin Nucl Med. 2014;44(6):461–78.
36. Dhamija E, Gulati M, Manchanda S, Singhal S, Sharma D, Kumar S, et al. Imaging in carcinoma cervix and revised 2018 FIGO staging system: implications in radiology reporting. Indian J Radiol Imaging. 2021 Jul;31(03):623–34.
37. Sun R, Koubaa I, Limkin EJ, Dumas I, Bentivegna E, Castanon E, et al. Locally advanced cervical cancer with bladder invasion: clinical outcomes and predictive factors for vesicovaginal fistulae. Oncotarget. 2018;9(10):9299–310.
38. Bhatla N, Berek JS, Cuello Fredes M, Denny LA, Grenman S, Karunaratne K, et al. Revised FIGO staging for carcinoma of the cervix uteri. Intl J Gynecol Obste. 2019;145(1):129–35.

Chapter 26
Evaluation and Staging of Endometrial Cancer

Abhishek Shinghal, Jhansi Pattanaik, and Prashasti Sharma

26.1 Introduction and Epidemiology

Endometrial cancer originates from the lining epithelium of the uterus. It is also called uterine corpus cancer or cancer of the corpus uterus. With the advent of a proper understanding of tumor biology now we can classify endometrial carcinoma into distinct histological subtypes and molecular phenotypes. According to GLOBOCAN 2022, there were 4,20,368 cases and 97,723 deaths due to endometrial cancer [1, 2]. Endometrial cancer accounts for 4.4% of all cancers seen in women worldwide. It is the fourth most commonly diagnosed cancer in women, and the mortality rate due to this cancer is increasing at a rate of 1% per year [3]. India has a relatively lower incidence, with 17,420 new cases and 6845 deaths as per GLOBOCAN 2022 [1]. The five population-based cancer registries (PBCRs) with the highest rates of cancer corpus uteri were located in the districts of Hyderabad, Chennai, Bangalore, Thiruvananthapuram, and Delhi, according to the reports issued in 2020 by NCDIR and ICMR as part of the national cancer registry program (2012–2016).

Carcinoma endometrium was previously regarded as a disease of the developed world, but the burden of carcinoma endometrium is increasing in India. The estimation by the national cancer registry shows a cumulative risk of 1 in 190 and a 5-year prevalence of 6.56 per 100,000 women [4]. The evaluation of endometrial cancer warrants a proper understanding of the disease pathology, indications for endometrial biopsy, various techniques for endometrial tissue sampling, imaging for proper diagnosis, and assessment of metastasis. Management of endometrial cancer is multimodal, which includes surgery and surgical staging, adjuvant treatment in the form

A. Shinghal (✉) · J. Pattanaik · P. Sharma
Department of Radiation Oncology, MPMMCC/HBCH, Varanasi, Units of Tata Memorial Centre and affliated with Homi Bhabha National institute, Mumbai, India

S. Pradhan et al. (eds.), *Evidence Based Handbook on Diagnosis and Staging in Oncology*, https://doi.org/10.1007/978-981-95-9701-7_26

of radiotherapy, chemotherapy, hormone therapy, and targeted therapy, along with post treatment timely follow-ups for early detection and salvage of recurrences.

26.2 Risk Factors

Uninterrupted endothelial proliferation culminates in the pathogenesis of endometrial cancer. The risk factors can be subdivided into environmental or genetic.

- *Environmental:*

Increasing age has been associated with increased risk of this cancer. Higher BMI increases the risk due to the conversion of adipocytes from adrenal-derived androstenedione to estrone, a weak circulating estrogen that increases the bioavailable estrogens in the circulation and the endometrial tissue. Obesity and hyperinsulinemia, a common feature of insulin-resistant type II diabetes, lower the levels of sex hormone binding globulin (SHBG) to result in higher circulating levels of free estrogen. The higher the BMI, the more is the risk of endometrial cancer [5] (relative risk with increasing BMI as follows: 30–34.9 the RR-2.53; 35–39.9 the RR-2.77; $\geq$ 40 the RR −6.25). Diabetes mellitus (RR-1.89) and metabolic syndrome (1.89), anovulation (OR-1.22), and nulliparity (OR-1.76) are linked to endometrial cancer [6–9]. Early menarche or late menopause increases estrogenic exposure and endometrial cancer risk. Estrogen-secreting, ovarian tumors, and polycystic ovaries (PCO), which interfere with regular ovulation and menstruation, result in elevated levels of free estrogens leading to endometrial hyperplasia [6]. History of breast cancer (RR-1.6) and long-term use of tamoxifen (RR-2.3) are associated with increased risk [7, 8]. Tamoxifen has an antiestrogenic action in premenopausal women, but a mild estrogenic impact in post-menopausal women because estrogen receptors are upregulated in this age group. Tamoxifen's risk of endometrial cancer, including the duration of usage, must be balanced against its effectiveness in lowering breast cancer mortality. Hypertension, family history of endometrial cancer, and prior pelvic irradiation also increase the risk of development of endometrial cancer.

- *Genetics:*

Endometrial cancer can be one of the first presentations of an undiagnosed genetic syndrome. Many genetic mutations have been discovered in the past 5 decades which have helped us in better understanding of tumor biology as well as hereditary syndromes. Lynch syndrome, MMR-deficient hereditary diseases, and any familial history of endometrial, colorectal, ovarian, and other cancers increase endometrial cancer risk [9]. Hereditary nonpolyposis colorectal cancer (HNPCC) may cause <5% of endometrial cancer cases [10]. DNA mismatch repair gene germline mutations cause Lynch syndrome, which has autosomal dominant inheritance. MLH1 or MSH2 mutation carriers had 25% to 60% risk of endometrial cancer, MSH6 carriers 16% to 20%, and PMS2 carriers 15%. Most of these endometrial

Table 26.1 Syndromes linked to endometrial cancer

Syndrome	Lifetime risk of developing endometrial carcinoma	Gene mutation
Lynch syndrome or HNPCC [13]	40–60%	MLH1, MSH2, MSH6, PSM2, EPCAM
Muir-Torre syndrome [14]	20–60%	MSH2, MLH1
Cowden syndrome ([15]	28%	PTEN

cancers involve the lower uterine segment and are diagnosed at the age of 50, compared to 61 in sporadic cases [11]. In Lynch syndrome, endometrioid is the commonest histology, but clear cell carcinoma, serous carcinoma, and carcinosarcoma have been reported. Aberrant PTEN mutations may also increase endometrial and other tumor risks [12]. Table 26.1 summarizes different genetic syndromes associated with endometrial carcinoma and the gene mutations involved.

26.3 Screening and Prevention

Screening is defined as the presumptive diagnosis of an unrecognized disease in a healthy population to initiate appropriate intervention for prevention or delay in the onset of disease and for effective management of one particular disease. As a part of primordial prevention, modifiable risk factors should be avoided and awareness should be there in the community regarding the association of these risk factors with the inception of endometrial cancer. As primary prevention, increasing parity, decreasing inter-childbirth intervals, and increasing intervals between the last birth and menopause decrease the risk of endometrial cancer reduces occurrence of endometrial cancer [16]. Further, breastfeeding has been shown to decrease the risk of endometrial cancer; 11% lower risk with breastfeeding has been shown, and it has been shown to have a pooled odds ratio (OR) of 0.89 with 95% CI 0.81–0.98) [17]. Combination contraceptive pills have a preventive effect against the development of endometrial cancer. As a part of secondary prevention, multiple screening methods are available. The transvaginal sonography to measure endometrial thickness, sonohysterography or saline infusion sonography to localize abnormal sites in the endometrium, and endometrial sampling can be used as secondary screening methods to diagnose at early stages. The American Cancer Society (ACS) recommends informing women of the average and increased risk of endometrial cancer, its risks and symptoms (especially, abnormal bleeding and spotting), at the onset of menopause. The American College of Obstetricians and Gynecologists (ACOG) along with the Society of Gynecologic Oncology (SGO) together recommend that all females with endometrial cancer should be screened for the association of Lynch syndrome [18]. The European Society of Medical Oncology, European Society of Gynaecological Oncology, and the European Society of Radiotherapy and Oncology (ESMO/ESGO/ESTRO) have proposed a consensus guideline that recommends annual surveillance by using transvaginal sonography (TVS) and biopsy starting from the age of 35 until hysterectomy for all patients with Lynch syndrome mutation [19]. All these guidelines have been explained in detail in the following.

- *ACS recommendation of screening in average and increased risk women:*
  - To inform women of the average and increased risk of carcinoma endometrium; its risks and symptoms (especially, unexpected bleeding and spotting), at the onset of menopause.
  - Annual screening with transvaginal ultrasound and endometrial biopsy starting at age 35 for women who possess or are related to HNPCC carriers [20]. Endometrial cancer risk can be greatly reduced in patients with HNPCC undergoing hysterectomy and bilateral salpingo-oophorectomy (BSO) prophylactically after the end of childbearing age [21].
- *The ACOG/SGO recommendations for surveillance for lynch syndrome in women with endometrial cancer:*
  - To perform colonoscopy every 1–2 years, starting at the age of 20–25.
  - To perform endometrial sampling every 1–2 years starting at the age of 30–35.
  - To perform hysterectomy and bilateral salpingo-oophorectomy prophylactically in women in their early to mid-40 s.
- *The ESMO/ESGO/ESTRO recommendation for all women who are lynch syndrome mutation carriers:*
  - Annual screening to begin at the age of 35.
  - Regular hysteroscopy and endometrial biopsies.
  - Any premalignant disease should be treated (e.g., atypical endometrial hyperplasia or endometrial intraepithelial neoplasia).
  - To perform hysterectomy and bilateral oophorectomy.

All the above-mentioned guidelines have not defined screening in asymptomatic individuals. For the Indian population, the incidence is not a major health problem to initiate population-based screening programs, hence ICMR has not recommended any specific guidelines. Hence, currently there is no recommendation for screening in asymptomatic individuals.

26.4 Pre-invasive Lesions

The current consensus is that the majority of the endometrioid endometrial carcinomas result from uninterrupted endometrial proliferation. The endometrial proliferation is stimulated by endogenous or exogenous estrogen, which is unopposed by progesterone or progestins. It progresses through simple endometrial hyperplasia and then to complex endometrial hyperplasia types, finally becoming endometrial carcinoma. There are four distinct forms of endometrial hyperplasia, as defined by the World Health Organization: simple hyperplasia, complex hyperplasia, simple atypical

Table 26.2 The risk of endometrial cancer in different subgroups of hyperplasia

WHO 1994	WHO 2014	Risk of co-existent endometrial cancer	Progression to invasive carcinoma
Simple	Hyperplasia without atypia	<1%	RR:1.01–1.03
Complex			
Simple hyperplasia with atypia	Atypical hyperplasia	25–33%	RR:14–45
Complex hyperplasia with atypia			

hyperplasia, and complex atypical hyperplasia. Atypical hyperplasia can lead to endometrial intraepithelial neoplasia (EIN), which can progress to become endometrioid carcinoma with stromal and/or myometrial invasion. Table 26.2 describes the risk of development of endometrial cancer with different types of hyperplasia.

26.5 The Pattern of Spread

Endometrial carcinoma (EC) begins as a pre-invasive lesion, as we have already discussed, which progresses to show atypia and finally becomes invasive carcinoma, which spreads to the endometrial stroma and then penetrates the myometrium. Endometrial cancer spreads by direct infiltration or via lymphatic, transtubal, peritoneal seeding, or hematogenous routes. After entering the myometrium, it spreads through the serosa to directly invade the parametrium, bowel or bladder. The location of lymph node metastases occurs according to the portion of the uterus involved by the cancer as lymphatic channels follow the corresponding vessels. The parametrial, paracervical, and the obturator lymph nodes are involved when the tumor is located in the middle and lower third of the uterus. The tumor in the upper corpus or fundus of the uterus spreads to the common iliac and obturator lymph nodes. Low-grade tumors usually remain confined to the uterus and warrant favorable prognosis; whereas high-grade tumors often metastasize either through the lymphatic system or through the fallopian tubes resulting in dissemination in the abdomen and pelvis resulting in advanced stage and poor prognosis.

26.6 Staging

In 1988, surgical staging supplanted the clinical staging for determining the severity of endometrial cancer. After that, several new insights into the pathologic and molecular aspects of endometrial cancer have been discovered since the previous update to the FIGO staging system in 2009 [22]. The outcomes and biological behaviors of the many histological kinds have expanded greatly in recent years. Since the release of TCGA data, the pace of molecular and genetic discoveries has increased, shedding light on the varied biological characteristics and prognostic outcomes of this group of endometrial malignancies. The complexity of the multiple types of endometrial carcinoma and its underlying biologic behavior is reflected in the updated 2023 staging of endometrial cancer, which encompasses histomorphological categories, tumor patterns, and molecular categorization.

26.7 Histological Types of Endometrial Carcinoma

Histological tumor type is of great prognostic significance. EC can be categorized into histological subtypes and molecular phenotypes. In 1983, Bokhran described two risk types of endometrial carcinoma and categorized them into Type I and Type II. Type I is associated with stimulation by unopposed estrogen. It comprises of low-grade cells that are more common and have a favorable prognosis. Type II carcinomas are not driven by estrogen, comprising high-grade cells. This type is less common and has an unfavorable prognosis. Type I ECs include grade I or grade II endometrioid adenocarcinomas, whereas Type II ECs mostly show grade III endometrioid adenocarcinomas, serous clear cell, undifferentiated, and carcinosarcomas. However, this risk grouping could not explain diversity in tumor biology and their clinical outcomes. According to the fifth edition of WHO classification of tumors of the female genital tract, following histological types have been recognized. These types differ in their molecular features, microscopic appearance, precursor lesions, and natural history.

1. Endometrioid carcinoma (EEC), of low grade (grades 1 and 2) or high grade (grade 3).
2. Serous carcinoma (SC).
3. Clear cell carcinoma (CCC).
4. Mixed-cell type carcinoma (MC).
5. Undifferentiated carcinoma (UC).
6. Carcinosarcoma (CS).
7. Other unusual types.
8. Gastrointestinal mucinous type carcinomas.

26.8 Grading of Endometrial Carcinoma

All serous adenocarcinomas, clear cell adenocarcinomas, gastrointestinal-like mucinous endometrial carcinoma, undifferentiated carcinomas are of high grade. In case of endometrioid carcinoma, the percentage of solid non-glandular component determines the grade.

- Grade 1: solid non-glandular growth <= 5%.
- Grade 2: solid non-glandular growth 6%–50%.
- Grade 3: solid non-glandular growth >50% [23].

26.9 Clinical Features

Unlike other gynecological cancers, most individuals with uterine cancer experience symptoms and present with post-menopausal bleeding, which leads to an early diagnosis and better prognosis.

Common symptoms include the following:

- AUB: One of the most common signs of endometrial cancer is abnormal uterine bleeding (AUB). Irregular uterine bleeding in women in their fifth decade should be treated with strong suspicion for endometrial cancer.
- Post-menopausal bleeding: 10% of post-menopausal bleeding is related to endometrial cancer.
- Less frequent symptoms: Discharge from uterus, pelvic pain, constipation, or diarrhea.
- Abnormal Pap smear.
- Increased endometrial thickness in routine examination.
- Symptoms associated with metastatic disease include cough, diffuse abdominal pain, ascites, cough, chest pain, and bone pain depending on the sites of metastasis.

26.10 Workup

- *History and Clinical Assessment:*

Proper history and physical examination are crucial in the initial evaluation. History should include presenting symptoms, risk factors, family history with pedigree, and lifestyle habits. A meticulous family cancer history should be obtained in cases with suspected genetic syndrome. BMI should be evaluated at the baseline as higher BMI in young females increases the risk. Clinical assessment should be performed with head-to-toe examination, per abdominal and pre vaginal examination along with all the systemic examinations.

- *Laboratory Studies:*

Complete hemogram should be done to rule out anemia and other hematolymphoid abnormalities. Biochemical profile should be done to ensure proper functioning of the kidney and liver, pregnancy tests (serum/urine) to rule out bleeding due to implantation or miscarriage; Coagulation profile, to rule out any bleeding disorders and as a prerequisite before any invasive diagnostic or therapeutic procedure. Other routine blood investigations like viral markers, blood grouping to establish baseline fitness of the patient. Cancer antigen 125 (CA-125) serum levels should be tested as it could be elevated in patients with endometrial cancer. However, unlike in the case of ovarian cancer, the relevance of cancer antigen 125 (CA-125) in endometrial cancer patients is not well defined.

- *Endometrial Biopsy.*

Endometrial biopsy is an office based diagnostic tool. Tissue diagnosis is essential and cannot be replaced by imaging techniques for confirming a diagnosis. The procedure of endometrial sampling includes endometrial aspiration with a pipelle or syringe and a dilatation and curettage with or without hysteroscopic guidance. It is indicated in post-menopausal bleeding. Any instance of vaginal bleeding in a post-menopausal woman should be investigated with a prompt endometrial assessment to rule out the presence of hyperplasia and malignancy. All women with AUB with more than 35 years of age should undergo an endometrial assessment in order to rule out hyperplasia or malignancy and evaluation for endocrinopathies, as well as evaluation for systemic and iatrogenic causes [24]. Endometrial sampling has a sensitivity of 99.6% in women of post-menopausal age group, whereas the sensitivity decreases to 91.1.% in younger women, and for both the age groups, the specificity is 98%. It is used for (i) evaluation for endometrial neoplasia or precancerous hyperplasia, (ii) surveillance in previously diagnosed cases of endometrial hyperplasia or cancer, (iii) evaluation of uterine response to hormone therapy, and (iv) evaluation of abnormal endometrial thickness on imaging. Endometrial thickness < 4 mm does not warrant endometrial biopsy, where transvaginal ultrasonography is a reliable option with a negative predictive value (NPV) of 99%. However, when the endometrial thickness (ET) is more than 4 mm in a post-menopausal female, it is advised that the endometrial biopsy should be obtained. Even in post-menopausal female patients with endometrial thickness < 4 mm if post-menopausal bleeding persists, then it requires further evaluation. In premenopausal women, the endometrial thickness keeps fluctuating across the menstrual cycle; however, ET > 12 mm with features of AUB should be considered for Endometrial Biopsy [25].

26.11 Imaging Studies

Transvaginal ultrasonography is the initial imaging modality of choice in women with history of PMB/AUB. Diagnosis is done by measuring endometrial thickness with sensitivity-96% [26] and specificity-61% [26] for assessment of endometrial thickness. Sensitivity and specificity for deep myometrial invasion are 68–100% and 71–90%, respectively [27]. Heterogenous echotexture and irregularity warrant strong suspicion for malignancy. It does not expose the patient to any ionizing radiation, but it also has its disadvantages in terms of operator dependence, limited field of view, limited role in metastatic workup, and overestimation of myometrial invasion. Color Doppler doesn't show any additional benefit, because there is no significant difference in the pattern of blood flow between benign and malignant endometrial tissue. Endometrial cancers appear as a hypoattenuating and hypoenhancing mass in the endometrial cavity in computed tomography (CT), which lacks specificity for the diagnosis of endometrial cancer. It is not useful for local staging owing to the limited soft tissue differentiation. In evaluating myometrial invasion, the sensitivity and specificity of CT are 40–83% and 42–75%, respectively [28], whereas the sensitivity and specificity of multidetector CT are 95% and 81%, respectively [29]. CT is mainly used to evaluate nodal disease status and distant metastases.

Magnetic resonance imaging is the imaging modality of choice to know accurate disease parameters owing to its excellent soft tissue delineation. The endometrial cancer appears hypo to isointense on T1-weighted image (T1W) and shows intermediate signal intensity on T2W image; on dynamic post-contrast images, there is more enhancement of endometrial cancer compared to the myometrium. Dynamic contrast-enhanced MRI has a sensitivity of 81% and specificity of 72%, whereas the sensitivity and specificity of T2W image are 87% and 58%, respectively. In terms of cervical invasion, MRI has a sensitivity and specificity of 100% and 87% respectively; post contrast T1W image provides 100% sensitivity and specificity [30]. Lymph node metastases are better identified on CT compared to MRI; MRI has a sensitivity and specificity of 44% and 98% respectively. Comparison between diffusion weighted image (DWI) and dynamic contrast imaging showed better sensitivity, specificity, PPV, and NPV in DW images [31]. With the advent of PETCT now we can find both anatomic and metabolic information, which has made this an essential tool for diagnosis and staging. In terms of detection of nodal metastases, FDG PETCT has sensitivity, specificity, and accuracy of 53%, 99%, and 98%, respectively [32]. Compared to MRI, PETCT has better sensitivity and specificity to detect pelvic and para-aortic lymph nodes. DWI MRI is compared with PETCT; DWI showed higher sensitivity (83% vs. 38%) and lower specificity (51% vs. 96%) [33]. PET MRI inculcates the advantage of MRI's soft tissue delineation to improve local assessment of tumor along with the strength of PET in staging nodal and distant metastasis [34]. However, there is no published data yet indicating the use of PET/MR in the workup of endometrial cancer. Table 26.3 shows the comparison between different imaging modalities.

Table 26.3 Different imaging modalities in the staging workup of endometrial cancer

Modality	Depth of myometrial invasion		Cervical invasion	Lymph node metastasis	Advantage	Disadvantage
	Sensitivity	Specificity				
USG	68–100%	71–90%	–	Not detected	Initial imaging modality of choice Higher sensitivity in detecting endometrial thickness > 5 mm (96%) No exposure to ionizing radiation	Operator dependent Limited role in myometrial invasion Specificity in detecting endometrial thickness > 5 mm is 63%
CT	40–83%	42–75%	–	Detects lymph node metastasis	Evaluate nodal disease and distant metastasis	Exposure to ionizing radiation
MRI	DCE-81% T2WI-87%	DCE-72% T2WI-58%	Sensitivity-100% Specificity-87% Post contrast T1WI-100% sensitivity and specificity	Sensitivity-44% Specificity-98%	Excellent soft tissue delineation Accurate local staging No exposure to ionizing radiation	Cannot be used in claustrophobic patients
PETCT	–	–	–	Sensitivity-53% Specificity-99%	Better in detecting pelvic and para-aortic lymph nodes	Exposure to ionizing radiation

26.12 Surgical Staging

The FIGO staging of endometrial cancer was clinical staging before 1988. In 1984, the Gynecologic Oncology Group (GOG) performed a study to evaluate clinico-pathologic factors and recurrence pattern in stage I endometrial cancer. The shift from clinical staging to surgical staging was partly due to the results from the GOG 33 [35]. The result of this study was incorporated into FIGO staging. Surgery is the mainstay of the management of endometrial cancer. The GOG surgical manual has described the comprehensive surgical staging of endometrial cancer which includes the following:

- Extra-fascial total hysterectomy with bilateral salpingo-ophorectomy.
- Inspection of the pelvic and abdominal cavities.
- Biopsy of any suspicious extrauterine lesions.
- Peritoneal washings in most cases.
- Surgical assessment of lymph node:

  Palpation and biopsy of suspicious nodes.
  Sentinel lymph node biopsy/pelvic ± para-aortic lymphadenectomy.

- Omental biopsy—in clear cell/serous carcinoma and carcinosarcoma histology.

26.13 Risk-Based Stratification

The proper estimation of the risk of metastases at diagnosis and the risk of recurrence in the future confers the selection of best management and improves prognosis by reducing the side effects of adjuvant treatment modalities, which are unnecessary. Since the publication by Bokhman et al. [36] in 1983, endometrial cancer has been divided into two histological types as has been described earlier in this chapter. Later, these subtypes were found to have been associated with different molecular aberrations which account for diversity in the prognostic outcomes even in similar histological types. As per the findings from the PORTEC-1 [37], patients with at least 2 of 3 risk factors, i.e., age > 60 years, Grade 3 histology, and > 50% myometrial invasion, were defined as high-risk categories. They found to have an increased risk of locoregional relapse, hence showed the highest absolute benefit of pelvic radiotherapy post-surgery. The 10-year locoregional relapse rates (LRR) in this "high-risk" category were 4.6% and 23.1% in the RT group and control group, respectively. In the year 2004 came the GO-99 study which defined the high-intermediate risk group category based on the prognostic factors, including age, tumor grade, myometrial invasion, and the presence of LVSI [38]. Based on these findings, the FIGO staging was revised in 2009 which included myometrial invasion in staging. The SEPAL study, which was published in 2010, incorporated LVSI in risk stratification [39]. In 2016, the ESMO-ESGO-ESTRO consensus provided a new histomorphological classification defining 4 risk groups, taking into account the stage, histology, grade, myometrial invasion, and lymphovascular invasion [40].

However, these histomorphological classifications could not explain the grade and stage migration from the endometrial biopsy specimens of 15–30% of patients, and the significant discordance among pathologists, hence poor reproducibility in identifying multiple pathologic features. In addition to this, identifying patients requiring adjuvant treatment remained a tremendous challenge. The updated revised FIGO staging 2023 categorizes low-grade (grades 1 and 2) endometrioid endometrial carcinomas (EECs) as non-aggressive, while high-grade (grade 3) EECs, SCs, CCCs, MCs, UCs, and CSs, as well as mesonephric-like and gastro-intestinal-type mucinous carcinomas, are classified as aggressive. High-grade EEC grade 3 can be further classified according to molecular perturbations, which have prognostic significance and help in the management of the disease [41]. The first molecular classification was proposed by The Cancer Genome Atlas (TCGA). It includes the detection of the POLE gene mutation. According to this classification, after genomic sampling, if POLE super-mutation is present, then it is regarded as POLE-mutant. Those samples which did not show POLE mutation, the MSI sequencing was done at four gene loci, including MLH1, MSH2, MSH6, and PMS2. The presence of mutations in one of these genes is defined to be MSI-H. On the basis of presence or absence of p53 gene mutations, it was categorized as Copy Number-high (CN) and CN-low, respectively. The steps involved in sample processing for TCGA classification has been shown in the flowchart (Fig. 26.1).

There are certain caveats in the methods incorporated in molecular testing as proposed by TCGA, which makes it impractical to use in routine practice. TCGA risk stratification needs fresh frozen tissue for analysis and gene sequencing as an integral part which results in logistic and financial constraints for its global implementation. Hence, subsequent studies, particularly the PORTEC group and the ProMisE group, came up with development and validation of molecular surrogates based on three immunohistochemical markers (p53, MSH6, and PMS2) and a molecular test (analysis for mutation in POLE gene). Surrogate tests have been used to classify patients into four molecular prognostic categories: POLE mutation, mismatch repair (MMR) deficiency, p53 abnormality, and "no specific molecular profile"(NSMP) [42]. This is more practical and could be done on standard formalin-fixed and paraffin-embedded samples and use IHC for testing as a surrogate for TCGA classification. Integrating molecular markers added more objectivity to the risk stratification (Table 26.4).

The ESGO/ESTRO/ESP guidelines have proposed two alternative approaches to stratify the risk in endometrial carcinoma, on the basis of available molecular classification shown in Table 26.5. The current recommendation focuses on the distribution as well as the prognostic value of the TCGA groups in each histotype.

The refinements in the molecular-based risk stratification proposed by the new guideline have helped in risk-based therapeutic approaches. Future studies are focused on establishing their predictive role in planning treatment for a tailored approach in all endometrial cancers.

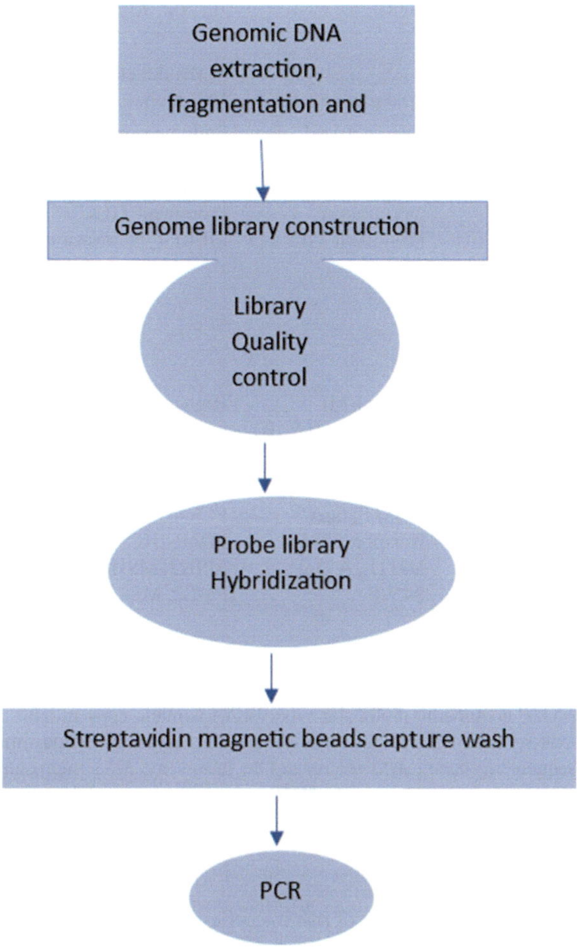

Fig. 26.1 Steps involved in TCGA classification/ sample processing [41, 42]

Table 26.4 Molecular and clinicopathological features of endometrial carcinoma molecular subgroups—combined comparison based on TCGA and ProMisE groups [43, 44]

Molecular subgroups	Pole mutation	MMR deficiency/ MSI high	NSMP/ P53 wild type/ low copy number	P53 abnormal/ high copy number
Prevalence (%)	5–15	25–30	30–40	5–15
Molecular features	>100 mut/Mb, SCNA-very low, MSS	10–100 mut/ Mb, SCNA-low, MSI	<10 mut/Mb, SCNA-low, MSS	<10 mut/Mb, SCNA-high, MSS

(continued)

Table 26.4 (continued)

Molecular subgroups	Pole mutation	MMR deficiency/ MSI high	NSMP/ P53 wild type/ low copy number	P53 abnormal/ high copy number
Histological features	Endometrioid, often high grade Ambiguous morphology Prominent TILs and TLSs	Endometrioid, often high grade LVSI substantial Prominent TILs MELF-type invasion	Mostly low grade Notable absence of TILs Squamous differentiation ER/PgR diffuse	All histological subtypes Mostly high grade High cytonuclear atypia Low levels of TILs
Associated clinical features	Lower BMI Early stage (IA-IB) Early onset	Higher BMI Lynch syndrome	Higher BMI	Lower BMI Advanced stage Late onset
Diagnostic test	NGS/ Sanger/ Hotspot: P286R, V411L, A456P, S459F	PCR-based tests MMR-IHC: MLH1, MSH2, MSH6, PMS2, MSI assay		PCR-based tests p53-IHC Mutant-like/ abnormal staining
Prognosis	Excellent	Intermediate	Intermediate Stage-dependent	Poor

NSMP no specific molecular type, *SCNA* somatic copy number alteration, *TIL* tumor-infiltrating leukocytes, *LVSI* lymphovascular space invasion, *BMI* body mass index, *NGS* next generation sequencing panel, *MSI* microsatellite instability, *MSS* microsatellite stable, *MELF* microcystic, elongated and fragmented, *MMR* mismatch repair, *IHC* immunohistochemistry, *ER* estrogen receptor, *PgR* progesterone receptor

Table 26.5 Distribution of risk categories according to stage and histology [43, 44]

Risk group	Molecular classification known	Molecular classification unknown
Low risk	Stage I-II POLEmut Stage IA MMRd/NSMP low-grade EEC with no or focal LVS	Stage IA endometrioid + low grade LVSI negative or focal
Intermediate risk	Stage IB MMRd/NSMP low-grade EEC with no or focal LVSI Stage IA MMRd/NSMP high-grade EEC with no or focal LVSI Stage IA p53abn EEC with no myometrial invasion Stage IA non-endometrioid with no myometrial invasion	Stage IB endometrioid + low grade Stage IA endometroid + high grade, LVSI negative or focal Stage IA non- endometrioid

(continued)

Table 26.5 (continued)

Risk group	Molecular classification known	Molecular classification unknown
High-intermediate risk	Stage IB MMRd/NSMP low-grade EEC with no or focal LVSI Stage IA MMRd/NSMP high-grade EEC with no or focal LVSI Stage IA p53abn EEC with no myometrial invasion Stage IA non-endometrioid with no myometrial invasion	Stage I endometrioid + substantial LVSI regardless of grade and depth of invasion Stage IB endometrioid high grade regardless of LVSI status Stage II
High risk	Stage III–IVa EEC with no residual disease Stage I–IVa p53abn EEC with myometrial invasion and no residual disease Stage I–IVa non-endometrioid [a] with myometrial invasion and no residual disease	Stage III-IVA with no residual disease Stage I-IVA non-endometrioid
Very high risk	Stage III–Iva with residual disease Stage IVb[a]	Stage III-IVA with residual disease Stage Ivb

[a]For stage III–IVA POLEmut endometrial carcinoma and stage I–IVA MMRd or NSMP clear cell carcinoma with myometrial invasion, insufficient data are available to allocate these patients to a prognostic risk group in the molecular classification

References

1. Sung H, Ferlay J, Siegel RL, Laversanne M, Soerjomataram I, Jemal A, et al. Global cancer statistics 2020: GLOBOCAN estimates of incidence and mortality worldwide for 36 cancers in 185 countries. CA Cancer J Clin. 2021;71(3):209–49.
2. GLOBOCAN 2022: Latest global cancer data shows rising incidence and stark inequities | UICC [Internet]. [cited 2024 Jun 15]. Available from: https://www.uicc.org/news/globocan-2022-latest-global-cancer-data-shows-rising-incidence-and-stark-inequities
3. Siegel RL, Miller KD, Wagle NS, Jemal A. Cancer statistics, 2023. CA Cancer J Clin. 2023;73(1):17–48.
4. Mathur P, Sathishkumar K, Chaturvedi M, Das P, Sudarshan KL, Santhappan S, et al. Cancer statistics, 2020: report from National Cancer Registry Programme, India. JCO Global Oncol [Internet]. 2020;6. [cited 2020 Dec 8]; Available from: http://www.ncbi.nlm.nih.gov.elibraryaiimsdelhi.remotexs.in/pmc/articles/PMC7392737/
5. Renehan AG, Zwahlen M, Egger M. Adiposity and cancer risk: new mechanistic insights from epidemiology. Nat Rev Cancer. 2015;15(8):484–98.
6. Amant F, Moerman P, Neven P, Timmerman D, Limbergen EV, Vergote I. Endometrial cancer. Lancet. 2005;366(9484):491–505.
7. Fisher B, Costantino JP, Redmond CK, Fisher ER, Wickerham DL, Cronin WM, et al. Endometrial cancer in tamoxifen-treated breast cancer patients: findings from the National Surgical Adjuvant Breast and bowel project (NSABP) B-14 *. JNCI J Natl Cancer Inst. 1994;86(7):527–37.
8. Magriples U, Naftolin F, Schwartz PE, Carcangiu ML. High-grade endometrial carcinoma in tamoxifen-treated breast cancer patients. JCO. 1993;11(3):485–90.

9. Lynch HT, Lanspa S, Shaw T, Casey MJ, Rendell M, Stacey M, et al. Phenotypic and genotypic heterogeneity of Lynch syndrome: a complex diagnostic challenge. Fam Cancer. 2018;17(3):403–14.
10. Meyer LA, Broaddus RR, Lu KH. Endometrial cancer and Lynch syndrome: clinical and pathologic considerations. Cancer Control. 2009;16(1):14–22.
11. Ring KL, Modesitt SC. Hereditary cancers in gynecology: what physicians should know about genetic testing, screening, and risk reduction. Obstet Gynecol Clin N Am. 2018;45(1):155–73.
12. Predicting PTEN mutations: an evaluation of Cowden syndrome and Bannayan-Riley-Ruvalcaba syndrome clinical features – PubMed [Internet]. [cited 2023 Oct 28]. Available from: https://pubmed.ncbi.nlm.nih.gov/21659347/
13. Simpkins SB, Bocker T, Swisher EM, Mutch DG, Gersell DJ, Kovatich AJ, et al. MLH1 promoter methylation and gene silencing is the primary cause of microsatellite instability in sporadic endometrial cancers. Hum Mol Genet. 1999;8(4):661–6.
14. Lynch HT, Bardawil WA, Harris RE, Lynch PM, Guirgis HA, Lynch JF. Multiple primary cancers and prolonged survival: familial colonic and endometrial cancers. Dis Colon Rectum. 1978;21(3):165–8.
15. Mester JL, Moore RA, Eng C. PTEN germline mutations in patients initially tested for other hereditary cancer syndromes: would use of risk assessment tools reduce genetic testing? Oncologist. 2013;18(10):1083–90.
16. Setiawan VW, Yang HP, Pike MC, McCann SE, Yu H, Xiang YB, et al. Type I and II endometrial cancers: have they different risk factors? J Clin Oncol. 2013;31(20):2607–18.
17. Jordan SJ, Na R, Johnatty SE, Wise LA, Adami HO, Brinton LA, et al. Breastfeeding and endometrial cancer risk: an analysis from the epidemiology of endometrial cancer consortium. Obstet Gynecol. 2017;129(6):1059–67.
18. SGO Clinical Practice Endometrial Cancer Working Group, Burke WM, Orr J, Leitao M, Salom E, Gehrig P, et al. Endometrial cancer: a review and current management strategies: part I. Gynecol Oncol. 2014;134(2):385–92.
19. Concin N, Matias-Guiu X, Vergote I, Cibula D, Mirza MR, Marnitz S, et al. ESGO/ESTRO/ESP guidelines for the management of patients with endometrial carcinoma. Int J Gynecol Cancer. 2021;31(1):12–39.
20. Smith RA, Andrews KS, Brooks D, Fedewa SA, Manassaram-Baptiste D, Saslow D, et al. Cancer screening in the United States, 2017: a review of current American Cancer Society guidelines and current issues in cancer screening. CA Cancer J Clin. 2017;67(2):100–21.
21. Schmeler KM, Lynch HT, May CL, Munsell MF, Soliman PT, Clark MB, et al. Prophylactic surgery to reduce the risk of gynecologic cancers in the Lynch syndrome. N Engl J Med. 2006;354(3):261–9.
22. Abu-Rustum NR, Zhou Q, Iasonos A, Alektiar KM, Leitao MM, Chi DS, et al. The revised 2009 FIGO staging system for endometrial cancer: should the 1988 FIGO Stage IA and IB be altered? Int J Gynecol Cancer. 2011;21(3):511–6. https://doi.org/10.1097/IGC.0b013e31820cc305.
23. Berek JS, Matias-Guiu X, Creutzberg C, Fotopoulou C, Gaffney D, Kehoe S, et al. FIGO staging of endometrial cancer: 2023. Int J Gynaecol Obstet. 2023;162(2):383–94.
24. Dijkhuizen FP, Mol BW, Brölmann HA, Heintz AP. The accuracy of endometrial sampling in the diagnosis of patients with endometrial carcinoma and hyperplasia: a meta-analysis. Cancer. 2000;89(8):1765–72.
25. Giri SK, Nayak BL, Mohapatra J. Thickened endometrium: when to intervene? A clinical conundrum. J Obstet Gynecol India. 2021;71(3):216–25.
26. Smith-Bindman R, Kerlikowske K, Feldstein VA, Subak L, Scheidler J, Segal M, et al. Endovaginal ultrasound to exclude endometrial cancer and other endometrial abnormalities. JAMA. 1998;280(17):1510–7.

27. Epstein E, Blomqvist L. Imaging in endometrial cancer. Best Pract Res Clin Obstet Gynaecol. 2014;28(5):721–39.
28. Hardesty LA, Sumkin JH, Hakim C, Johns C, Nath M. The ability of helical CT to preoperatively stage endometrial carcinoma. AJR Am J Roentgenol. 2001;176(3):603–6.
29. Tsili AC, Tsampoulas C, Dalkalitsis N, Stefanou D, Paraskevaidis E, Efremidis SC. Local staging of endometrial carcinoma: role of multidetector CT. Eur Radiol. 2008;18(5):1043–8.
30. Murakami T, Kurachi H, Nakamura H, Tsuda K, Miyake A, Tomoda K, et al. Cervical invasion of endometrial carcinoma--evaluation by parasagittal MR imaging. Acta Radiol. 1995;36(3):248–53.
31. Rechichi G, Galimberti S, Signorelli M, Perego P, Valsecchi MG, Sironi S. Myometrial invasion in endometrial cancer: diagnostic performance of diffusion-weighted MR imaging at 1.5-T. Eur Radiol. 2010;20(3):754–62.
32. Kitajima K, Murakami K, Yamasaki E, Kaji Y, Sugimura K. Accuracy of integrated FDG-PET/contrast-enhanced CT in detecting pelvic and paraaortic lymph node metastasis in patients with uterine cancer. Eur Radiol. 2009;19(6):1529–36.
33. Kitajima K, Yamasaki E, Kaji Y, Murakami K, Sugimura K. Comparison of DWI and PET/CT in evaluation of lymph node metastasis in uterine cancer. World J Radiol [Internet]. 2012;4(5) [cited 2024 Jun 17]. Available from: https://pubmed.ncbi.nlm.nih.gov/22761980/
34. Kitajima K, Suenaga Y, Ueno Y, Kanda T, Maeda T, Takahashi S, et al. Value of fusion of PET and MRI for staging of endometrial cancer: comparison with ^{18}F-FDG contrast-enhanced PET/CT and dynamic contrast-enhanced pelvic MRI. Eur J Radiol. 2013;82(10):1672–6.
35. Creasman WT, Morrow CP, Bundy BN, Homesley HD, Graham JE, Heller PB. Surgical pathologic spread patterns of endometrial cancer. A Gynecologic Oncology Group Study. Cancer. 1987;60(8 Suppl):2035–41.
36. Bokhman JV. Two pathogenetic types of endometrial carcinoma. Gynecol Oncol. 1983;15(1):10–7.
37. Scholten AN, Van Putten WLJ, Beerman H, Smit VTHBM, Koper PCM, Lybeert MLM, et al. Postoperative radiotherapy for stage 1 endometrial carcinoma: long-term outcome of the randomized PORTEC trial with central pathology review. Int J Radiat Oncol Biol Phys. 2005;63(3):834–8.
38. Keys HM, Roberts JA, Brunetto VL, Zaino RJ, Spirtos NM, Bloss JD, et al. A phase III trial of surgery with or without adjunctive external pelvic radiation therapy in intermediate risk endometrial adenocarcinoma: a Gynecologic Oncology Group study. Gynecol Oncol. 2004;92(3):744–51.
39. Todo Y, Kato H, Kaneuchi M, Watari H, Takeda M, Sakuragi N. Survival effect of para-aortic lymphadenectomy in endometrial cancer (SEPAL study): a retrospective cohort analysis. Lancet. 2010;375(9721):1165–72.
40. Colombo N, Creutzberg C, Amant F, Bosse T, González-Martín A, Ledermann J, et al. ESMO-ESGO-ESTRO Consensus Conference on Endometrial Cancer: diagnosis, treatment and follow-up. Ann Oncol. 2016;27(1):16–41.
41. Bosse T, Nout RA, McAlpine JN, McConechy MK, Britton H, Hussein Y, et al. Molecular classification of grade 3 endometrioid endometrial cancers identifies distinct prognostic subgroups. Am J Surg Pathol. 2018;42(5):561–8.
42. Levine DA. Integrated genomic characterization of endometrial carcinoma. Nature. 2013;497(7447):67–73.
43. Kandoth C, Schultz N, Cherniack AD, et al. Integrated genomic characterization of endometrial carcinoma. Nature. 2013;497(7447):67–73. https://doi.org/10.1038/nature12113.
44. Talhouk A, McConechy MK, Leung S, et al. Confirmation of ProMisE: a simple, genomics-based clinical classifier for endometrial cancer. Cancer. 2017;123(5):802–13. https://doi.org/10.1002/cncr.30496.

Chapter 27
Presentation and Evaluation of Ovarian Cancer

Anuj Gupta, Bipinesh Sansar, Avradeep Datta, and Shubham Dokania

27.1 Epidemiology

Ovarian cancer is the third most commonly diagnosed gynecologic malignancy worldwide [1]. It ranks fourth in overall global incidence with an age-standardized rate of 6.6 per 100,000 women. According to the Global Cancer Observatory (GLOBOCAN) 2022, it ranks 14th in overall cancer-associated deaths and second in gynecological cancer-associated deaths. The burden is higher in Western and Central Europe, reflecting geographic variation. In India, ovarian cancer ranks ninth in overall incidence and tenth in cancer-related mortality, and is the second most common gynecologic malignancy, underscoring its national relevance [2].

The lifetime risk of a woman developing ovarian cancer by the age of 95 is approximately 1.1%, a modest individual risk with substantial population-level implications [3]. Incidence increases with age, and the disease is most frequently diagnosed in postmenopausal women [4]. Distinct histologic subtypes show age-specific patterns: high-grade serous ovarian carcinoma (HGSOC) typically presents in women in their sixth to seventh decades, low-grade endometrioid tumors occur more often between 45 and 50 years, and clear-cell carcinoma (CCC) is commonly diagnosed between 55 and 60 years [5]. Epidemiology also varies by ethnicity, with non-Hispanic White women exhibiting the highest incidence of HGSOC and endometrioid cancers, while Asian and Pacific Islander women show a higher prevalence of CCC. Non-Hispanic Black women have the lowest incidence across subtypes.

A. Gupta (✉) · B. Sansar · A. Datta · S. Dokania
Department of Medical Oncology, MPMMCC & HBCH Varanasi, Units of Tata Memorial Centre and affliated with Homi Bhabha National institute, Mumbai, India

S. Pradhan et al. (eds.), *Evidence Based Handbook on Diagnosis and Staging in Oncology*, https://doi.org/10.1007/978-981-95-9701-7_27

More than 50% of patients present with advanced-stage disease, which has a profound impact on survival. Five-year survival exceeds 93.1% in early-stage disease but falls to approximately 30.8% in advanced stages, with recurrence rates rising from <10% in stage I to nearly 90% in stage IV disease, highlighting the importance of early detection and optimized management strategies [3].

27.2 Risk Factors and Etiopathogenesis

Factors that increase lifetime ovulatory cycles, such as nulliparity and early menarche or late menopause, are associated with an elevated risk of ovarian cancer. However, the precise biological mechanisms are still not fully understood [6]. Conversely, the factors that reduce ovulation, including multiparity, breastfeeding, late menarche, and early menopause, confer a protective effect [7]. Chronic inflammatory conditions like endometriosis and obesity further increase risk, potentially through mechanisms involving oxidative stress, hormonal imbalance, and DNA damage [8, 9]. A personal or familial history of breast or ovarian cancer substantially increases the susceptibility, with germline BRCA1 and BRCA2 mutations representing the most well-established genetic risk factors. Other inherited mutations associated with increased risk include ATM, PALB2, and NF1. Lynch syndrome (HNPCC), caused by defects in DNA mismatch repair genes (MLH1, MSH2, MSH6, PMS2) and rarer hereditary syndromes such as Cowden syndrome (PTEN mutation) and Peutz–Jeghers syndrome (STK11 mutation) [10].

At the somatic level, TP53 mutations are nearly ubiquitous in high-grade serous ovarian carcinoma (HGSOC), while alterations in BRCA1/2, PTEN, PIK3CA, KRAS, and BRAF are observed across different histologic subtypes [11]. In addition, epigenetic dysregulation, including aberrant DNA methylation, plays an important role in ovarian carcinogenesis. Although population-based screening has not shown a clear survival benefit, risk-adapted surveillance and preventive strategies are recommended for women with a hereditary predisposition [3, 12].

Ovarian cancer spreads primarily via the transcoelomic route, with the peritoneum and omentum serving as common metastatic sites. Lymphatic spread follows ovarian and tubal drainage pathways, initially involving para-aortic and paracaval nodes, followed by pelvic nodal chains. Hematogenous metastasis is uncommon in early disease but may occur in advanced stages [13]. Emerging evidence supports a fallopian tube origin for many serous carcinomas, particularly HGSOC and low-grade serous ovarian cancers (LGSOC), arising from precursor lesions such as tubal intraepithelial carcinoma (TIC) [14]. Given the frequent overlap between ovarian, fallopian tube, and primary peritoneal cancers, the International Federation of Gynecology and Obstetrics (FIGO) staging system incorporates all three sites within a unified staging system [15].

27.3 Histopathology and Immunohistochemistry (IHC)

The histological classification of ovarian tumors has been illustrated in Fig. 27.1. Epithelial ovarian cancers constitute around 90%. Epithelial ovarian malignancies are subdivided by cytopathology, IHC markers, and molecular studies. The clinical behavior, management, and outcomes vary significantly among subtypes. The primary subtypes of ovarian cancer include HGSOC, LGSOC, CCC, endometrioid, and mucinous carcinomas [16]. The grading for non-serous epithelial ovarian cancers is based on histologic architecture, while grading for serous carcinoma is determined by tumor biology [14].

27.3.1 IHC Classification of Epithelial Ovarian Cancers

The WT1 immunohistochemical marker helps distinguish high-grade and low-grade serous tumors from clear-cell and mucinous subtypes, as WT1 is absent in the latter. The p53 abnormal (p53abn) marker can also differentiate high-grade serous tumors from low-grade ones. Endometrioid subtypes show paint positive results for ER/PR and beta-catenin. 10% to 15% of endometrioid tumors may exhibit positive staining for both WT1 and p53abn markers. Positive immunohistochemical stains for napsin A and HNF1B, alongside negative staining for progesterone receptors, typically indicate CCC. A flowchart for the diagnostic algorithm is shown in Fig. 27.2.

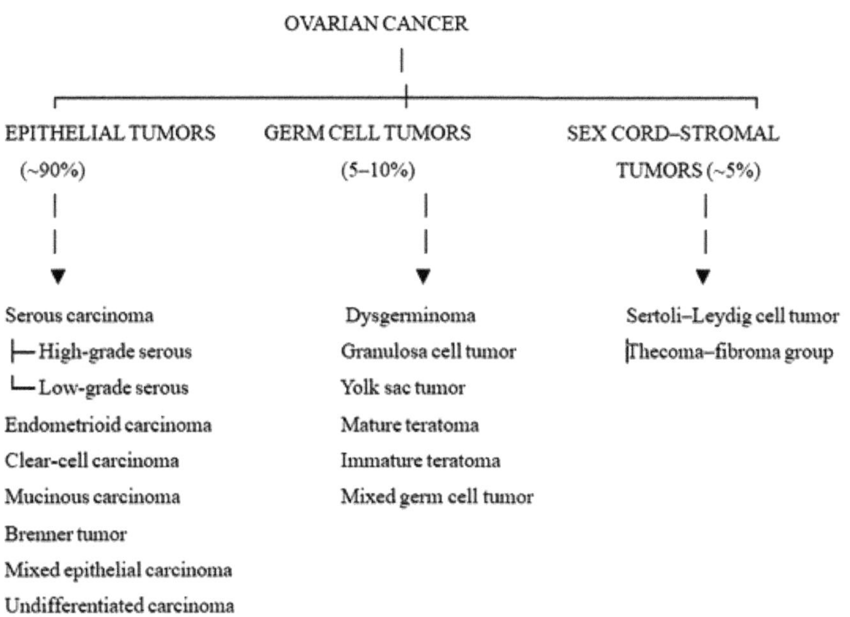

Fig. 27.1 Classification of ovarian tumors

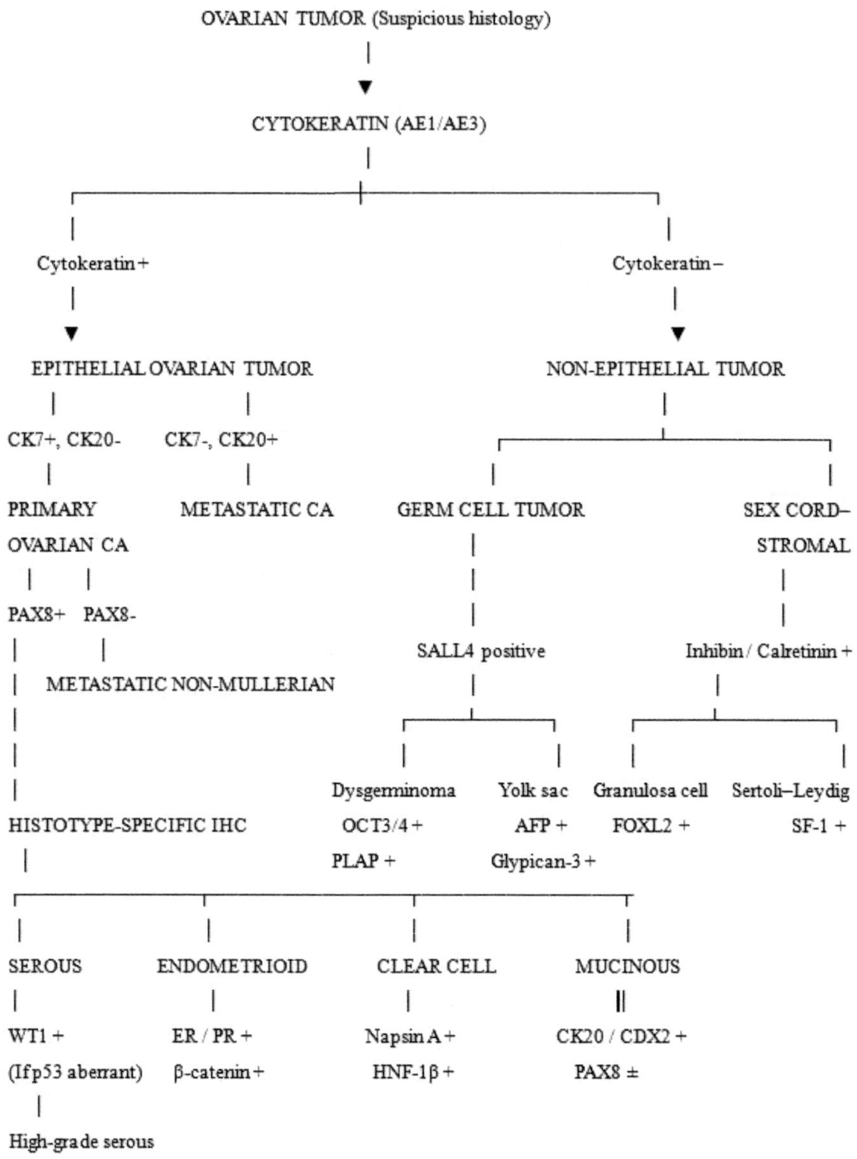

Fig. 27.2 Flowchart showing the diagnostic algorithm of ovarian cancers using IHC markers

27.4 Workup

27.4.1 Clinical History

Epithelial ovarian cancer is occasionally detected incidentally in asymptomatic women; however, most patients present with vague, nonspecific symptoms, leading to diagnostic delay. These symptoms may include abdominal fullness, bloating, nausea, abdominal distention, early satiety, fatigue, changes in bowel movements, urinary symptoms, back pain, dyspareunia, and weight loss. Notably, abnormal uterine bleeding is not typically a symptom of ovarian cancer [17].

27.4.2 Physical Examination

A thorough physical examination should be performed with informed verbal consent, ensuring privacy and the presence of a female attendant. Pelvic examination should include visual inspection of the perineum, cervix, and vagina, along with performing a bimanual examination. This examination aims to detect any pelvic or abdominal masses. Features suggestive of malignancy include irregular, firm, fixed, or nodular adnexal masses, masses in the Pouch of Douglas, and the presence of ascites, warranting further imaging [3]. Examination should also include supraclavicular lymph node palpation, abdominal and breast examination, pulmonary auscultation, and rectovaginal assessment with an empty bladder. Rarely, a firm umbilical or paraumbilical nodule, known as a Sister Mary Joseph nodule, may be palpable due to metastasis. The Lesar-Trélat sign, characterized by a sudden increase in seborrheic keratosis, can serve as a clinical indicator of occult cancer [18]. Other paraneoplastic syndromes, such as subacute cerebellar degeneration (ataxia, dysarthria, nystagmus, vertigo) and hypercalcemia (altered mental status, fatigue, constipation, abdominal pain), although very rare, may occasionally precede diagnosis and should raise suspicion of occult malignancy [18, 19].

27.4.3 Investigations

27.4.3.1 Baseline Fitness Assessment

Blood investigations (complete blood count, liver function test, kidney function test, serum electrolytes, coagulation profile), and chest X-ray.

27.4.3.2 Serum Tumor Biomarkers

Tumor markers are typically measured alongside imaging studies in patients suspected of having ovarian cancer. Cancer antigen 125 (CA-125) remains the most widely used biomarker for suspected epithelial ovarian cancer. It is elevated in the majority of advanced-stage cases but in only about half of early-stage disease, with higher specificity in postmenopausal women. A value >35 U/mL in this group is suggestive of pelvic pathology and warrants further investigation. Although elevations may occur in malignancies, they may also occur in benign and inflammatory conditions (e.g., acute pelvic inflammatory disease, adenomyosis, and endometriosis) [20].

Human epididymis protein 4 (HE4) demonstrates high specificity and greater sensitivity in early-stage disease, while CA-125 performs better in advanced stages. However, HE4 is not diagnostic and may be elevated in other malignancies, such as endometrial cancer and lung adenocarcinomas [20].

In women below 40 years of age with suspected ovarian cancer, beta-human chorionic gonadotropin (b-hCG), alpha-fetoprotein (AFP), and lactate dehydrogenase (LDH) should be tested to rule out germ-cell tumors [21]. Ca 19.9 may be elevated in mucinous carcinomas arising from the ovary or peritoneum and needs to be documented to follow the response to treatment.

27.4.3.3 Imaging

Transvaginal ultrasonography (TVS) is the preferred first-line modality for evaluation of an adnexal mass, as it reliably differentiates benign from malignant features. Sonographic findings suggestive of ovarian malignancy include solid or papillary components, irregular morphology, ascites, and increased Doppler vascularity. Approximately 20% of lesions remain indeterminate on ultrasound and require further assessment with magnetic resonance imaging (MRI) [3, 22]. Risk stratification is challenging, as overestimation may result in unnecessary interventions and patient anxiety, while underdiagnosis can delay treatment and adversely affect outcomes. The Ovarian-Adnexal Reporting and Data System (O-RADS) offers a standardized, ultrasound-based risk stratification system to guide management and identify patients requiring gynecologic oncology referral [22, 23]. O-RADS scores with respective interpretation and management have been tabulated in Table 27.1.

Several risk prediction models have been developed to estimate the probability of epithelial ovarian cancer using serum tumor markers, with or without transvaginal ultrasonography. The Risk of Malignancy Index (RMI) integrates CA-125 level, ultrasound features, and menopausal status [18]. An RMI greater than 200, particularly in postmenopausal women, is associated with a high risk of malignancy with a reported specificity exceeding 96%. The risk of ovarian malignancy algorithm (ROMA) employs a mathematical model incorporating HE4 and CA-125 levels, adjusted for menopausal status, to estimate the risk of malignancy [24]. However, these marker-based models are generally less accurate than imaging-based risk stratification systems for characterizing adnexal masses [20].

Table 27.1 Ovarian-Adnexal Reporting and Data System (O-RADS)

O-RADS category	Estimated risk of malignancy	Interpretation	Recommended management
O-RADS 0	Not applicable	Incomplete evaluation	Repeat or additional imaging (targeted US/MRI)
O-RADS 1	0%	Normal ovary	Routine care; no follow-up required
O-RADS 2	<1%	Almost certainly benign lesion (e.g., simple cyst, hemorrhagic cyst, classic dermoid, endometrioma)	Routine follow-up or no follow-up, depending on size and symptoms
O-RADS 3	1–<10%	Low risk of malignancy	MRI or USG by a specialist; gynecologic referral
O-RADS 4	10–<50%	Intermediate risk of malignancy	Gynecologic oncology referral; consider MRI or USG by a specialist
O-RADS 5	≥50%	High risk of malignancy	Prompt referral to a gynecologic oncologist; definitive surgical management

In patients with indeterminate ultrasound findings or normal CA-125 levels, magnetic resonance imaging (MRI) provides valuable additional characterization due to its high specificity for malignancy [25]. Analogous to ultrasound-based stratification, the O-RADS MRI (AdnexMR) system classifies adnexal masses into five risk categories based on defined MRI features, thereby guiding preoperative decision-making regarding the need for surgery and extent of intervention [22, 26]. Recommended MRI protocols include axial T1- and T2-weighted sequences, with and without fat suppression, supplemented by post-contrast T1-weighted imaging [26]. O-RADS MRI stratifies adnexal masses into the following categories based on specific criteria:

- AdnexMR 1: no adnexal lesion is visualized.
- AdnexMR 2: benign.
- AdnexMR 3: likely benign.
- AdnexMR 4: indeterminate risk of being malignant.
- AdnexMR 5: high risk of malignancy.

Computed tomography (CT) of the thorax, abdomen, and pelvis (TAP) is widely used in patients with nonspecific symptoms to evaluate differential diagnoses and assess disease burden, owing to its broad availability and rapid acquisition. Although magnetic resonance imaging (MRI) is preferred as a second-line modality after USG for detailed adnexal characterization, CT TAP remains indispensable for staging and preoperative planning, particularly in evaluating lymph node involvement, which may preclude surgical intervention in select patients [21]. Positron emission tomography–CT (PET-CT) offers incremental value over CT alone in detecting nodal and peritoneal metastases and in the assessment of recurrent disease [27].

27.4.3.4 Homologous Recombination Deficiency (HRD) and Germline BRCA (gBRCA) Testing

HRD (Homologous Recombination Deficient) and gBRCA (germline BRCA) testing constitute a cornerstone of contemporary ovarian cancer management, with significant prognostic and therapeutic implications. HRD, reflecting impaired repair of DNA double-strand breaks, is identified in approximately 50% of HGSOC and is frequently associated with BRCA1/2 and related pathway mutations [28]. gBRCA mutations are present in 15–20% of cases, with an additional 5–7% attributable to somatic BRCA alterations. Tumors harboring BRCA mutations demonstrate enhanced sensitivity to platinum-based chemotherapy and poly (ADP-ribose) polymerase inhibitors (PARPi), translating into improved clinical outcomes [29]. HRD testing broadens the scope for PARPi eligibility by identifying non-BRCA HRD-positive tumors, which account for approximately 20–30% of BRCA–wild-type HGSOC.

The National Comprehensive Cancer Network (NCCN) guidelines recommend testing for ovarian cancer susceptibility genes (including BRCA1, BRCA2, ATM, BRIP1, PALB2, and MMR genes) in all patients with epithelial ovarian cancer (including fallopian tube cancer or peritoneal cancer) and selected non-epithelial ovarian cancers (sex-cord tumors with annular tubules and small cell carcinoma of the ovary) [30].

The American Society of Clinical Oncology (ASCO) guidelines recommend offering testing for gBRCA1, gBRCA2, and other ovarian cancer susceptibility genes to all women diagnosed with epithelial ovarian cancer [31]. Somatic tumor testing for BRCA1 and BRCA2 is advised when gBRCA 1/2 mutations are absent. Additionally, for patients with clear cell, endometrioid, or mucinous ovarian cancer subtypes, mismatch repair defect (MMRd) testing should be offered. However, no recommendations could be made supporting routine testing for HRD using currently available HRD assays.

27.5 Staging

Ovarian tumors are staged surgically. The FIGO staging is used for staging.

References

1. 25-ovary-fact-sheet.pdf [Internet]. [cited 2026 Jan 29]. Available from: https://gco.iarc.who.int/media/globocan/factsheets/cancers/25-ovary-fact-sheet.pdf
2. 356-india-fact-sheet.pdf [Internet]. [cited 2026 Jan 29]. Available from: https://gco.iarc.who.int/media/globocan/factsheets/populations/356-india-fact-sheet.pdf
3. Burke W, Barkley J, Barrows E, Brooks R, Gecsi K, Huber-Keener K, et al. Executive summary of the ovarian cancer evidence review conference. Obstet Gynecol. 2023;142(1):179–95.

4. Sambasivan S. Epithelial ovarian cancer: review article. Cancer Treat Res Commun. 2022;33:100629.
5. Phung MT, Pearce CL, Meza R, Jeon J. Trends of ovarian cancer incidence by histotype and race/ethnicity in the United States 1992–2019. Cancer Res Commun. 2023;3(1):1–8.
6. Jelovac D, Armstrong DK. Recent progress in the diagnosis and treatment of ovarian cancer. CA Cancer J Clin. 2011;61(3):183–203.
7. Flaum N, Crosbie EJ, Edmondson RJ, Smith MJ, Evans DG. Epithelial ovarian cancer risk: a review of the current genetic landscape. Clin Genet. 2020;97(1):54–63.
8. Varier L, Sundaram SM, Gamit N, Warrier S. An overview of ovarian cancer: the role of cancer stem cells in chemoresistance and a precision medicine approach targeting the Wnt pathway with the antagonist sFRP4. Cancers (Basel). 2023;15(4):1275.
9. Friedenreich CM, Ryder-Burbidge C, McNeil J. Physical activity, obesity and sedentary behavior in cancer etiology: epidemiologic evidence and biologic mechanisms. Mol Oncol. 2021;15(3):790–800.
10. Hereditary cancer syndromes and risk assessment: ACOG COMMITTEE OPINION, Number 793. Obstet Gynecol. 2019;134(6):e143–9.
11. Liberto JM, Chen SY, Shih IM, Wang TH, Wang TL, Pisanic TR. Current and emerging methods for ovarian cancer screening and diagnostics: a comprehensive review. Cancers (Basel). 2022;14(12):2885.
12. Shih IM, Wang Y, Wang TL. The origin of ovarian cancer species and precancerous landscape. Am J Pathol. 2021;191(1):26–39.
13. de Oliveira LRLB, Horvat N, Andrieu PIC, Panizza PSB, Cerri GG, Viana PCC. Ovarian cancer staging: what the surgeon needs to know. Br J Radiol. 2021;94(1125):20210091.
14. Berek JS, Renz M, Kehoe S, Kumar L, Friedlander M. Cancer of the ovary, fallopian tube, and peritoneum: 2021 update. Int J Gynaecol Obstet. 2021;155(Suppl 1):61–85.
15. Prat J. FIGO'S staging classification for cancer of the ovary, fallopian tube, and peritoneum: abridged republication. J Gynecol Oncol. 2015;26(2):87–9.
16. Köbel M, Kang EY. The evolution of ovarian carcinoma subclassification. Cancers (Basel). 2022;14(2):416.
17. Berek JS, Kehoe ST, Kumar L, Friedlander M. Cancer of the ovary, fallopian tube, and peritoneum. Int J Gynaecol Obstet. 2018;143(Suppl 2):59–78.
18. Smith CG. A resident's perspective of ovarian cancer. Diagnostics (Basel). 2017;7(2):24.
19. Renjen PN, Chaudhari DM, Shilpi US, Zutshi D, Ahmad K. Paraneoplastic cerebellar degeneration associated with ovarian adenocarcinoma: a case report and review of literature. Ann Indian Acad Neurol. 2018;21(4):311–4.
20. Zhang R, Siu MKY, Ngan HYS, Chan KKL. Molecular biomarkers for the early detection of ovarian cancer. Int J Mol Sci. 2022;23(19):12041.
21. Fotopoulou C, Hall M, Cruickshank D, Gabra H, Ganesan R, Hughes C, et al. British Gynaecological Cancer Society (BGCS) epithelial ovarian/fallopian tube/primary peritoneal cancer guidelines: recommendations for practice. Eur J Obstet Gynecol Reprod Biol. 2017;213:123–39.
22. Sadowski EA, Rockall AG, Maturen KE, Robbins JB, Thomassin-Naggara I. Adnexal lesions: imaging strategies for ultrasound and MR imaging. Diagn Interv Imaging. 2019;100(10):635–46.
23. Andreotti RF, Timmerman D, Strachowski LM, Froyman W, Benacerraf BR, Bennett GL, et al. O-RADS US risk stratification and management system: a consensus guideline from the ACR ovarian-adnexal reporting and data system Committee. Radiology. 2020;294(1):168–85.
24. Moore RG, McMeekin DS, Brown AK, DiSilvestro P, Miller MC, Allard WJ, et al. A novel multiple marker bioassay utilizing HE4 and CA125 for the prediction of ovarian cancer in patients with a pelvic mass. Gynecol Oncol. 2009;112(1):40–6.
25. Zhang Q, Dai X, Li W. Systematic review and meta-analysis of O-RADS ultrasound and O-RADS MRI for risk assessment of ovarian and adnexal lesions. AJR Am J Roentgenol. 2023;221(1):21–33.

26. Thomassin-Naggara I, Poncelet E, Jalaguier-Coudray A, Guerra A, Fournier LS, Stojanovic S, et al. Ovarian-adnexal reporting data system magnetic resonance imaging (O-RADS MRI) score for risk stratification of sonographically indeterminate adnexal masses. JAMA Netw Open. 2020;3(1):e1919896.
27. Patel PR, De Jesus O. CT scan. In: StatPearls [Internet]. Treasure Island: StatPearls Publishing; 2025. [cited 2026 Jan 28]. Available from: http://www.ncbi.nlm.nih.gov/books/NBK567796/.
28. Cancer Genome Atlas Research Network. Integrated genomic analyses of ovarian carcinoma. Nature. 2011;474(7353):609–15.
29. Moore K, Colombo N, Scambia G, Kim BG, Oaknin A, Friedlander M, et al. Maintenance Olaparib in patients with newly diagnosed advanced ovarian cancer. N Engl J Med. 2018;379(26):2495–505.
30. genetics_bopp.pdf [Internet]. [cited 2026 Jan 31]. Available from: https://www.nccn.org/professionals/physician_gls/pdf/genetics_bopp.pdf
31. Konstantinopoulos PA, Norquist B, Lacchetti C, Armstrong D, Grisham RN, Goodfellow PJ, et al. Germline and somatic tumor testing in epithelial ovarian cancer: ASCO guideline. J Clin Oncol. 2020;38(11):1222–45.

Chapter 28
Evaluation and Staging of Ewing Sarcoma and Rhabdomyosarcoma

Ajay S. Krishnan and Jhansi Pattanaik

28.1 Introduction and Epidemiology

Ewing sarcoma is a malignant neoplasm of bone characterized histologically by sheets of small round blue cells. The tumor was first identified in 1921 by James Ewing, who originally described it as an endothelioma of bone. Ewing sarcoma (ES), along with Ewing-like sarcomas, represents a group of highly aggressive round-cell tumors of mesenchymal origin that predominantly affect children and young adults. Although the exact cell of origin remains uncertain, these tumors are believed to arise from primitive mesenchymal cells with neuroectodermal differentiation.

Ewing sarcoma most frequently develops in close association with bone and is therefore traditionally classified as a primary bone malignancy. However, tumors with identical histological, immunohistochemical, and cytogenetic features may also arise in soft tissues. Both skeletal and extra-skeletal forms are collectively referred to as the *Ewing Sarcoma Family of Tumors (ESFT)* [1].

Despite its potential to occur at any age, Ewing sarcoma is primarily a disease of childhood and adolescence, with the majority of cases diagnosed before 20 years of age [2]. It is the second most common primary malignant bone tumor in children and adolescents and accounts for nearly 3% of all pediatric malignancies [3].

A. S. Krishnan (✉) · J. Pattanaik
Department of Radiation Oncology, MPMMCC/HBCH Varanasi, Units of Tata Memorial Centre, and Homi Bhabha National Institute, Mumbai, India

S. Pradhan et al. (eds.), *Evidence Based Handbook on Diagnosis and Staging in Oncology*, https://doi.org/10.1007/978-981-95-9701-7_28

28.1.1 Epidemiology

- Approximately 80% of ESFT cases occur within the first two decades of life, and nearly 80% originate in the skeletal system [4].
- Ewing sarcoma ranks as the second most frequent bone malignancy in adolescents and young adults.
- Around 250 new cases are diagnosed annually in the United States.
- The incidence is very low in children under five years of age (about 0.6 per million) but increases during puberty, reaching a peak incidence of approximately 5 per million.
- A slight male predominance is observed, with a male-to-female ratio of about 1.3:1.
- The disease is more commonly seen in individuals of White ethnicity compared with Asians and Hispanics, and is extremely rare in individuals of African descent.
- Extra-skeletal Ewing sarcoma (EES) accounts for 15–20% of all ESFT cases, with an estimated incidence of nearly one case per million population in the United States.
- While skeletal Ewing sarcoma is more common in children, extra-skeletal tumors constitute more than half of ESFT cases diagnosed in adults.

28.1.2 Indian Perspective

- In India, Ewing sarcoma accounts for approximately 15% of all malignant bone tumors.
- Nearly 68% of cases occur in the 0–19-year age group, with tumors more frequently involving the appendicular skeleton; limb bones are affected about 1.6 times more often than other skeletal sites.
- The highest incidence rate is observed in children aged 10–14 years.
- A marked male predominance is noted, with incidence rates of approximately 1.6 in males compared to 1.0 in females.
- About 12% of cases are reported in individuals aged 30 years or older [5].

28.1.3 Risk Factors

- Syndromes:
    - Li-Fraumeni syndrome (LFS).
    - Retinoblastoma predisposition syndrome.
    - Bloom syndrome.
    - Fanconi anemia.

    - Constitutional mismatch repair deficiency syndrome (CMMRD).
    - Multiple endocrine neoplasia type 2A (MEN2A) [6, 7].
- Environmental factors.
    - Parental exposure to pesticides, solvents, and farming or agricultural occupation.

28.1.4 Clinical Features

- Ewing Sarcoma Family of Tumors (ESFT) typically presents as a solitary, rapidly enlarging mass and may arise in almost any anatomical location, involving either bone or soft tissue, at superficial or deep sites. Clinical manifestations are variable and largely depend on the size, location, and extent of the lesion, with symptoms resulting from compression or invasion of adjacent structures. Localized pain or tenderness is a common presenting complaint and is influenced by the primary site of origin.
- Certain ESFT subtypes may be associated with systemic or constitutional symptoms such as fever, loss of appetite, and unintentional weight loss, which can obscure the clinical picture and contribute to delays in diagnosis. Regional lymph node involvement is uncommon; however, when present, it may manifest as clinically detectable lymphadenopathy.

28.1.5 Diagnostic Evaluation

- Diagnosis of ESFT requires a systematic approach that includes detailed clinical history taking and thorough physical examination, followed by pathological confirmation.

28.1.6 Histopathological Assessment

- Definitive diagnosis is established through biopsy of the primary lesion [8]. Percutaneous biopsy should be carefully planned and performed in coordination with the surgeon responsible for definitive local treatment, as the biopsy tract must be incorporated into the surgical excision field or included within the radiotherapy volume.
- Pre-procedural imaging plays a critical role in selecting the optimal biopsy pathway, ensuring preservation of anatomical tissue planes and maintaining future reconstructive options. Given that extra-skeletal Ewing sarcoma often demonstrates areas of necrosis or hemorrhage, imaging guidance is essential to target

the most viable and metabolically active regions of the tumor, typically identified by contrast enhancement or increased fluorodeoxyglucose (FDG) uptake.
- For percutaneous sampling, the use of a biopsy needle of at least 18-gauge is recommended, as longer core specimens—preferably measuring 10 mm or more—are associated with improved diagnostic yield. A minimum of three core samples should be obtained to ensure adequate material for histopathological evaluation, immunohistochemistry, and molecular genetic studies.
- On gross examination, untreated Ewing sarcoma typically appears as a soft, gray-white mass with frequent areas of hemorrhage and necrosis. Microscopically, the tumor exhibits a solid growth pattern composed of uniform small round cells with scant cytoplasm and round nuclei.
  - Bone marrow Biopsy is indicated in case PET CT is not available or PET CT gives unclear findings.
- Radiological Examination
  - Plain X-ray.
    - Osteolytic damage created by the tumor mass in the diaphyseal-metaphyseal bone.
    - Radiographically, it is commonly an ill-defined large intramedullary, mostly lytic lesion with multilayered periosteal reaction. The periosteal reaction is either laminated or perpendicular in form.
    - Rarely, the lesions are sclerotic.
  - Contrast-enhanced MRI ± CT of primary site.
  - Chest CT.
  - FDG-PET/CT.
  - Bone scan.
- Cytogenetics and/or molecular studies: [9].
- The *2020 World Health Organization (WHO) Classification of Tumors of Soft Tissue and Bone* categorizes round cell sarcomas into four distinct molecular and pathological entities: classic Ewing sarcoma (EwS), round cell sarcomas harboring *EWSR1::non-ETS gene fusions*, *CIC-rearranged sarcomas*, and *sarcomas characterized by BCOR gene alterations*.

28.1.7 Classic Ewing Sarcoma

- Conventional Ewing sarcoma is histologically defined by diffuse sheets of uniform small round cells exhibiting indistinct cytoplasmic borders, scant pale or clear cytoplasm, and round nuclei with finely dispersed chromatin. Immunohistochemically, these tumors demonstrate strong and diffuse membranous expression of *CD99*, along with nuclear positivity for *NKX2.2* and *FLI1*.
- The hallmark molecular abnormality in Ewing sarcoma is a *FET::ETS fusion*, most commonly *EWSR1::FLI1*, which is identified in approximately 70–80% of

cases. Other less frequent translocations include *EWSR1 or FUS::ERG* (around 15%), followed by *EWSR1 or FUS::FEV* (approximately 5%) and rare fusions involving *EWSR1::ETV1 or ETV4* (about 1%).

28.1.7.1 Round Cell Sarcoma with EWSR1:: non-ETS Fusions

- Sarcomas characterized by *EWSR1:: non-ETS rearrangements* represent a small but distinct subset of round cell sarcomas. In a large contemporary cohort, these tumors accounted for nearly 6% of 240 patients with round cell sarcomas harboring EWSR1 or FUS fusions. The presence of alternative EWSR1 fusion partners creates significant diagnostic challenges and carries therapeutic relevance. These findings also underscore the limitations of relying solely on *EWSR1 break-apart FISH* assays for molecular confirmation.

28.1.8 CIC-Rearranged Sarcoma

- CIC-rearranged sarcomas are defined by the presence of the *CIC::DUX4 fusion*, most commonly arising from either t(4;19) or t(10;19) chromosomal translocations. This genetic alteration is detected in approximately two-thirds of FET-negative round cell sarcomas. These tumors typically affect young adults and are associated with a poorer clinical outcome, including reduced five-year survival rates.
- Pathologically, CIC-rearranged sarcomas show a preference for soft tissue involvement and exhibit heterogeneous morphology, with round cell areas admixed with epithelioid or spindle cell components within a myxoid stroma. Immunohistochemistry frequently demonstrates positivity for *WT1* and *ETV4*, with variable expression of *CD99*.

28.1.8.1 Sarcomas with BCOR Gene Alterations

- Round cell sarcomas with *BCOR genetic alterations* represent another distinct entity with characteristic clinical behavior. Tumors harboring *BCOR::CCNB3 fusions* generally display a relatively favorable prognosis. In contrast, round cell sarcomas associated with *BCOR internal tandem duplication (ITD)* demonstrate highly aggressive biological behavior and poorer outcomes.
- Given the diagnostic complexity and therapeutic implications of these molecular subtypes, the *National Comprehensive Cancer Network (NCCN)* guidelines strongly recommend that sarcoma pathology be reviewed at specialized centers with access to advanced immunohistochemical and molecular diagnostic testing.
- Blood Investigations:
  - Complete hemogram.
  - Liver function test.

- Kidney function test.
- Coagulation profile.
- Anemia profile.

• Fertility consultation: [10]

- All cancer patients of reproductive age should receive complete oncofertility counselling as early as possible in the treatment planning process, irrespective of type and stage of disease.
- This should include discussion of:

  • Patients' current or future family desire.
  • Their health and prognosis.
  • The potential impact of the disease and/or proposed anticancer treatment on their fertility and gonadal function.
  • Chances of future conception.
  • Pregnancy outcomes and offspring.
  • The need for effective contraception in the context of systemic anticancer treatment.
  • Should be individualized based on patient/couple- and disease/treatment-related factors, with patient interest and age as well as type of treatment being the most important.

- Male patients:

  • Sperm cryopreservation.
  • Gonadal shielding during RT.
  • Medical gonadoprotection.

- Female patients.

  • Oocyte and embryo cryopreservation.
  • Ovarian tissue cryopreservation.
  • Ovarian transposition and gonadal shielding during RT.
  • Medical gonadoprotection.

28.2 Magnetic Resonance Imaging (MRI) [1, 2]

Magnetic resonance imaging is the preferred modality for the evaluation of soft tissue components of Ewing sarcoma and related tumors. On MRI, lesions typically demonstrate low to intermediate signal intensity on T1-weighted sequences and high signal intensity on T2-weighted images, with heterogeneous enhancement following contrast administration. MRI provides precise assessment of tumor depth, size, and local extension, and is particularly useful in confirming the absence of intramedullary marrow involvement.

MRI should be performed prior to biopsy to guide optimal selection of the biopsy site and to minimize interpretative errors caused by post-procedural hemorrhage or edema. It is also recommended for pre-operative restaging before definitive local control, as tumor dimensions and extent may change during neoadjuvant chemotherapy. The reported diagnostic performance of MRI includes a sensitivity of approximately 95%, specificity of 84%, positive predictive value of 85%, and negative predictive value of 85%.

Due to its superior soft tissue contrast resolution and avoidance of ionizing radiation, MRI is used more frequently than CT for local disease evaluation. Post-chemotherapy MRI findings play a critical role in planning definitive local treatment. MRI can accurately determine transphyseal spread, joint involvement, encasement or displacement of adjacent neurovascular structures, and invasion of surrounding musculature.

28.3 Recommended MRI Protocol

- Long-axis imaging using T1-weighted and/or short tau inversion recovery (STIR) sequences covering the entire involved bone to evaluate tumor extent and identify skip lesions.
- Axial fast spin-echo T2-weighted sequences with fat suppression or STIR through the tumor to delineate relationships with adjacent soft tissues and vascular structures.
- Gradient echo sequences may be added to confirm vascular flow when vessel involvement is suspected.
- Post-gadolinium T1-weighted fat-suppressed sequences are useful for identifying areas of necrosis; limited field-of-view imaging in at least two planes is recommended for accurate assessment of joint involvement.

28.3.1 Computed Tomography (CT) [11]

On computed tomography, Ewing sarcoma typically appears as a large, well-defined soft tissue mass with attenuation equal to or slightly lower than that of adjacent skeletal muscle. Following contrast administration, tumors exhibit marked and heterogeneous enhancement, with hypodense regions frequently corresponding to areas of intratumoral necrosis. Calcifications are uncommon, occurring in approximately 10% of cases, and are usually faint and amorphous in appearance.

Studies have shown no statistically significant difference between CT and MRI in assessing local tumor extent [12]. However, CT is superior to conventional radiography for the detection of pulmonary metastases and remains the imaging modality of choice for thoracic staging.

28.3.2 CT Imaging Protocol

High-resolution chest CT using a spiral technique with collimation of 5 mm or less, acquired during a single breath-hold, is the preferred protocol. Intravenous contrast is generally unnecessary unless there is suspected involvement of the chest wall, hilar, or mediastinal structures requiring improved anatomical delineation. Chest CT should ideally be performed before biopsy, as post-anesthetic atelectasis may mimic metastatic lesions.

Pulmonary metastatic deposits typically appear as round or ovoid, well-circumscribed nodules, most often located in the peripheral lung fields. Sharply marginated nodules measuring greater than 5 mm in diameter, particularly when multiple, are considered highly suggestive of metastatic disease. Criteria for the diagnosis of pulmonary and pleural metastases are defined by the *EURO--E.W.I.N.G.* protocol.

- *X-Ray*
  - Osteolytic damage created by the tumor mass in the diaphyseal-metaphyseal bone.
  - Radiographically, it is commonly an ill-defined large intramedullary, mostly lytic lesion with multi-layered periosteal reaction. The periosteal reaction is either laminated or perpendicular in form.
  - Rarely, the lesions are sclerotic.
- *Bone Scan*
  - Recommended for detection of bone metastasis at presentation.
  - If regions of increased uptake are noted on the scan, radiographs are performed to further confirm the presence of metastasis.
- *FDG PETCT*

28.3.3 FDG–Positron Emission Tomography (FDG-PET)

Fluorodeoxyglucose positron emission tomography has demonstrated greater sensitivity than conventional bone scintigraphy for the detection of osseous metastatic disease [13]. In addition to its role in staging, FDG-PET has shown value as a non-invasive modality for evaluating response to chemotherapy and for identifying recurrent disease during follow-up. Although FDG-PET is recommended as part of the imaging work-up in Ewing sarcoma, its use is not considered mandatory in all cases.

28.3.4 Positron Emission Tomography–Magnetic Resonance Imaging (PET-MRI)

The introduction of hybrid PET-MRI systems allows for the simultaneous acquisition of metabolic information from PET and high-resolution morphologic and functional data from MRI. This integrated approach offers the potential for comprehensive characterization and staging of primary bone tumors within a single imaging examination [14]. An important advantage of PET-MRI is the absence of additional ionizing radiation from the MRI component.

However, a notable limitation of integrated PET-MRI is its reduced sensitivity for the detection and characterization of pulmonary nodules, largely due to inherent constraints of MRI in lung imaging.

Clinical Pathway & Radiological Protocols for suspected Ewing Sarcoma

CLINICAL MILESTONE	MANDATORY RADIOLOGICAL PROTOCOLS
1. Suspicion of Malignant Bone Lesion	• Conventional plain radiography (minimum 2 orthogonal views). • Local Anatomic Staging: High-resolution contrast-enhanced MRI encompassing the entire involved anatomical compartment and adjacent joints. Mandatory sequences include: T1-weighted, T2-weighted, T1 + Contrast Medium (CM), native T1, and Short Tau Inversion Recovery (STIR). • Systemic Metastatic (M) Staging: Whole-body imaging (PET CT) or Computed Tomography (CT) of the chest to rule out pulmonary macrometastases.
2. Histopathological Confirmation	• Image-guided or open biopsy targeted directly to the primary local lesion site. • Image-guided FNAC or biopsy of the metastatic lesions when uncertain regarding its nature • Complete all core staging imaging sequences before introducing any cytotoxic treatment components to avoid therapeutic artifact contamination.
3. Induction Chemotherapy (CTX)	• Interval Therapeutic Assessment: Targeted local MRI of the primary tumor site to precisely calculate volumetric response and change in nature. • Systemic Staging: Repeat targeted systemic M-staging to monitor for potential early disease progression or micrometastatic evolution.
4. Pre-Local Therapy Evaluation	• Surgical / Radiotherapy Planning: Full repetition of baseline anatomical sequences (T1, T2, T1 + CM, STIR) to map viable tumor margins, neurovascular involvement, and boundaries for local control.
5. Local Control Intervention	• Definitive local treatment execution via radical surgical resection, radiotherapy, or a combined modality approach. • Postoperative Baseline Staging: Early localized MRI of the operative bed or structural reconstruction to establish a new definitive baseline for long-term tracking.
6. Consolidation Chemotherapy	• Surveillance local MRI of the primary treated site and systemic M-staging at regular intervals to ensure continuous remission status.
7. Post-Therapy Follow-Up	• Long-Term Multi-Year Surveillance Protocol: Structured, serial tracking utilizing high-resolution local MRI and targeted systemic staging to capture early recurrence or late systemic relapse. • Initiation of second-line chemotherapy regimens if surveillance tracking indicates disease recurrence.

Diagnostic Algorithm for Undifferentiated Small Round Cell Sarcomas

CD99-POSITIVE DIFFERENTIAL DIAGNOSES:
Membranous CD99 expression is not entirely specific to Ewing sarcoma. When encountering non-typical round cell morphology, pathologists must systematically rule out the following mimics via targeted marker panels:

1. Lymphoma/Leukemia (evaluate CD45, CD79a, CD20, CD3, TdT)
2. Rhabdomyosarcoma (evaluate Desmin)
3. Small Cell Carcinoma (evaluate Cytokeratin, TTF1)
4. Synovial Sarcoma (evaluate TLE1, or SS18/SYT FISH)
5. Clear Cell Sarcoma (evaluate S-100, MelanA, HMB45, SOX10)
6. Myxoid/Round Cell Liposarcoma (evaluate DDIT3 FISH)
7. Neuroblastoma (evaluate NB84 reactivity)

2. Stepwise Histomolecular Matrix

INITIAL MORPHOLOGY	IMMUNOHISTOCHEMISTRY (IHC)	MOLECULAR PATHOLOGY	DEFINITIVE CLINICAL DIAGNOSIS
Typical Round Cell Morphology Granular PAS positivity Sparse/few reticulin fibers	Diffuse, consistent membranous CD99+ NKX2-2 strong positive Variable NSE and Synaptophysin positivity	EWSR1 break-apart positivity OR rarely FUS break-apart confirmation Confirmed via RT-PCR or RNA Sequencing for fusion partner mapping	**Classic Ewing Sarcoma**
Non-Typical Variant Morphology Heightened cytological variability Prominent spindle cell or epitheloid architectural patterns	Heterogeneous or completely negative CD99 expression WT-1 positive ETV4 positive	CIC break-apart alteration OR confirmed via targeted RNA Sequencing panels	**CIC-Rearranged Sarcoma**
Non-Typical Variant Morphology Heightened cytological variability Prominent spindle cell or epitheloid architectural patterns	Heterogeneous or completely negative CD99 expression Cyclin B3 positive BCOR strong positive	BCOR-CCNB3 RT-PCR positive OR BCOR-ITD PCR amplification Confirmed via high-throughput RNA Sequencing	**Sarcoma with BCOR Genetic Alteration**
Non-Typical Variant Morphology Heightened cytological variability Prominent spindle cell or epitheloid architectural patterns	CD99 strong positive Variable/focal NKX2-2 expression EMA positive	EWSR1 break-apart positivity Confirmed via RNA Sequencing identifying unique non-ETS partners (e.g., NFATc2)	**Round Cell Sarcoma with EWSR1-NFATc2 Fusion**

References

1. Campbell K, Shulman D, Janeway KA, DuBois SG. Comparison of epidemiology, clinical features, and outcomes of patients with reported Ewing sarcoma and PNET over 40 years justifies current WHO classification and treatment approaches. Sarcoma. 2018;2018:1712964.
2. Daniel A, Ullah E, Wahab S, Kumar V. Relevance of MRI in prediction of malignancy of musculoskeletal system–a prospective evaluation. BMC Musculoskelet Disord. 2009;10:125.

3. Ludwig JA. Ewing sarcoma: historical perspectives, current state-of-the-art, and opportunities for targeted therapy in the future. Curr Opin Oncol. 2008;20(4):412–8.
4. Wright A, Desai M, Bolan CW, Badawy M, Guccione J, Rao Korivi B, et al. Extraskeletal Ewing sarcoma from head to toe: multimodality imaging review. Radiographics. 2022;42(4):1145–60.
5. Chakraborty D, Rangamani S, Kulothungan V, Chaturvedi M, Stephen S, Das P, et al. Trends in incidence of Ewing sarcoma of bone in India – evidence from the National Cancer Registry Programme (1982–2011). J Bone Oncol. 2018;12:49–53.
6. Holly EA, Aston DA, Ahn DK, Kristiansen JJ. Ewing's bone sarcoma, paternal occupational exposure, and other factors. Am J Epidemiol. 1992;135(2):122–9.
7. Valery PC, Williams G, Sleigh AC, Holly EA, Kreiger N, Bain C. Parental occupation and Ewing's sarcoma: pooled and meta-analysis. Int J Cancer. 2005;115(5):799–806.
8. Zöllner SK, Amatruda JF, Bauer S, Collaud S, de Álava E, DuBois SG, et al. Ewing sarcoma-diagnosis, treatment, clinical challenges and future perspectives. J Clin Med. 2021;10(8):1685.
9. Shulman DS, Whittle SB, Surdez D, Bailey KM, de Álava E, Yustein JT, et al. An international working group consensus report for the prioritization of molecular biomarkers for Ewing sarcoma. npj Precis Onc. 2022;6(1):1–11.
10. Lambertini M, Peccatori FA, Demeestere I, Amant F, Wyns C, Stukenborg JB, et al. Fertility preservation and post-treatment pregnancies in post-pubertal cancer patients: ESMO clinical practice guidelines†. Ann Oncol. 2020;31(12):1664–78.
11. Manaster BJ, Dalinka MK, Alazraki N, Berquist TH, Daffner RH, DeSmet AA, et al. Follow-up examinations for bone tumors, soft tissue tumors, and suspected metastasis post therapy. American College of Radiology. ACR appropriateness criteria. Radiology. 2000;215(Suppl):379–87.
12. Meyer JS, Nadel HR, Marina N, Womer RB, Brown KLB, Eary JF, et al. Imaging guidelines for children with Ewing sarcoma and osteosarcoma: a report from the children's oncology group bone tumor committee. Pediatr Blood Cancer. 2008;51(2):163–70.
13. Aryal A, Kumar VS, Shamim SA, Gamanagatti S, Khan SA. What is the comparative ability of 18F-FDG PET/CT, 99mTc-MDP skeletal scintigraphy, and whole-body MRI as a staging investigation to detect skeletal metastases in patients with osteosarcoma and Ewing sarcoma? Clin Orthop Relat Res. 2021;479(8):1768–79.
14. Chodyla M, Barbato F, Dirksen U, Kirchner J, Schaarschmidt BM, Schweiger B, et al. Utility of integrated PET/MRI for the primary diagnostic work-up of patients with Ewing sarcoma: preliminary results. Diagnostics (Basel). 2022;12(10):2278.

28.4 Rhabdomyosarcoma

28.4.1 Introduction and Epidemiology

Soft tissue sarcomas constitute approximately 7% of all malignancies diagnosed in the pediatric population and about 1% of cancers in adults [1]. Among these, *rhabdomyosarcoma (RMS)* represents the most frequently occurring soft tissue sarcoma in children. It is a high-grade malignant tumor arising from primitive embryonal mesenchymal cells with the potential for skeletal muscle differentiation. Although uncommon overall, RMS is a significant pediatric malignancy and remains the most prevalent soft tissue sarcoma of childhood.

The estimated incidence of RMS is approximately 4.5 cases per million individuals younger than 20 years, with more than half of diagnoses occurring during the first decade of life [2, 3]. The incidence is comparatively lower in several Asian populations, including Japanese, Indian, and Chinese cohorts, where rates slightly above 2 cases per million have been reported [4]. Data from hospital-based cancer registries across seven Indian cities indicate that RMS accounts for roughly 1–4.5% of all childhood cancers, with a higher incidence observed in males than females [5].

Given its origin from embryonal mesenchyme, RMS can arise at virtually any anatomical site. The disease demonstrates a bimodal age distribution, with peak incidence in early childhood (2–5 years) and adolescence (12–17 years). The two principal histological subtypes are *embryonal* and *alveolar rhabdomyosarcoma.* Embryonal RMS is commonly associated with oncogenic alterations involving pathways such as *RAS* and *TP53*, whereas alveolar RMS is characterized by specific chromosomal translocations resulting in *PAX3–FOXO1* or *PAX7–FOXO1* fusion genes [6].

Multimodal treatment incorporating systemic chemotherapy along with surgery and/or radiotherapy has led to favorable outcomes in patients with localized disease, achieving an approximate five-year overall survival rate of 80%. Survival outcomes vary widely by risk group, ranging from about 50.6% (95% CI: 39.7–60.5) in very high-risk patients to nearly 100% in low-risk categories. In contrast, patients presenting with metastatic disease have a significantly poorer prognosis, with five-year survival rates declining to approximately 35% [7–10].

28.4.2 Risk Factors

Defining risk factors for this rare disease remains difficult. However, extensive literature supports the idea that genetic susceptibility and environmental influences contribute to the development of RMS (Table 28.1).

- Genetic:
  - The majority of cases are sporadic.
  - Syndromes associated with increased risk include:
    - Li-Fraumeni syndrome [11].
    - Neurofibromastosis type-1 syndrome [11, 12].

Table 28.1 Syndromes with increased risk of RMS

Syndrome	Associated genes
Li-Fraumeni syndrome	TP53
Neurofibromatosis type-1	NF1
DICER1	DICER1
Costello	HRAS
Noonan	BRAF, KRAS,PTPN11, RAF, SOS1
Beckwith-Wiedemann	IGF2, CDKN1C,H19, KCNQ10T1

  - Beckwith-Wiedeman syndrome [13].
  - Costello syndrome [14].
  - Noonan syndrome [15].
  - DICER1 syndrome [16].

- Environmental:
  - Paternal cigarette smoking (RR = 3.9) [17].
  - Advanced maternal age [18].
  - X-ray exposure in utero [18].
  - Maternal antibiotics use (RR = 2.7) [17].
  - Use of antibiotics in children after birth (RR = 6.8) [19].
  - Maternal recreational drug use (RR = 3.1) [20].
- Congenital anomalies are more frequently observed in children and adolescents with RMS compared to the general population (32% vs. 3%) [21].

28.4.3 *Clinical Features*

RMS can occur in any anatomic location because of its origin from embryonal mesenchyme. Head and neck RMS can be either parameningeal or non-parameningeal. Parameningeal locations include the middle ear, nasal cavity, paranasal sinuses, nasopharynx, and infratemporal fossa. Non-parameningeal sites encompass the scalp, parotid gland, oral cavity, pharynx, thyroid and parathyroid glands, and neck. Typically, these tumors present as an asymptomatic mass; however, as the disease progresses, specific signs and symptoms related to the tumor's location may develop. Patients with parameningeal RMS often experience nasal, aural, or sinus blockage, cranial nerve palsies, and headaches. Conversely, those with genitourinary RMS may present with hematuria, urinary obstruction, and constipation. The clinical signs and symptoms vary according to the tumor's site of origin (Fig. 28.1).

28.4.4 *Diagnosis*

Investigations in patients with suspected rhabdomyosarcoma should be directed toward establishing a definitive diagnosis, completing disease staging, and performing baseline assessments prior to initiation of chemotherapy.

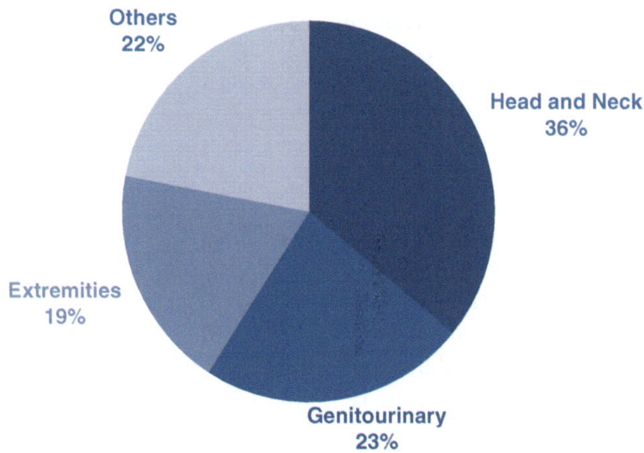

Fig. 28.1 Site of origin and frequency of presentation [22]

28.4.4.1 Baseline Evaluation

Baseline investigations are essential to identify pre-existing comorbidities, metabolic abnormalities, or coagulation disorders that may influence treatment planning and tolerance. Any abnormalities detected should be appropriately managed before starting tumor-directed therapy to ensure the patient's fitness for systemic chemotherapy, radiotherapy, and surgical intervention. Routine baseline assessments include complete blood count, renal and hepatic function tests, serum electrolytes including uric acid levels, coagulation profile, and baseline cardiac evaluation using two-dimensional echocardiography.

28.4.4.2 Diagnostic Investigations

Cross-sectional imaging of the primary tumor is recommended using contrast-enhanced computed tomography (CT) or magnetic resonance imaging (MRI). MRI is particularly preferred for tumors located at parameningeal, paraspinal, or pelvic sites, including rhabdomyosarcomas involving the bladder and prostate. Pathological confirmation is obtained through histopathological examination of tissue obtained via Tru-Cut biopsy or from an excised specimen. Cytogenetic and molecular studies are performed to identify characteristic chromosomal abnormalities and fusion genes that aid in diagnosis, classification, and risk stratification.

28.4.4.3 Staging Investigations

Assessment for metastatic disease includes contrast-enhanced CT of the thorax to evaluate pulmonary involvement and radionuclide bone scintigraphy to detect skeletal metastases. Bilateral bone marrow aspiration and trephine biopsy are routinely performed to assess marrow involvement. In cases of parameningeal rhabdomyosarcoma, cerebrospinal fluid examination is indicated to detect malignant cells. Where available, positron emission tomography–computed tomography (PET-CT) may be used as part of staging, although it should be complemented by bone marrow examination.

28.4.5 Radiologic Evaluation

28.4.5.1 Magnetic Resonance Imaging (MRI)

MRI is the imaging modality of choice for detailed assessment of tumor morphology and its relationship to surrounding anatomical structures. The imaging field should include the primary lesion, locoregional extension, and regional lymph node basins. European imaging guidelines recommend MRI protocols incorporating standard sequences such as T1-weighted, T2-weighted, post-contrast images, along with diffusion-weighted imaging (DWI).

MRI is particularly valuable in detecting perineural spread in head and neck rhabdomyosarcoma, especially at parameningeal sites, and is superior in identifying intracranial extension. Advanced multiparametric MRI techniques, including DWI, chemical shift imaging, and dynamic contrast-enhanced (DCE) MRI, provide improved tumor characterization, allow assessment of treatment response, and aid in detecting residual or recurrent disease following surgical intervention (Table 28.2).

Table 28.2 Multiparametric MRI techniques and type of information provided [23]

Multiparametric MRI technique	Type of information provided
DWI	Cellularity
DCE imaging	Vascularization
Chemical shift imaging	Fat
MRS	Metabolism

28.4.5.2 USG: Ultrasonography [24]

It may serve as a starting point in the diagnostic process. In the USG, rhabdomyosarcoma typically appears as a well-defined, slightly hypoechoic, inhomogeneous mass that may exhibit increased blood flow. It is easily accessible and provides critical information about the mass

28.4.5.3 CT: Computed Tomography [25]

Computed tomography (CT) reveals a large, well-defined mass with density at or below that of nearby muscle. Following contrast injection, the lesion shows intense, heterogeneous enhancement, often with hypodense regions caused by intratumoral necrosis. Calcification occurs in only about 10% of cases, typically faint and irregular. CT is particularly effective at detecting bony erosion, especially in the head and neck area, including the skull base. Importantly, apparent bone erosion from orbital primary tumors may lead to reclassification of orbital rhabdomyosarcoma into a less favorable para-meningeal category. For accurate assessment of metastatic spread, a chest CT performed at maximum inspiration is recommended to effectively identify lung nodules

28.4.5.4 Bone Scan

It is recommended for the detection of bone metastasis at presentation. If regions of increased uptake are noted on the scan, further imaging is performed to confirm the presence of metastasis

28.4.5.5 PETCT

Emerging evidence indicates that PET-CT scans could be more precise than traditional imaging methods for staging children with RMS. PET-CT has the potential to enhance initial staging accuracy and is more effective at detecting nodal disease and distant metastases(Table 28.3). However, there is limited data on the use of PET-CT for assessing treatment response or post-treatment evaluation. However, as depicted in Table 28.4, diagnostic CT has a higher sensitivity than PET/CT for detecting pulmonary metastases [26]

28.4.5.6 Histopathology

The cell of origin of RMS is the unsegmented, undifferentiated mesoderm. Myogenesis involves the differentiation of mesenchymal fibroblasts into skeletal muscle under the control of MyoD protein family and the halting of cell

Table 28.3 Comparison of PET/CT and diagnostic CT detection parameters for nodal and distant metastases [27]

		Sensitivity	Specificity	PPV	NPV
Detecting nodal Mets	PETCT	100	85	96.7	100
	CT	71	93	88	86.7
Detecting distant Mets	PETCT	98	86.5	96.5	93
	CT	75.5	60	94	11

Table 28.4 Comparison of PET/CT and diagnostic CT detection parameters for nodal and distant metastases

	Sensitivity	PPV
PETCT	92.5	96.3
Conventional	100	93

cycling and subsequent differentiation. It has been proposed that rhabdomyosarcoma represents an aberrant stage of normal muscle development [28]. RMS cells demonstrate little myogenesis, including undifferentiated mesenchymal cells, elongated myoblasts, and poorly differentiated myofibers [29]. The diagnosis of RMS requires examination of tumor tissue obtained via incisional, excisional, or core needle biopsies, followed by detailed histologic and molecular pathology studies

Previously, RMS was categorized into two main groups: embryonal and alveolar, based on their histological differences. The latest 2020 WHO classification now identifies four primary subtypes: embryonal, alveolar, spindle or sclerosing cell, and pleomorphic. Some variants previously unspecified have also been incorporated [30]. Morphologically, RMS cells vary in shape, including undifferentiated round, ovoid, "tadpole-like," and spindle-shaped cells, and fully differentiated rhabdomyoblasts [31]. These cells often display features of the skeletal muscle lineage and differentiation, as assessed by light or electron microscopy, immunohistochemistry (IHC), or molecular markers of skeletal muscle gene expression, such as muscle-specific actin, myosin, desmin, myoglobin, Z-band proteins, and transcription factors like MyoD1 or myogenin. Nonetheless, cellular morphology and tissue architecture remain essential for accurate diagnosis, as myogenic proteins can also be expressed in other childhood tumors like Wilms tumor and malignant rhabdoid tumor [32]

Alveolar RMS

Alveolar RMS constitutes 15–20% of cases. It is more frequently found in the extremities, trunk, perineal, and perianal areas. The prognosis is generally poor, particularly if metastasis is present at diagnosis (6). This subtype can be classified further based on the presence of PAX3–FOXO1 or PAX7–FOXO1 fusion transcripts. About 60% of ARMS patients have PAX3–FOXO1, 20% have PAX7–FOXO1, and the remaining 20% are fusion-negative, which correlates with a better prognosis than fusion-positive RMS. Genome-wide mRNA expression analyses reveal that ERMS and fusion-negative ARMS tumors have very similar profiles, which are distinct from those of PAX3–FOXO1-positive and PAX7–FOXO1-positive ARMS tumors [33]

Embryonal RMS

Embryonal histology represents 70–80% of cases. It includes classical embryonal, botryoid, and spindle cell subtypes. ERMS consists of immature "rhabdomyoblasts" set against a less dense, stroma-rich background, lacking an alveolar pattern. These tumors mainly develop in the head and neck or the genitourinary tract. The botryoid variant often affects the vagina, urinary bladder, biliary tract, and nasopharynx. The spindle cell variant is frequently found in the paratesticular area. Both the botryoid and spindle cell variants generally have a favorable prognosis

28.4.5.7 Pleomorphic RMS

Pleomorphic RMS is a rare adult variant of RMS distinguished by unique histological features. It comprises classic, round cell, and spindle cell types, based on overall morphology. The pleomorphic rhabdomyoblasts characteristic of this subtype express various skeletal muscle proteins identifiable through immunohistochemistry, aiding in differentiating it from adult pleomorphic sarcoma (32). Typically, pleomorphic RMS appears in older adults, more often in males, and frequently affects the lower extremities [34]. Because of its rarity, specific molecular abnormalities in this disease are not well established (Table 28.5)

28.4.5.8 Risk Stratification

Risk stratification is crucial for assessing a patient's prognosis and tailoring our treatment decisions. Risk stratification involves pretreatment staging, clinical grouping, age, and histology (Fig. 28.2). For RMS, it relies on pre-treatment (TNM) staging, surgical/pathologic clinical group, and tumor histology, each independently linked to outcomes [35, 36]. The IRSG first introduced the concept that RMS disease status can be described in terms of both "stage" and clinical "group" [35]. The TNM system evaluates tumor size, invasiveness, nodal status, primary site, and distant metastases. The clinical group considers residual tumor after surgery, regional lymph node involvement, and distant metastases [37]. There are two approaches to risk stratification based on the treatment allocation in clinical trials: the North American approach, defined by the Intergroup Rhabdomyosarcoma Study Group (IRS) I-IV (Table 28.6), and the European approach, defined by the European risk stratification for localized RMS used in the recent European Paediatric Soft Tissue sarcoma Group (EpSSG) [38]

Table 28.5 Rhabdomyosarcoma staging and clinical group classification systems [35]

Stage	Sites	Criteria
1	Orbit, head and neck (head and neck) (non-Para meningeal), GU (non-bladder, non-prostate), biliary	Tumor may be confined to organ of origin or extend to surrounding tissues with any size and presence or absence of regional lymph nodes/ unknown nodes
2	Bladder, prostate, extremities, para meningeal, other	Tumor may be confined to organ of origin or extend to surrounding tissues with size <5 cm and regional lymph node negative or unknown
3	Bladder, prostate, extremities, para meningeal, other	Tumor may be confined to organ of origin or extend to surrounding tissues with size >5 cm and/or regional lymph node positive
4	Any	Presence of metastases
Clinical group as per surgical staging		
I	Completely resected, localized disease	
II	Grossly complete resection with microscopic residual or involved regional nodes	
III	Biopsy or partial resection	
IV	Distant metastatic disease	

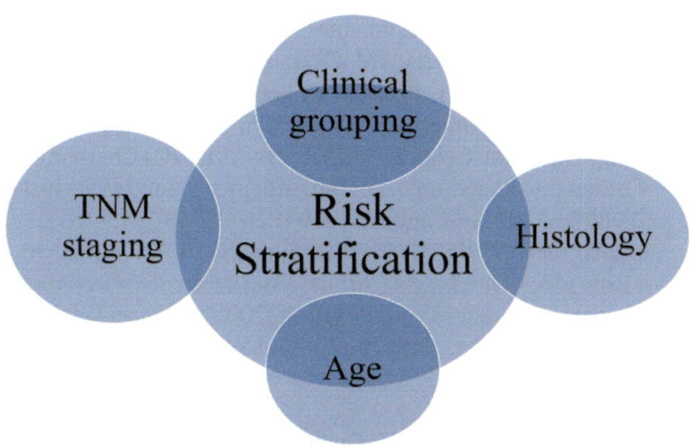

Fig. 28.2 Risk stratification in RMS

Table 28.6 Rhabdomyosarcoma risk stratification as per the Children's Oncology Group [39]

Risk group	Stage and clinical group	Other essential factors including molecular
Low	Stage and group I or II and Stage I, group III Orbit	FOXO1 fusion negative
Intermediate	All except low and high risk criteria	
High	Stage IV and group IV	Age >10 years or FOXO1 fusion positive[a]

[a]Either factor in stage IV, group IV makes it high risk; If both absent, then intermediate risk

28.5 Conclusion

The diagnosis and treatment of RMS necessitate a proper multidisciplinary team approach. Prompt diagnosis is essential for lowering mortality in rhabdomyosarcoma. Delayed diagnoses can lead to a higher rate of advanced-stage cancers and worse outcomes. Thus, a collaborative approach among healthcare professionals that enhances access to diagnostic and treatment modalities facilitates better communication and is vital for improving outcomes. Accurate staging and risk assessment are also key to more effective management of RMS

References

1. Hawkins DS, Spunt SL, Skapek SX, COG Soft Tissue Sarcoma Committee. Children's oncology group's 2013 blueprint for research: soft tissue sarcomas. Pediatr Blood Cancer. 2013;60(6):1001–8.
2. US Department of Health and Human Services; National Cancer Institute. Cancer incidence and survival among children and adolescents: United States SEER program 1975–1995 [Internet]. 1999 [cited 2026 Feb 1]. Available from: http://www.crossref.org/deleted_DOI.html
3. Panda SP, Chinnaswamy G, Vora T, Prasad M, Bansal D, Kapoor G, et al. Diagnosis and management of rhabdomyosarcoma in children and adolescents: ICMR consensus document. Indian J Pediatr. 2017;84(5):393–402.
4. Stiller CA, Parkin DM. International variations in the incidence of childhood soft-tissue sarcomas. Paediatr Perinat Epidemiol. 1994;8(1):107–19.
5. Ognjanovic S, Linabery AM, Charbonneau B, Ross JA. Trends in childhood rhabdomyosarcoma incidence and survival in the United States (1975–2005). Cancer. 2009;115(18):4218–4226. Google Search [Internet]. [cited 2026 Feb 1]. Available from: https://www.google.com/search?q=Ognjanovic+S%2C+Linabery+AM%2C+Charbonneau+B%2C+Ross+JA.+Trends+in+Childhood+Rhabdomyosarcoma+Incidence+and+Survival+in+the+United+States+(1975%E2%80%932005).+Cancer.+2009+Sep+15%3B115(18)%3A4218%E2%80%9326.&rlz=1C1UEAD_enIN927IN927&oq=Ognjanovic+S%2C+Linabery+AM%2C+Charbonneau+B%2C+Ross+JA.+Trends+in+Childhood+Rhabdomyosarcoma+Incidence+and+Survival+in+the+United+States+(1975%E2%80%932005).+Cancer+2009+Sep+15%3B115(18)%3A4218%E2%80%9326.+&gs_lcrp=EgZjaHJvbWUyBggAEEUYOTIHCAEQIRiPAjIHCAIQIRiPAjIHCAMQIRiPAtIBCTE2NjFqMGoxNagCCLACAfEFYdde4Yu2iDc&sourceid=chrome&ie=UTF-8.
6. Sorensen PHB, Lynch JC, Qualman SJ, Tirabosco R, Lim JF, Maurer HM, et al. PAX3-FKHR and PAX7-FKHR gene fusions are prognostic indicators in alveolar rhabdomyosarcoma: a report from the children's oncology group. J Clin Oncol. 2002;20(11):2672–9.
7. de Vries ISA, van Ewijk R, Adriaansen LME, Bohte AE, Braat AJAT, Fajardo RD, et al. Imaging in rhabdomyosarcoma: a patient journey. Pediatr Radiol. 2023;53(4):788–812.
8. Bisogno G, De Salvo GL, Bergeron C, Gallego Melcón S, Merks JH, Kelsey A, et al. Vinorelbine and continuous low-dose cyclophosphamide as maintenance chemotherapy in patients with high-risk rhabdomyosarcoma (RMS 2005): a multicentre, open-label, randomised, phase 3 trial. Lancet Oncol. 2019;20(11):1566–75.
9. Bergeron C, Jenney M, De Corti F, Gallego S, Merks H, Glosli H, et al. Embryonal rhabdomyosarcoma completely resected at diagnosis: the European paediatric soft tissue sarcoma study group RMS2005 experience. Eur J Cancer. 2021;146:21–9.

10. Schoot RA, Chisholm JC, Casanova M, Minard-Colin V, Geoerger B, Cameron AL, et al. Metastatic rhabdomyosarcoma: results of the European paediatric soft tissue sarcoma study group MTS 2008 study and pooled analysis with the concurrent BERNIE study. J Clin Oncol. 2022;40(32):3730–40.
11. Malkin D, Li FP, Strong LC, Fraumeni JF, Nelson CE, Kim DH, et al. Germ line p53 mutations in a familial syndrome of breast cancer, sarcomas, and other neoplasms. Science. 1990;250(4985):1233–8.
12. Sung L, Anderson JR, Arndt C, Raney RB, Meyer WH, Pappo AS. Neurofibromatosis in children with rhabdomyosarcoma: a report from the intergroup rhabdomyosarcoma study IV. J Pediatr. 2004;144(5):666–8.
13. Smith AC, Squire JA, Thorner P, Zielenska M, Shuman C, Grant R, et al. Association of alveolar rhabdomyosarcoma with the Beckwith-Wiedemann syndrome. Pediatr Dev Pathol. 2001;4(6):550–8.
14. Hennekam RCM. Costello syndrome: an overview. Am J Med Genet C Semin Med Genet. 2003;117C(1):42–8.
15. Kratz CP, Rapisuwon S, Reed H, Hasle H, Rosenberg PS. Cancer in Noonan, Costello, cardiofaciocutaneous and LEOPARD syndromes. Am J Med Genet C Semin Med Genet. 2011;157C(2):83–9.
16. Doros L, Yang J, Dehner L, Rossi CT, Skiver K, Jarzembowski JA, et al. DICER1 mutations in embryonal rhabdomyosarcomas from children with and without familial PPB-tumor predisposition syndrome. Pediatr Blood Cancer. 2012;59(3):558–60.
17. Grufferman S, Wang HH, DeLong ER, Kimm SY, Delzell ES, Falletta JM. Environmental factors in the etiology of rhabdomyosarcoma in childhood. J Natl Cancer Inst. 1982;68(1):107–13.
18. Grufferman: In utero X-ray exposure and risk of childhood... – Google Scholar [Internet]. [cited 2024 June 9]. Available from: https://scholar.google.com/scholar_lookup?journal=Paediatr+Perinat+Epidemiol&title=In+utero+x-ray+exposure+and+risk+of+childhood+rhabdomyosarcoma&volume=5&publication_year=1991&pages=A6&
19. Hartley AL, Birch JM, McKinney PA, Teare MD, Blair V, Carrette J, et al. The Inter-Regional Epidemiological Study of Childhood Cancer (IRESCC): case control study of children with bone and soft tissue sarcomas. Br J Cancer. 1988;58(6):838–42.
20. Grufferman S, Schwartz AG, Ruymann FB, Maurer HM. Parents' use of cocaine and marijuana and increased risk of rhabdomyosarcoma in their children. Cancer Causes Control. 1993;4(3):217–24.
21. Ruymann FB, Maddux HR, Ragab A, Soule EH, Palmer N, Beltangady M, et al. Congenital anomalies associated with rhabdomyosarcoma: an autopsy study of 115 cases. A report from the intergroup rhabdomyosarcoma study committee (representing the children's cancer study group, the pediatric oncology group, the United Kingdom children's cancer study group, and the pediatric intergroup statistical center). Med Pediatr Oncol. 1988;16(1):33–9.
22. Sultan I, Qaddoumi I, Yaser S, Rodriguez-Galindo C, Ferrari A. Comparing adult and pediatric rhabdomyosarcoma in the surveillance, epidemiology and end results program, 1973 to 2005: an analysis of 2,600 patients. J Clin Oncol. 2009;27(20):3391–7.
23. Inarejos Clemente EJ, Navallas M, Martínez B, de la Torre I, Suñol M, Munuera Del Cerro J, Torner F, et al. MRI of rhabdomyosarcoma and other soft-tissue sarcomas in children. Radiographics. 2020;40(3):791–814.
24. Jacobson JA, Middleton WD, Allison SJ, Dahiya N, Lee KS, Levine BD, et al. Ultrasonography of superficial soft-tissue masses: Society of Radiologists in ultrasound consensus conference statement. Radiology. 2022;304(1):18–30.
25. Manaster BJ, Dalinka MK, Alazraki N, Berquist TH, Daffner RH, DeSmet AA, et al. Follow-up examinations for bone tumors, soft tissue tumors, and suspected metastasis post therapy. American College of Radiology. ACR appropriateness criteria. Radiology. 2000;215(Suppl):379–87.
26. Chambers G, Frood R, Patel C, Scarsbrook A. ^{18}F-FDG PET-CT in paediatric oncology: established and emerging applications. BJR. 2019;92(1094):20180584.

27. kholy EE, Rezk M. 18F-FDG PET/CT in staging pediatric rhabdomyosarcoma; added benefits in comparison to conventional imaging. The Egyptian journal. Nuclear Med. 2019;18(1):25–39.
28. Hettmer S, Wagers AJ. Muscling in: uncovering the origins of rhabdomyosarcoma. Nat Med. 2010;16(2):171–3.
29. Parham DM, Barr FG. Classification of rhabdomyosarcoma and its molecular basis. Adv Anat Pathol. 2013;20(6):387–97.
30. Rudzinski ER, Anderson JR, Hawkins DS, Skapek SX, Parham DM, Teot LA. The World Health Organization classification of skeletal muscle tumors in pediatric rhabdomyosarcoma. Arch Pathol Lab Med. 2015;139(10):1281–7.
31. Dziuba I, Kurzawa P, Dopierała M, Larque AB, Januszkiewicz-Lewandowska D. Rhabdomyosarcoma in children – current pathologic and molecular classification. Pol J Pathol. 2018;69(1):20–32.
32. Skapek SX, Ferrari A, Gupta AA, Lupo PJ, Butler E, Shipley J, et al. Rhabdomyosarcoma. Nat Rev Dis Primers. 2019;5(1):1.
33. Ruiz-Mesa C, Goldberg JM, Coronado Munoz AJ, Dumont SN, Trent JC. Rhabdomyosarcoma in adults: new perspectives on therapy. Curr Treat Options in Oncol. 2015;16(6):27.
34. Furlong MA, Mentzel T, Fanburg-Smith JC. Pleomorphic rhabdomyosarcoma in adults: a clinicopathologic study of 38 cases with emphasis on morphologic variants and recent skeletal muscle-specific markers. Mod Pathol. 2001;14(6):595–603.
35. Malempati S, Hawkins DS. Rhabdomyosarcoma: review of the children's oncology group (COG) soft-tissue sarcoma committee experience and rationale for current COG studies. Pediatr Blood Cancer. 2012;59(1):5–10.
36. Meza JL, Anderson J, Pappo AS, Meyer WH, Children's Oncology Group. Analysis of prognostic factors in patients with nonmetastatic rhabdomyosarcoma treated on intergroup rhabdomyosarcoma studies III and IV: the children's oncology group. J Clin Oncol. 2006;24(24):3844–51.
37. Lawrence W, Anderson JR, Gehan EA, Maurer H. Pretreatment TNM staging of childhood rhabdomyosarcoma: a report of the intergroup rhabdomyosarcoma study group. Children's cancer study group. Pediatric oncology group. Cancer. 1997;80(6):1165–70.
38. Yechieli RL, Mandeville HC, Hiniker SM, Bernier-Chastagner V, McGovern S, Scarzello G, et al. Rhabdomyosarcoma. Pediatr Blood Cancer. 2021;68(Suppl 2):e28254.
39. Haduong JH, Heske CM, Rhoades WA, Xue W, Teot LA, Rodeberg DA, et al. An update on rhabdomyosarcoma risk stratification and the rationale for current and future children's oncology group clinical trials. Pediatr Blood Cancer. 2022;69(4):e29511.

Chapter 29
Evaluation and Staging of Wilms Tumor

Sambit Swarup Nanda, Satyendra Narayan Singh, and Narapareddy Venkata Dinesh Reddy

Wilms tumor, also known as nephroblastoma, is the most common renal tumor of childhood and infancy. Clinical presentation of Wilms' tumor in children may vary from an asymptomatic abdominal mass to gross hematuria and pressure effects over surrounding structures. Of Wilms' tumor cases, 90% are brought by parents with an asymptomatic abdominal mass noticed while bathing, clothing, or playing with the child. Since Wilms' tumor is retroperitoneal, it can grow into a large mass unhampered by any strict anatomical boundaries. Imaging studies should be obtained promptly if a renal tumor is suspected, due to a mass or unexplained hematuria. The initial aim is to identify if a tumor is present and, if present, to know its origin. Once there is a confirmed tumor, the aim will be to stage the tumor. Diagnostic imaging in suspected Wilms tumor can include renal ultrasound for initial study and abdominal and Chest CT. This chapter will explain in detail the workup and staging of Wilms tumor.

29.1 Introduction

Wilms tumor, also known as nephroblastoma, is the most common renal tumor of childhood and infancy [1]. It was named after German Surgeon, Max Wilms, who first described the tumor in 1899. Being the fourth most common tumor in children after Leukemia, CNS tumors, and Neuroblastoma, 75% of Wilms tumors are seen below 5 years of age, with a peak at 2–3 years [2].

S. S. Nanda (✉) · N. Venkata Dinesh Reddy
Department of Radiation Oncology, MPMMCC/ HBCH Varanasi, Units of Tata Memorial Centre; Also affliated with Homi Bhabha National Institute, Mumbai, India

S. N. Singh
Department of Radio-diagnosis, MPMMCC/ HBCH Varanasi, Units of Tata Memorial Centre; Also affliated with Homi Bhabha National Institute, Mumbai, India

S. Pradhan et al. (eds.), *Evidence Based Handbook on Diagnosis and Staging in Oncology*, https://doi.org/10.1007/978-981-95-9701-7_29

As the name nephroblastoma indicates, Wilms tumor arises from embryonic renal precursor cells (nephrogenic rests) that fail to undergo normal differentiation. Wilms tumor can occur sporadically or as a part of specific genetic syndromes. Of Wilms tumor cases, 8–10% have bilateral presentation with syndromes that frequently include genitourinary malformation or overgrowth. With an overall age-standardized incidence rate of 7.9 per million person-years worldwide, incidence rates vary across various regions of the globe (Fig. 29.1). The incidence of Wilms is three times higher among Africans and African Americans than among East Asians. Mean age at diagnosis varies with gender and laterality, with boys about 6 months earlier than girls and bilateral tumors earlier than unilateral tumors. The mean age of diagnosis is 41.6 months in boys and 46.9 months in girls for unilateral tumors. While the mean age at diagnosis for bilateral disease is 29.5 months in boys and 32.6 months in girls. Age at diagnosis for unilateral multifocal tumors was found to be intermediate between unilateral and bilateral disease [3].

The renal system develops from the urogenital ridge. Intermediate mesoderm forms nephrotomes that join into a pro-nephric duct. The pronephric duct induces nearby intermediate mesoderm to form mesonephric tubules, which receive tufts of capillaries, allowing filtration of blood and draining into the mesonephric duct. Caudally, the mesonephric duct sprouts the ureteric bud that induces the development of the metanephric blastema, which forms the metanephric system. Loss of inductive capacity of the ureteric bud occurs after 36 weeks, leading to the disappearance of metanephric blastemal cells completely 4–6 weeks prior to birth. Nephrogenic rest is a cluster of these cells that persists even after birth. If multiple cell rests are present. Two types of nephrogenic rests have been described by Beckwith et al.: [4] (1) perilobar rests, which are common in infants below 3 months of age, and (2) intralobar rests, which are rare except in cases of Wilms' tumor.

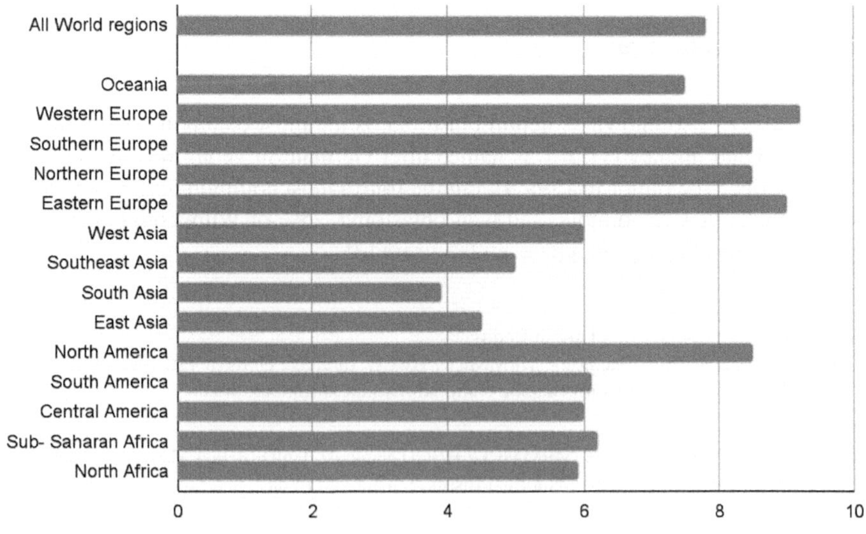

Fig. 29.1 Age-standardized incidence rates per million persons per year of Wilms tumor

Wilms' tumor consists of three components: blastemal, epithelial, and stromal components displaying varying differentiation of stem cells, sometimes with anaplastic features. Histology is defined partly by underlying genetic defects. Genetic factors so far known to cause Wilms' tumor include mutations of WT1, CTNNB1, WTX, loss of 1p and 16q, gain of 1q, and loss of H19-IGF2 imprinting. Around 17% of Wilms tumors occur with genetic malformation syndromes [5]., which include WAGR syndrome, Denys–Drash syndrome, Beckwith–Wiedemann syndrome, Li–Fraumeni syndrome, and other syndromes (Table 29.1).

Of Wilms' tumor cases, 10–15% are known to be caused by genetic variations or epigenetic alterations that occur during embryogenesis [6]. Of affected individuals, 2% have a family history of Wilms' tumor

Clinical presentation of Wilms' tumor in children may vary from an asymptomatic abdominal mass to gross hematuria and pressure effects over surrounding structures. Of Wilms' tumor cases, 90% are brought by parents with an asymptomatic abdominal mass noticed while bathing, clothing, or playing with the child. Since Wilms' tumor is retroperitoneal, it can grow into a large mass unhampered by any strict anatomical boundaries. Apart from Wilms' tumor, other conditions may also present with an abdominal mass (Table 29.2). Symptoms are found only in less than 20% children with new onset Wilms' tumor, which may include pain, hematuria, fever, urinary tract infection, weight loss, constipation, and other constitutional symptoms. Due to tumoral hemorrhage, patients can have signs and symptoms of anemia [7].

Of patients, 15–18% present with hematuria, which can be seen due to extension of the tumor within the renal pelvis or, rarely, renal vein thrombosis, and 25% present with abdominal pain, which is due to an expanding mass, subcapsular hemorrhage, and mass effects of the tumor. In 1977, Ramsay described three cases of Wilms tumor with acute hemorrhage causing a rapidly growing abdominal mass, hypertension, anemia, and fever—Ramsay's triad.

Table 29.1 Various syndromes associated with increased risk of Wilms' tumor and clinical features

Syndrome	Genetic defect	Features	Risk of WT
WAGR	11p13 deletion [WT1 gene]	Wilms tumor, aniridia, genitourinary anomalies, range of developmental delays	50%
Denys–Drash	Point mutation in the zinc finger region of WT1	Triad of diffuse mesangial sclerosis (nephrotic syndrome), ambiguous genitalia, and Wilms' tumor	75%
Beckwith–Wiedemann	Loss/dysregulation of H19–IGF2 imprinting	Overgrowth syndrome (organomegaly, macroglossia, omphalocele, hemihypertrophy, neonatal hypoglycemia)	0.2–24%
Li–Fraumeni	TP53 mutations [17p13]	Familial predisposition to cancer	Fewer cases reported
Frasier	Point mutation in WT1 [11p13]	Ambiguous genitalia, focal segmental glomerulo-sclerosis, diffuse mesangial sclerosis	A few case reports
Fanconi anemia	13q12 mutation	Short stature, bone marrow failure, and other heterogeneous features	20–40%

Table 29.2 Differential diagnosis of abdominal mass in children

Tumor	Age	Clinical features
Wilms' tumor	<5 years	U/L flank pain, aniridia, hematuria, thrombocytosis
Neuroblastoma	<5 years	GI/ GU obstruction, raccoon eye, diarrhea, raised VMA
Non-Hodgkin lymphoma	>1 year	Intussusception, raised LDH, pancytopenia
Rhabdomyosarcoma	All ages	GI/GU obstruction, vaginal bleeding/paratesticular mass, hypercalcemia
Germ cell tumor	<5 years, teenage	Abdominal pain, vaginal bleeding in females Testicular mass, hydrocele in males Raised ß- HCG, AFP
Hepatoblastoma	<3 years	Right upper quadrant mass, jaundice, raised AFP

In about 25% cases, hypertension can be a presenting sign and may accompany complaints of headache or pain. This is probably due to ischemic effects of the surrounding renal tissue from the expanding mass [8].. A rapidly growing tumor causes a compression effect on renal vasculature, which causes activation of the Renin-Angiotensin system, leading to hypertension and secondary hyperaldosteronism. In rare cases, hypertension can be severe, causing encephalopathy and retinal hemorrhage, but it usually resolves quickly following nephrectomy.

If an expanding tumor obstructs the venous drainage of the left spermatic cord, it may lead to dragging pain in the left sacrum and left-sided varicocele. Rarely, in right-sided tumors, due to tumor extension through the inferior vena cava to the right atrium or thromboembolism, cardiac manifestations, including arrhythmias, may be the presenting symptoms. Acute abdominal crisis, which includes acute abdominal pain, anemia, and hypotension, is an acute emergency that can occur due to rupture of a tumor secondary to abdominal trauma.

During physical examination on palpation, a mass that is typically smooth and eccentrically located towards the flank can be noted. Wilms' tumor mass should be distinguished from other abdominal masses, such as a palpable spleen that moves with respiration, and neuroblastoma, which is more frequently central and typically immobile. Complete top-to-toe examination to be done to rule out aniridia, Dysmorphic face, genital abnormalities, varicocele, and other features of syndromic Wilms' tumor.

Bilateral Wilms tumor is seen in 5–7% during presentation, of which synchronous disease is the majority at diagnosis, and 1.2% develop metachronous contralateral kidney involvement within 4 years of primary diagnosis.

29.2 Pathology

Wilms tumor presents as a large, rounded, multinodular, unifocal mass with a pseudocapsule. Wilms tumor arising from anywhere from renal parenchyma, compresses adjacent normal renal tissue, can extend to renal pelvis to renal vein and even to

Inferior vena cava and Right atrium. In the Botryoid-type Wilms tumor, the tumor extends in a polypoidal fashion into the pelvicalyceal system. Wilms tumor is classically described by Max Wilms as a triphasic tumor of both epithelial and stromal lineages. Blastemal component shows round cells, with a high nucleo-cytoplasmic ratio, scant cytoplasm, and coarse chromatin, arranged in a diffuse or nested pattern. Diffuse blastemal pattern is aggressive, but classified under favorable histology as it responds well to chemotherapy. Nested blastemal patterns include several organizational patterns, such as serpentine, nodular, or basaloid patterns. The epithelial component can differ from ill-formed, less aggressive papillary formations to well-formed glomeruloid structures. Stromal components include myxoid, spindled mesenchymal, smooth muscle, and fibroblast differentiation or heterologous differentiation. Rhabdomyoblastic differentiation is the most common heterologous differentiation.

Anaplasia, first described by Beckwith and Palmer, is the presence of enlarged, hyperchromatic nuclei with atypical multipolar mitotic figures [9]. Presence of anaplasia is the criteria for unfavorable histology. In some types of histology, enlarged hyperchromatic nuclei lacking atypical multipolar mitotic figures, but not severe enough to be labelled as anaplasia, are known as nuclear unrest. Wilms with nuclear unrest lies between favorable histology and anaplastic histology.

Children's Oncology Group (COG)	Histological type
Favorable histology	No anaplasia
Unfavorable histology	Focal anaplasia: Discrete foci of well-circumscribed anaplasia within the primary tumor No nuclear unrest outside anaplastic foci
	Diffuse anaplasia Non-localized anaplasia Localized anaplasia with severe nuclear unrest elsewhere Anaplastic foci outside the tumor capsule/involving vascular spaces Metastatic sites showing anaplastic cells

Chemotherapy-induced histology changes: Chemotherapy is an efficient and essential modality of Wilm's treatment. Chemotherapy reduces tumor burden, chances of tumor rupture, and accidental spill during surgery. Chemotherapy can bring maturation of all 3 components, and changes can be seen in the form of necrosis, fibrosis, and the presence of xanthomatous or hemosiderin-laden histiocytes. Immature, mitotically active blastemal cells undergo extensive necrosis, whereas epithelial and stromal components show poor response. In post-chemotherapy specimens, a large proportion of blastemal component signifies a worse prognosis.

Problems in the pathology of post-chemotherapy Wilms tumor [10]:

- *Completely necrotic tumor*: Look for nephrogenic nests (specific for Wilms). If none found, assume it is WT, as other renal tumors don't respond so well to preoperative chemotherapy.

- *Small stromal foci in a completely necrotic tumor*: Classify as low risk (completely necrotic).
- *No clear-cut viable tumor*: If tumor cells are dying but nuclear morphology is vaguely recognizable, regard such areas as non-viable.
- *Hypocellular tumor stroma*: Difficult to distinguish from chemotherapy-induced changes. Then see for rhabdomyoblasts, which indicate viable tumor stroma, or foamy macrophages, which represent chemo-induced changes.
- *Blastema %*: If >66% then blastemal type (high risk) vs <66% in mixed type (intermediate risk).
- *Anaplasia*: If meeting all three criteria, which includes atypical/ multipolar mitotic figures, marked nuclear enlargement (diameter > 3 times those of the same type adjacent cells), and hyperchromatic nuclei.

Wilms' tumor histological subtyping

Tumor type	Chemotherapy-induced changes [%]	Histological features [% of tumor]		
		Epithelium	Stroma	Blastema
Blastemal	≤65	≤33	≤33	>65
Stromal	≤65	≤33	>65	≤10
Epithelial	≤65	>65	≤33	≤10
Mixed	≤65	≤65	≤65	≤65
Regressive	>65	≤33	≤33	≤33
Completely necrotic	100	0	0	0

29.3 Evaluation

Usual laboratory tests are not specific for Wilms' tumor, but are used to rule out other pathologies. And these should include as follows:

- Complete blood counts, with special attention to hematocrit and anemia.
- Renal function tests include a full panel of electrolytes, creatinine, and blood urea nitrogen. Renal tumors rarely have renal failure; rather have compression from mass effect. Also, it was observed that marked elevation of calcium was seen in renal tumors of infants.
- Coagulation studies, including PT & aPTT: rarely deranged if coagulopathy is caused by acquired von Willebrand disease.
- Urinalysis may show hematuria, which indicates invasion of the tumor into the renal pelvis or ureter.
- Urinary beta- fibroblastic growth factor might be elevated in some children with Wilms tumor. But not specific for Wilms' tumor.
- Cytogenetic studies to look for 1p and 16q deletion.

Imaging studies should be obtained promptly if a renal tumor is suspected, due to a mass or unexplained hematuria. The initial aim is to identify if a tumor is present and, if present, to know its origin. Once there is a confirmed tumor, the aim will be to stage the tumor.

Diagnostic imaging in suspected Wilms tumor can include the following:

- Renal ultrasound for initial study.
- Chest X-ray for ruling out lung metastases.
- If available, abdominal and chest CT will be better.

Ultrasonography is often the first modality of imaging in suspicious abdominal mas to differentiate if it is of renal or extra-renal origin, cystic or solid nature. Wilms tumor on USG is usually seen as a large, intrarenal, solid heterogeneous mass with a pseudo-capsule that can be detected. With USG Doppler, tumor extension into the inferior vena cava or surrounding tissue can be detected. USG Abdomen has an overall sensitivity of 76% in detecting Wilms tumor among children presenting with abdominal mass [11] (Fig. 29.2).

Computed Tomography [CT] of the abdomen is the second-line modality after USG for Wilms tumor. Usually, nonionic iodinated contrast at 2 ml/kg is used for a single portal venous phase image, obtained 65–70 s after contrast injection. Less enhancing, large, well-defined heterogeneous mass with a beak or claw sign suggests Wilms tumor. Exophytic growth with irregular contours suggests capsular invasion. Taking histopathology as the gold standard, it was found that CECT has a sensitivity of 90.36% and specificity of 51.72% with a positive predictive value of 68.18% and a negative predictive value of 82.42% [12] (Fig. 29.3).

Magnetic Resonance Imaging (MRI): Abdominal MRI is the preferred imaging modality as per the SIOP (International Society of Pediatric Oncology) UMBRELLA protocol.

- WT shows a well-defined heterogeneous lobulated mass with hypointensity on T1w and slight hyperintensity with necrosis and cystic changes on T2w images.
- If intratumoral hemorrhage is present, it shows T1 hyperintensity.
- Pseudocapsule seen as a hypointense rim on both T1 and T2w images.
- Positive beak or claw sign confirms that the tumor is of renal origin.

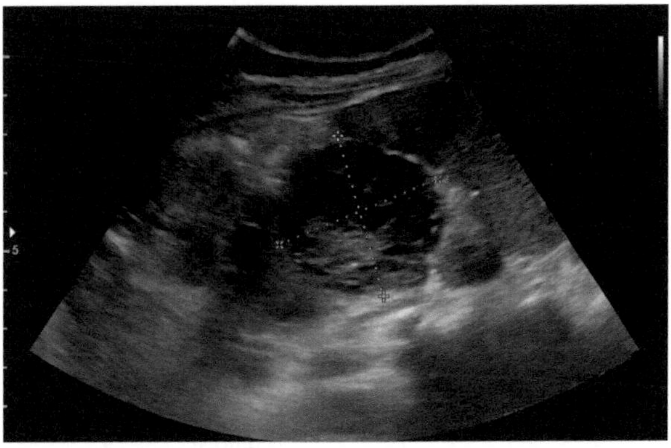

Fig. 29.2 USG images of a Wilms tumor diagnosed in a pediatric patient who presented with complaints of an abdominal lump

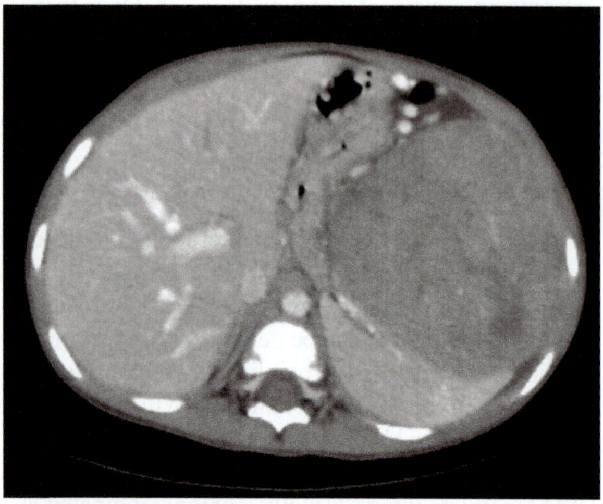

Fig. 29.3 CT images of a Wilms tumor diagnosed in a pediatric patient who presented with complaints of an abdominal lump

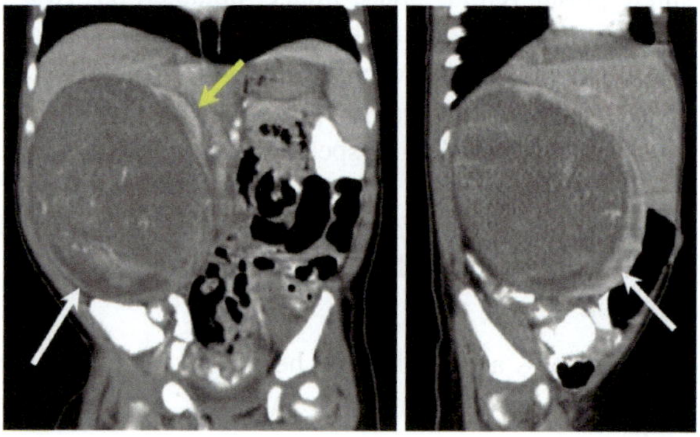

Fig. 29.4 CT images of a Wilms tumor diagnosed in a pediatric patient who presented with complaints of an abdominal lump

MRI can accurately evaluate the primary tumor size, regional spread, and extension of tumor thrombus into the vasculature. Small Wilms and nephrogenic rests can also be detected with gadolinium-enhanced MRI. MRI is also the imaging study of choice in bilateral WT [13]. DWI-MRI also helps in differentiating Wilms tumor from neuroblastoma with a sensitivity and specificity of around 80% and 100% [14] (Fig. 29.4).

Advantages and disadvantages of USG, CT, and MRI.

	Ultrasound	MRI	CT
Advantages	Non invasive No ionizing radiation Real time Easily available	No ionizing radiation Wide field of view Best for soft tissue resolution Functional imaging possible	Short imaging time No sedation required in older children Wide field of view
Disadvantages	Restricted field of view Operator dependent	Not easily available Long imaging time May need sedation and IV contrast	Ionizing radiation IV contrast required

29.4 Tumor Staging

- CT and MR have similar diagnostic performance in loco-regional staging of WT. [15]
- MRI can detect contralateral synchronous lesions; however, these are present in a very small number of cases.
- CT and MRI can both measure tumor size accurately.
- Local extent should be evaluated for.

  (a) Infiltration into adjacent structures.
  (b) Intravascular tumor extension.
  (c) Ureter invasion.
  (d) Regional lymph nodal involvement.
  (e) Signs of tumor rupture.
  (f) Peritoneal spread.

- Distant metastasis (via hematogenous spread), seen in 20% at initial presentation of WT, with the lungs being the most common site, followed by the liver.
- CT Chest is a mandatory evaluation of pulmonary metastasis, as per the new recommendations of the SIOP-UMBRELLA protocol. Baseline chest X-ray is also mandatory at initial diagnosis, so that it can be compared with chest X-rays during follow-up. [16]
- CT only nodules (small pulmonary nodules not seen in chest radiograph) if >3 mm in diameter, to be managed as metastatic stage IV disease.

29.5 PET-CT

Wilms tumor, being a metabolically active disease, Fluorodeoxyglucose gets accumulated and can be visualized in Positron emission tomography [PET] [17]. FDG PET can be useful in tumor staging, grading, and assessing preoperative chemotherapy response. It helps in directing biopsies from areas of active tumor activity. PET-CT also helps to distinguish lung nodules from benign lesions during diagnostic workup. However, due to the intrinsic limited resolution, FDG PET is not sensitive if lung nodules are less than 10 mm in diameter. FDG PET can be helpful in surveillance for detecting recurrences, predominantly at the postoperative bed, regional lymph nodes, distal urinary tract, lung, and liver, which may be missed by other imaging studies. Apart from the above, FDG PET can be used in the monitoring of tumor metabolic response to preoperative chemotherapy.

29.6 Diagnostic Biopsy

With collaborative working groups, particularly the International Society of Pediatric Oncology (SIOP) and the Children's Oncology Group (COG), the overall cure rate of Wilms' tumor is around 85% [18]. COG considers nephrectomy as the gold standard. But, biopsy preoperatively is recommended, especially if primary nephrectomy is contraindicated, which includes tumor thrombus extending to hepatic veins, surgery resulting in morbidity/ mortality, spillage, or incomplete resection. SIOP recommends induction chemotherapy in children aged 6 months or older without biopsy, purely based on imaging. Upfront nephrectomy is recommended in children below 6 months of age. Both COG and SIOP recommend a biopsy if there is any atypical radiology [19]. Avoid biopsy if the patient is unstable, suspected of rupture, or has any predisposing syndromes. Complications with biopsy include bleeding, rupture, and tract recurrences [20].

29.7 COG Staging [21]

Stage	Criteria
I	Tumor is limited to the kidney and completely excised; renal capsule is intact
II	Tumor is confined to the renal fossa; it can extend beyond the renal capsule and can extend into blood vessels, but the entire tumor can be resected en bloc. Does not include invasion of adjacent viscera or distant metastases
III	Tumor is not resected completely, which may occur by several means, including gross residual disease after surgery, local lymph node positivity, or tumor rupture
IV	Hematogenous metastases
V	Bilateral involvement at diagnosis

29.8 SIOP Staging System [21]

Stage	Criteria
I	A. Limited to the kidney and is completely resected. B. Tumor may be protruding into the pelvic system and dipping into the ureter (not infiltrating walls). C. No involvement of renal sinus. D. Involvement of intrarenal vessel.
II	● Extends beyond the kidney or penetrates through the renal capsule into the perirenal fat, but is completely resected. ● Infiltrates renal sinus and/or invades blood & lymphatic vessels outside renal parenchyma, but resected completely. ● Tumor infiltrates adjacent organs or vena cava, but is completely resected.

Stage	Criteria
III	A. Incomplete resection, extends beyond the resection margin. B. Any involvement of abdominal lymph nodes. C. Tumor rupture. D. Peritoneal surface penetrated by tumor. E. Tumor thrombus at the resection margin of vessels or ureter, transected or removed piecemeal by the surgeon. F. Tumor surgically biopsied prior to preoperative chemotherapy or surgery.
IV	Hematogenous or lymph node metastasis outside the abdominopelvic region
V	Bilateral renal tumors at presentation

References

1. Nakata K. Incidence of childhood renal tumours: an international population-based study. Int J Cancer. 2020;147(12):3313–27. https://doi.org/10.1002/ijc.33147.
2. https://www.cancer.org/cancer/types/cancer-in-children/types-of-childhood-cancers.html
3. Breslow N, Olshan A, Beckwith JB, Green DM. Epidemiology of Wilms tumour. Med Pediatr Oncol. 21(3):172–81. https://doi.org/10.1002/mpo.2950210305.
4. Beckwith JB, et al. Nephrogenic rests, nephroblastomatosis, and the pathogenesis of Wilms' tumour. Pediatr Pathol. 1990;10(1-2):1–36. https://doi.org/10.3109/15513819009067094.
5. Merks JHM, et al. High incidence of malformation syndromes in a series of 1,073 children with cancer. Am J Med Genet A. 2005;134A(2):132–43. https://doi.org/10.1002/ajmg.a.30603.
6. Mahamdallie S, et al. Identification of new Wilms tumour predisposition genes: an exome sequencing study. Lancet Child Adolesc Health. 3(5):322–31. https://doi.org/10.1016/S2352-4642(19)30018-5.
7. Ramsay NK, et al. Acute hemorrhage into Wilms tumor: a cause of rapidly developing abdominal mass with hypertension, anemia, and fever. J Pediatr. 91(5):763–5. https://doi.org/10.1016/s0022-3476(77)81035-4.
8. Maas MH, et al. Renin-induced hypertension in Wilms tumour patients. Pediatr Blood Cancer. 48v(5):500–3. https://doi.org/10.1002/pbc.20938.
9. National Wilms Tumour Study: An Update for Pathologists; https://doi.org/10.1007/s100249900010.
10. J Clin Pathol. 2010, 63:102e109. https://doi.org/10.1136/jcp.2009.064600.
11. Rahmani A, Sari N, Indriasari V. The role of ultrasonography for diagnosing Wilms tumor in developing country. IJHOSCR. 2021;15(3):145–51.
12. Amirali A, Darira J, Pathan H, Murtaza S, Irshad M. Assessment of imaging performance and accuracy for the diagnostic evaluation of Wilms tumor in kids in the ERA of contrast based CT scan with histopathological correlation: a Study in tertiary care hospital. Int J Innov Res Med Sci. 2021;6:668.
13. Imaging of Wilms tumor: an update; https://doi.org/10.1007/s00247-019-04423-3
14. Aslan M, Aslan A, Arıöz Habibi H, et al. Diffusion-weighted MRI for differentiating Wilms tumor from neuroblastoma. Diagn Interv Radiol. 2017;23:403–6.
15. Comparison of diagnostic performance of CT and MRI for abdominal staging of pediatric renal tumors: a report from the Children's Oncology Group; https://doi.org/10.1007/s00247-014-3138-2.
16. Current Role of Imaging in the Management of Children with Wilms Tumor According to the New UMBRELLA Protocol; Current Role of Imaging in the Management of Children with W | 25677 (longdom.org)

17. Shulkin BL, Chang E, Strouse PJ, Bloom DA, Hutchinson RJ. PET FDG studies of Wilms tumors. J Pediatr Hematol Oncol. 1997;19(4):334–8. https://doi.org/10.1097/00043426-199707000-00012.
18. Wilms tumor: “State-of-the-art” Update. 2016; https://doi.org/10.1053/j.sempedsurg.2016.09.003.
19. Surgery-Related Factors and Local Recurrence of Wilms Tumor in National Wilms Tumor Study 4; https://doi.org/10.1097/00000658-199902000-00019
20. Lee IS, et al. Needle tract seeding after percutaneous biopsy of Wilms tumor. J Urol. 1995;153(3 Pt 2):1074–6.
21. Erginel B. Wilms Tumor and Its Management in a Surgical Aspect. In: van den Heuvel-Eibrink MM, editor. Wilms Tumor [Internet]. Brisbane (AU): Codon Publications; 2016 Mar. Chapter 4. Available from: https://www.ncbi.nlm.nih.gov/books/NBK373361/ https://doi.org/10.15586/codon.wt.2016.ch4.

Chapter 30
Evaluation and Staging of Soft Tissue Sarcoma and Bone Sarcoma

Ashutosh Mukherji and Chandrima Mukherjee

30.1 Introduction

Malignant tumors arising in solid mesenchymal tissues are usually called *sarcomas* (Greek "*sarkoun*" = fleshy substance) [1]. These tumors arise from a diverse group of connective tissues and their derivatives, hence may display varying degrees of differentiation and genetic expression. However, they share a common embryologic origin, i.e., they are derived from the mesoderm.

Sarcomas can be broadly classified into sarcomas of the bone (~20%) and the soft tissue sarcomas (~80%) [2]. Their annual incidence is estimated to be 5 per 100,000 population [3, 4].

30.1.1 Bone Sarcomas

Primary bone tumors are rare, constituting <0.2% of all cancers.

Age incidence peaks between 10 and 20 years, with 60% occurring in this age group.

Eighty percent arise in long bones before epiphyseal closure; later, they emerge in the appendicular skeleton.

Prevalence order: *osteosarcoma* > *chondrosarcoma* > *Ewing's* > UPS/MFH of bone.

A. Mukherji (✉) · C. Mukherjee
Department of Radiation Oncology, MPMMCC/HBCH, Varanasi, Units of Tata Memorial Centre and affliated with Homi Bhabha National Institute (HBNI), Mumbai, India

S. Pradhan et al. (eds.), *Evidence Based Handbook on Diagnosis and Staging in Oncology*, https://doi.org/10.1007/978-981-95-9701-7_30

30.1.2 Staging

Two systems of staging are followed—AJCC and Enneking [13].

Malignant lesions are defined using Roman numerals (e.g., I, II, III).

Benign lesions are defined using Arabic numbers (1,2,3).

1 = Latent lesion, e.g., non-ossifying fibroma, enchondroma.
2 = Active lesion, e.g., ABC, UBC, chondromyxoid fibroma, chondroblastoma.
3 = Aggressive lesion, e.g., giant cell tumor of bone.

The prognosis of bone cancer depends on the following variables

- Stage of disease.
- Presence of metastasis.
- Skip (discontinuous) lesions within the same bone.
- Histologic grade.
- Tumor size.

30.2 Osteosarcoma

Osteosarcoma (OS) is a malignant neoplasm derived from primitive bone-forming (osteoid-producing) mesenchymal cells.

It is the most common primary (*no underlying bone pathology*) bone tumor in children and young adults. OS has a bimodal age distribution. The initial peak occurs in the 10–14-year age group (corresponding to pubertal growth spurt). The second peak is in adults aged >65 years [5].

The incidence rate of osteosarcoma in all races and genders is four cases per year per million people (3.5 to 4.6, 95% confidence interval).

Diabetes mellitus is a common association in these patients.

The 5-year overall survival rate is about 68%, regardless of sex [6].

30.3 Clinical Features

30.3.1 Symptoms and Physical Examination Findings of Osteosarcoma

30.3.1.1 Symptoms

Bone Pain:

Common presenting symptom, worsens with activity.

Often mistaken for sprains, arthritis, or growing pains, a history of musculoskeletal injury may or may not be present.

Pathologic Fractures: Telangiectatic osteosarcoma associated with fractures. May lead to limp and pain.

Swelling or Lump: Depends on tumor size and location.

Systemic Symptoms: Fever, night sweats (lymphoma-like symptoms) are rare.

Respiratory Symptoms: Rare, indicating extensive lung involvement.

Other additional symptoms uncommon due to rare metastases.

Physical Examination Findings:

Palpable Mass: Tender, warm, with/without pulsation or bruit. Nonspecific signs.

Joint Involvement: Decreased range of motion.

Lymphadenopathy: Local/regional (unusual).

Respiratory Findings: In metastatic settings.

30.4 Genetic Associations

Several genetic aberrations have been identified in a case of primary osteosarcoma [7] (Table 30.1).

Distribution of OS and sub-types [6].

OS most frequently occurs near the metaphysis of long bones of the appendicular skeleton.

Common locations of osteosarcoma and tumor distribution:

Femur: 42% occurrence—75% tumors in the distal portion.

Tibia: 19% occurrence—80% tumors in the proximal portion.

Humerus: 10% occurrence—90% tumors in the proximal portion (Table 30.2).

Table 30.1 Genetic syndromes associated with osteosarcoma

Syndrome	*Genetic association*	*Comment*
Hereditary RB	Autosomal dominant (AD) RB1 gene	Causes B/L retinoblastoma, absence of the "red reflex" in the eye or eyes of the affected child, increased risk of OS in later life
Li-Fraumeni syndrome	AD, p53 gene	
Rothmund-Thompson syndrome	Autosomal recessive (AR), RECQL4 gene	Predisposes to osteosarcoma as well as a characteristic infantile rash, dysplastic osseous structures, alopecia, premature cataracts, and chronic gastrointestinal distress
Bloom syndrome	AR, BLM gene	Predisposition to osteosarcoma and other cancers, these patients may also present with UV-induced rashes, short stature, and sparse subcutaneous fat
Werner syndrome	AR, WRN gene	Aka adult progeria, is characterized by premature aging, bilateral cataracts, osteoporosis, short stature, scleroderma-like skin changes, and a predilection for osteosarcoma

Table 30.2 Subtypes of osteosarcoma [14]

Subtypes of osteosarcomas	
Type	Description
Central (intramedullary)	
1. High-grade central	
a. Conventional	Classic appearance Spindle-like to polyhedral cells Variable nuclei, visible mitosis Osteoid, cartilaginous, fibrous matrix
i. Osteoblastoma-like	Resembles osteoblastoma Cellular atypia, local aggressiveness Osteoid matrix production
Ii. Chondroblastoma-like	Resembles chondroblastoma Cellular atypia, local aggressiveness Osteoid matrix production
Iii. Chondromyxoid fibroma-like	Resembles chondromyxoid fibroma Cellular atypia, local aggressiveness Osteoid matrix production
Iv. Malignant fibrous histiocytoma-like	Resembles malignant fibrous histiocytoma Cellular atypia, local aggressiveness Osteoid matrix production
v. Epithelioid	Poorly differentiated cells Difficulty distinguishing sarcoma/carcinoma origin
Vi. Giant cell	Benign multinucleated osteoclast-like giant cells
Vii. Clear cell	Numerous cells with clear/ground-glass cytoplasm and vacuoles
b. Telangiectatic	Blood-filled sinusoids mimic aneurysmal bone cyst Pleomorphic/atypical nuclei distinguish malignancy
c. Small cell	Combination of Ewing sarcoma and osteosarcoma Small round cells Minuscule osteoid matrix distinguishes variant
2. Low-grade central	
a. Fibrous dysplasia	Features a large volume of osseous matrix embedded in a small amount of fibrous stroma
b. Desmoplastic fibroma	Features a very small volume of osseous matrix embedded in a large amount of fibrous stroma.
Surface (periosteal/cortical)	
1. Low-grade surface	Parosteal—Outer periosteal surface of the bone, features ribbons of osseous trabeculae oriented in parallel, primarily composed of a chondroid matrix with only a minuscule amount of osteoid matrix.
2. Intermediate-grade surface	Periosteal—Between the cortex and the inner periosteal surface Parallel osseous trabeculae, chondroid matrix with more nuclear atypia
3. High-grade surface	High-grade surface—Identical to high-grade central, location confined to bone surface (dedifferentiated parosteal)

(continued)

Table 30.2 (continued)

Subtypes of osteosarcomas	
Type	Description
Extra-skeletal	
1. Low-grade	Similar to low-grade surface/central variants - can appear in soft tissues (thigh, buttocks, etc.)
2. High-grade	Similar to high-grade central variant - can appear in various extra-skeletal locations

30.5 Evaluation

This includes clinical history and physical examination.

Blood investigations, including LDH and ALP, serve as biochemical markers that aid osteosarcoma diagnosis and prognosis. Elevated ALP indicates osteoblastic activity, correlating with tumor burden and prognosis. Monitoring levels post-treatment tracks therapy response and recurrence risk [8].

-Diagnostic Imaging of Primary Tumor Site [8]:

- Radiographs: Conventional roentgenogram demonstrates medullary and cortical bone destruction, with "permeative or moth-eaten" appearance of the cortex. Classical signs include the "Sun-burst" (due to aggressive periostitis) or "Codman triangle" (due to elevation of periosteum away from bone), an ill-defined "fluffy" or "cloud-like" bony lesion, and classification produced due to formation of osteoid matrix by the tumor.
- Magnetic resonance imaging: MRI is a must for defining the extent of the disease. MRI of the entire affected bone is to be done, i.e., one joint above and below, to avoid missing "skip" lesions. MRI precisely assesses soft tissue involvement, joint involvement, physis crossing by the tumor, and proximity to nerves/vessels. MRI is used for pre-surgical assessment for limb-sparing resection to the degree of chemotherapy response in the form of tumor necrosis, shrinkage, and improved capsulation. In T1-weighted images, various components of osteosarcoma exhibit distinctive signal intensities. The non-ossified soft tissue component typically shows intermediate signal intensity, while the osteoid components appear with low signal intensity. Peri-tumoral edema demonstrates an intermediate signal intensity, and any scattered foci of hemorrhage display variable signal intensity depending on the stage of chronicity. In contrast, T2-weighted images reveal different patterns. The non-ossified soft tissue component manifests as high signal intensity, while osteoid components maintain low signal intensity. Peri-tumoral edema exhibits a high signal intensity in T2-weighted images. These signal characteristics play a crucial role in the radiological assessment of osteosarcoma.

- Computed tomography: CT is primarily used for assessment of distant metastases in the lungs. CT's value in primary tumor assessment follows that of radiography and MRI, unless the lesion is mainly lytic. Lytic lesions might hide some mineralized material on film and MRI.
- Positron emission tomography: PET is a newer imaging modality that detects highly metabolically active lesions. PET may aid in staging and recurrence detection. In a meta-analysis, the value of PET/CT in diagnosis and staging was summarized [12]. For the primary lesion, PET/CT showed 100% sensitivity. Pooled sensitivity and specificity for detecting lung metastases were 81% and 94%, respectively. For bone metastases, studies showed a pooled sensitivity of 93% and a pooled specificity of 97%. PET may be used instead of a CT scan where resources are available.
- Radionuclide bone scan: Technetium 99 methylenediphosphonate (Tc99 MDP) bone scan is an effective and readily available imaging modality for detecting bony metastasis. It is a less expensive but less specific alternative to PET imaging.
- Biopsy: The definitive surgical procedure must include resection of the biopsy tract. It should be tattooed for easy identification and to avoid recurrence due to potential seeding of this tract with cancer cells.

30.6 Chondrosarcoma

Chondrosarcomas are malignant neoplasms originating from cartilage. These account for 20% of all primary bone tumors. Most commonly occur in the pelvis or long bones of the extremities.

30.7 Types

Primary: Arising de novo in a normal bone.

Secondary: Occur in a preexisting enchondroma or osteochondroma.

Conventional	Non-conventional
Central	*Clear cell chondrosarcoma*
Periosteal	*Mesenchymal chondrosarcoma*
Peripheral	*Dedifferentiated chondrosarcoma*

30.7.1 Clinical Features

Deep, dull aching pain.

Night-time pain is characteristic.

Pain distinguishes malignancy from benign cartilaginous lesions.

Pain's reliability reduces in small hand/foot bones.
Lesions near neurovascular bundles may cause neural symptoms.
Pelvic lesions: Nerve dysfunction (lumbosacral plexus, sciatic, femoral nerves).
Proximity to joint: Limits joint range, disrupts function.

30.8 Evaluation

30.8.1 Plain X-ray (For Local Disease)

Initial evaluation employs plain radiography to identify the cartilaginous nature of the lesion and assess its aggressiveness.

In plain X-rays, common findings encompass lytic lesions in approximately 50% of cases, intralesional calcifications present in around 70% of cases (displaying characteristics such as *popcorn or rings and arcs calcification*), as well as indicators like endosteal scalloping and a permeative or moth-eaten appearance, particularly prominent in high-grade chondrosarcoma.

Additionally, plain X-rays reveal features such as cortical remodeling, thickening, and a periosteal reaction [9].

30.9 Computed Tomography

Computed tomography (CT) provides valuable insights. CT scans show matrix calcification in 94% of cases, along with the presence of endosteal scalloping. In about 90% of long bone chondrosarcomas, a cortical breach can be observed through CT imaging. Furthermore, CT scans frequently display heterogeneous contrast enhancement, enhancing their diagnostic utility [6].

30.10 Magnetic Resonance Imaging

Magnetic resonance imaging (MRI) showcases a distinct pattern of imaging. MRI typically reveals a lobulated lesion, characterized by a high signal on T2-weighted images and a low to intermediate signal on T1-weighted images [10].

30.11 Biopsy

Tissue biopsy plays a critical role in both diagnosing chondrosarcoma and distinguishing it from other bone tumors. The selection of the biopsy site is of paramount importance, and it is recommended to target the most aggressive region as identified through imaging techniques. This approach ensures that the biopsy sample provides representative information about the nature and characteristics of the tumor.

Macroscopic Findings
Chondrosarcomas: >4 cm, translucent lobular/blue-grey/white cut surface, myxoid/ mucoid/cystic areas, chalky calcium deposits, erosion into soft tissue.

Microscopic Findings
Abundant blue-grey cartilage matrix.

Irregular lobules of cartilage, variable size/shape, separated by fibrous bands.

Calcified areas suggesting pre-existing enchondroma.

Atypical chondrocytes, variable size/shape, enlarged hyperchromatic nuclei, and binucleation.

Chondroid matrix changes, necrosis, mitoses, permeation into cortical bone/marrow.

30.12 Grading

Grade I: Low-grade, resembles normal cartilage, "chondrosarcoma permeation pattern."
Grade II: More cellular, nuclear atypia, hyperchromasia, mitoses.
Grade III: Pleomorphic, atypical, detectable mitoses, less differentiation at lobule periphery.
Grade IV (dedifferentiated): High-grade, spindled/pleomorphic, lacks significant cartilage, poor prognosis.

Mesenchymal, clear cell chondrosarcomas are the least common types.

Immuno-phenotype: IDH1 mutations seen (20%): IDH1 R132H antibody identification.

**Ewing sarcoma is described in a separate chapter.*

30.13 Soft Tissue Sarcomas

30.13.1 Introduction

Soft tissue sarcomas (STS) are relatively rare tumors, comprising approximately 1% of all adult malignancies. It is a broad term that refers to a group of rare malignant tumors that arise from the mesenchymal tissues, which include muscle, fat, connective tissues, blood vessels, nerves, and other soft tissues in the body. Soft tissue sarcomas can occur in various parts of the body, such as the extremities, trunk, head and neck, abdomen, and retroperitoneum.

For the ease of understanding, we are going to divide STSs into Extremity Sarcoma & Visceral Sarcomas.

30.13.2 Epidemiology and Risk Factors

30.13.2.1 Incidence and Prevalence of Soft Tissue Sarcoma

Soft tissue sarcomas (STS) are relatively rare tumors, comprising approximately 1% of all adult malignancies. The incidence and distribution of soft tissue sarcomas in the US can vary based on factors such as age, race, and histological subtypes.

The estimated distribution of soft tissue sarcomas by histological subtypes in the US:

Undifferentiated pleomorphic sarcoma (formerly malignant fibrous histiocytoma): 20%.
Liposarcoma: 13%.
Leiomyosarcoma: 11%.
Gastrointestinal stromal tumors (GIST): 7%.
Synovial sarcoma: 6%.
Other subtypes: 43% (including fibrosarcoma, rhabdomyosarcoma, malignant peripheral nerve sheath tumor, etc.*)*

30.13.3 Age and Gender Distribution

Soft tissue sarcomas can occur in children and adolescents of various age groups, with the highest incidence observed in infants and young children. The peak incidence is seen in the age range of 0–4 years. Soft tissue sarcomas are relatively rare in adolescents and young adults [11].

Soft tissue sarcomas can occur in adults of all age ranges, but the incidence increases with age. The highest incidence is typically observed in middle-aged and older adults. Soft tissue sarcomas can affect both males and females. In general, soft tissue sarcomas have a slightly higher incidence in males compared to females.

30.13.4 Distribution of Primary as Per Location

Lower limb, including gluteal region: 45%.
Upper limb: 12%.
Head and neck: 10%.
Retroperitoneum: 13%.

30.13.5 Risk Factors and Genetic Predisposition

30.13.5.1 Risk Factors

- Previous history of radiation.
- Chronic lymphedema (Stewart Treves syndrome—angio or lymphangiosarcoma).
- Other possible risk factors include arsenic and phenoxy-herbicide exposure. Interestingly, > 90% STS are not associated with the above risk factors.

30.13.5.2 Genetic Syndrome Association

- < 3% STS associated with genetic syndrome
- Associated syndromes include Recklinghausen neurofibromatosis and bilateral retinoblastoma.

30.13.5.3 Clinical Presentation of STS

Given the heterogeneity of STS, it is difficult to define the clinical features of a presenting sarcoma. *Extremity STS*: Soft-tissue lumps showing any of the following clinical features are to be considered malignant and should be evaluated with biopsy: increasing size, >5 cm in size, location being deep-seated, and/or painful.

Retroperitoneal sarcomas: Patients with retroperitoneal sarcomas present late because when symptoms occur, they are nonspecific, such as abdominal pain and fullness, and are initially dismissed as being caused by other less serious causes.

30.13.6 Evaluation

Diagnosis of soft tissue sarcoma involves a combination of clinical evaluation, imaging studies (such as MRI, CT, or PET-CT), and histopathological examination of a tissue biopsy sample. Often the first imaging is an ultrasound which suggests a solid tumor and then the patient gets referred to an oncology centre

Imaging modalities for initial evaluation (MRI, CT, PET-CT)

30.13.7 MRI

MRI scans are routinely used to evaluate soft tissue masses. Lymph nodal imaging also to be done if biopsy shows rhabdoid tumor, clear cell sarcoma, alveolar soft part sarcoma or epitheloid sarcoma.

MRI scans of the affected region should include the anatomical compartment, involved site, and its adjacent joints.

Signs on MRI which can be indicative of a malignancy are a deep-seated large mass, heterogeneous signal, surrounding edema, and associated destruction of bone.

MRI plays an essential role in the local staging of tumors. No surgery is to be performed nor biopsy taken until an MRI is carried out. In T1 images, most solid tumors are hypointense at presentation. Pre-contrast fat suppressed T1 weighted imaging is recommended to identify hemorrhagic content in suspected STS. In benign peripheral nerve sheath tumors, 'split fat sign' and 'entering nerve sign is often seen. Interestingly synovial sarcoma shows 'triple sign' i.e. simultaneous presence of low, intermediate and high intensities. Sometimes on MRI, 'tail sign' is seen that suggests myxofibrosarcoma or undifferentiated pleomorphic sarcoma

30.13.8 Computed Tomography

CT is not routinely used for local staging; however, it is essential in systemic staging to exclude pulmonary metastatic disease in extremity STS.

Contrast enhanced CT is recommended for the evaluation of retroperitoneal sarcomas, as MRI leads to motion artefact.

30.13.9 PET CT

. In places where resources are available, PET CT may be used in place of CT for distant metastatic disease assessment. In patients with lung metastases diagnosed with CT, PET Ct can be used for monitoring progression of disease.

30.13.10 Role of Biopsy and Histopathological Analysis

Biopsy is vital in the diagnosis and management of soft tissue sarcoma due to various reasons. Inadequate biopsies can lead to delayed or incorrect diagnoses, compromising treatment decisions. Partial excisions before referral increase the risk of distant metastasis and necessitate extensive resections. Improperly placed biopsies may impede subsequent surgical resections, flap preparations, and cosmetic repairs. Furthermore, they may require larger surgeries to encompass the biopsy site during definitive resection. Thus, early referral to specialized centers with multidisciplinary sarcoma teams is recommended. Meticulous biopsy planning ensures accurate diagnoses, avoids partial excisions, preserves function, minimizes cosmetic impact, and reduces extensive surgeries, optimizing patient outcomes.

Table 30.3 STS, IHC, and Fusion Source

Tumor type	Fusion source	IHC marker
Synovial sarcoma	SSX1-SS18	TLE1
Alveolar soft part sarcoma	TFE3-ASPL	TFE3
Low grade fibro-myxoid sarcoma	FUS-CREB1L1	MUC4
Ewing's is like an undifferentiated sarcoma	BCOR-CCNB3	CCNB3

30.13.11 Ancillary Diagnostic Techniques (Immunohistochemistry, Molecular Testing)

The role of immunohistochemistry (IHC) in the diagnosis of sarcomas is crucial and has become an essential adjunct in their evaluation. IHC should be performed alongside morphological assessment, clinical information, and radiologic findings, serving as a complementary tool for accurate diagnosis. Immunohistochemistry offers valuable insights into the cell phenotype and proliferative activity of sarcomas. By utilizing a diverse panel of antibodies, pathologists can determine the lineage or differentiation of the tumor cells, aiding in classification and subtype identification. Certain antibodies function as molecular surrogates, providing information about specific genetic alterations or fusion proteins associated with particular sarcoma subtypes (Table 30.3).

Staging may be done as per the AJCC TNM staging

References

1. Helman LJ, Meltzer P. Mechanisms of sarcoma development. Nat Rev Cancer. 2003;3(9):685–94.
2. Warren D, Koch C, Parsons MS, Pérez-Carrillo GJG, Eldaya RW. Head and neck sarcoma tumor board survival guide for Neuroradiologists: imaging findings, history, and pathology. Curr Probl Diagn Radiol. 2023;52(4):275–88.
3. Prognostic factors for adult sarcomas of head and neck – ClinicalKey [Internet]. [cited 2023 Aug 21]. Available from: https://www.clinicalkey.com
4. Descriptive epidemiology of sarcomas in Europe: Report from the RARECARE project – ClinicalKey [Internet]. [cited 2023 Aug 21]. Available from: https://www.clinicalkey.com.
5. Prater S, McKeon B. Osteosarcoma. In: StatPearls [Internet]. Treasure Island: StatPearls Publishing; 2023. [cited 2023 Aug 23]. Available from: http://www.ncbi.nlm.nih.gov/books/NBK549868/.
6. Ottaviani G, Jaffe N. The epidemiology of osteosarcoma. Cancer Treat Res. 2009;152:3–13.
7. Hameed M, Mandelker D. Tumor syndromes predisposing to osteosarcoma. Adv Anat Pathol. 2018;25(4):217–22.
8. Kundu ZS. Classification, imaging, biopsy and staging of osteosarcoma. Indian J Orthop. 2014;48(3):238–46.

9. Ollivier L, Vanel D, Leclère J. Imaging of chondrosarcomas. Cancer Imaging. 2003;4(1):36–8.
10. Chondrosarcoma: MR imaging with pathologic correlation – PubMed [Internet]. [cited 2023 Aug 24]. Available from: https://pubmed.ncbi.nlm.nih.gov/1636034/
11. https://seer.cancer.gov/archive/csr/1975_2018/results_merged/sect_05_soft_tissue_sarcomas.pdf
12. Oh C, Bishop MW, Cho SY, Im HJ, Shulkin BL. ^{18}F-FDG PET/CT in the Management of Osteosarcoma. J Nucl Med. 2023;64(6):842–51.
13. Enneking WF. A system of staging musculoskeletal neoplasms. Clin Orthop Relat Res. 1986;204:9–24.
14. Choi J, Ro J. The 2020 WHO classification of tumors of bone: an updated review. Adv Anat Pathol. Publish Ahead of Print. 2021; https://doi.org/10.1097/PAP.0000000000000293.

Chapter 31
Evaluation of Skin and Adnexal Malignancy

Ninad Patil and Pritam Mondal

31.1 Skin Anatomy [1, 2]

The skin is the largest organ in the body. It's made up of three main layers: the outer epidermis, middle dermis, and the hypodermis.

31.1.1 Epidermis

It is made with the following layers from deep to superficial.

Stratum basale—It is the deepest layer, and by the basement membrane, it separates from the dermis. The cell acts as a stem cell and produces keratinocytes continuously. This layer also contains melanocytes.

Stratum spinosum—It consists of 8–10 cell layers. Cells have cytoplasmic processes called "spines." This layer also contains dendritic cells.

Stratum granulosum—It consists of 3–5 cell layers. Cells are diamond-shaped and contain keratohyalin and lamellar granules.

Stratum lucidum—It consists of 2–3 cell layers. Found in thicker skin.

Stratum corneum—It is the uppermost layer of the epidermis. It consists of 20–30 cell layers (Figs. 31.1 and 31.2).

N. Patil (✉) · P. Mondal
Department of Radiation Oncology, MPMMCC/ HBCH Varanasi, Units of Tata Memorial Centre, and Homi Bhabha National Institute, Mumbai, India

S. Pradhan et al. (eds.), *Evidence Based Handbook on Diagnosis and Staging in Oncology*, https://doi.org/10.1007/978-981-95-9701-7_31

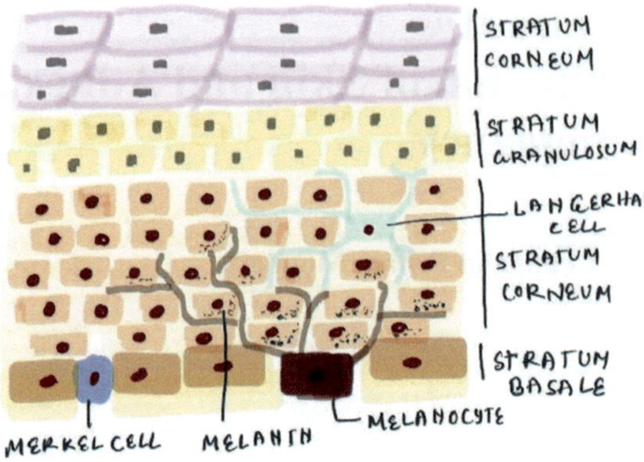

Fig. 31.1 Layers of epidermis

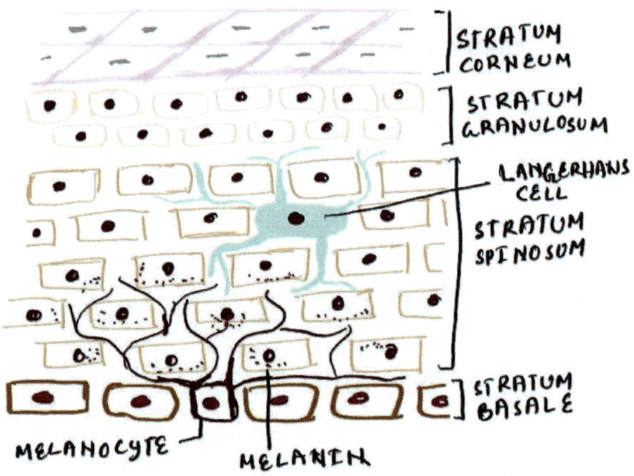

Fig. 31.2 Various cells in the epidermis

31.1.2 Cells Present in the Epidermis

Keratinocytes—It is the predominant cell type. They originate from the basal layer and produce keratin.

Melanocytes—It is derived from neural crest cells. They produce melanin, which is responsible for skin pigmentation. They are seen in the basal layer.

Langerhans' cells and dendritic cells—They are antigen-presenting cells that act as the skin's first line of defense. They are derived from mesenchyme.

Merkel cells—It is oval-shaped cells found in the stratum basale. They act as mechanoreceptors for light touch.

31.1.3 Dermis

It started below the basement membrane of the epidermis. It consists of two layers, a papillary layer and a reticular layer. The papillary layer is the upper layer; it is thinner and made of loose connective tissue. The reticular layer is deeper, it is thicker, and made of dense connective tissue. Dermis contains sweat glands, muscles, hair follicles, sensory neurons, and blood vessels.

31.1.4 Hypodermis

It is deep to the dermis, also called subcutaneous tissue. Mostly contains adipose tissue and skin appendages like blood vessels, sensory nerves, and hair follicles.

31.2 Types of Skin Cancers

Three main types

1. Basal cell carcinoma
2. Squamous cell carcinoma
3. Melanoma

   Others

1. Kaposi sarcoma
2. Markel cell carcinoma
3. Sebaceous gland carcinoma
4. Dermatofibrosarcoma protuberance
5. Langerhans cells histiocytosis

31.3 Epidemiology

In India, according to *ICMR* (Indian Council of Medical Research) data, melanoma of the skin is highest in northern India, for males 1.62 and females 1.21 for 1 lakh population. Overall Incidence of non-melanoma and other skin cancers is highest in northeast India, for men 5.14 and women 3.98, for 1 lakh population.

Worldwide, melanoma skin cancer incidents are highest in the Western Pacific region, and its incidence is 36.9 per lakh population; in Europe, the incidence is 31.7 per lakh population. Non-melanoma skin cancer incidents in the Western Pacific region and their incidence are 225.4 for men and 68.6 for women for 1 lakh population.

31.4 Risk Factors of Skin Cancers

Light-colored skin tone (melanin protects against UV rays-induced DNA damage) [3], with blonde or red hair or freckled skin

Tan or use of a tanning bed or excessive exposure to sunlight

Irregular-shaped moles

Easily sunburn or a history of that

Heavy family history

Prolonged contact with carcinogens (i.e., arsenic)

31.4.1 Signs and Symptoms

Any new mole or previous mole that is irregular in shape, changes color, or bleeds.

Pearly white or pinkish waxy bump over the skin.

Pinkish-red or reddish-brown colored patch or bump.

New onset skin dystrophies, such as scars.

Pinkish-reddish or reddish-brown dry scaly crusting, sometimes oozing or bleeding, may sometimes be itchy.

Long-time non-healing ulcer or recurrent ulcer in the same site, irregular margin, rolled out edge, Necrotic base, and around the ulcer, dark brown skin changes.

31.5 How to Differentiate a Benign Skin Lesion from a Malignant One!

"**ABCDE**" thumb-rule

Asymmetry—irregular shape

Border—irregular shape edges

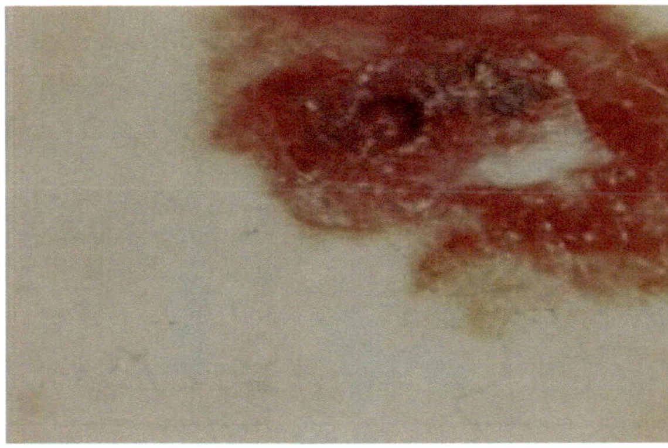

Fig. 31.3 "ABCDE" for melanoma

Color—non-uniform color or change in color

Diameter—generally more than 6 mm

Evolution—Rapidly enlarging, change in shape and size, color change (Most important sign of malignancy) (Fig. 31.3).

31.6 How Sunburn Causes Skin Cancer!

When excessive exposure to sunlight or use of a tanning bed, ultraviolet (UV) rays of sunlight burn skin tissue, which leads to premature aging and DNA damage. If enough DNA damage builds up over time, it can cause uncontrolled cell growth, leading to cancer.

[UV A&B → oxidative damage → cell cycle change → cyclopyrimidine dimers → base modification → strand breaks → mutations → 6-4photoproducts → accumulation of photoproducts → uncontrolled cell proliferation → skin cancer] [4, 5].

UV rays are of three types

UVA (90%–95%)—reaches deeper layer of skin (dermis), leading to aging.

UVB (5%–10%)—reaches the superficial layer of skin (epidermis) and leads to sunburn.

UVC—completely blocked by the ozone layer of the atmosphere (Figs. 31.4 and 31.5).

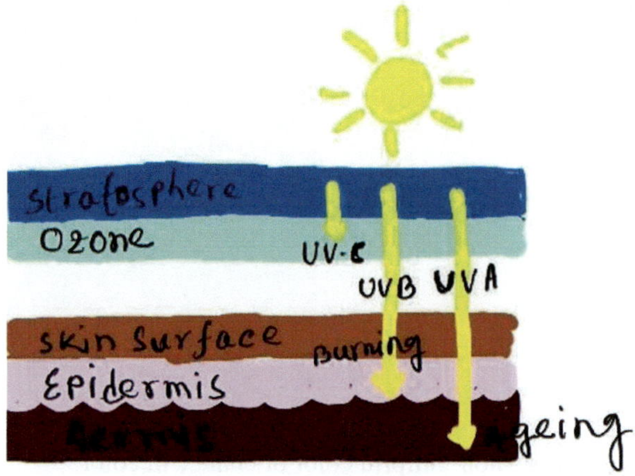

Fig. 31.4 Various UV rays and their penetration power

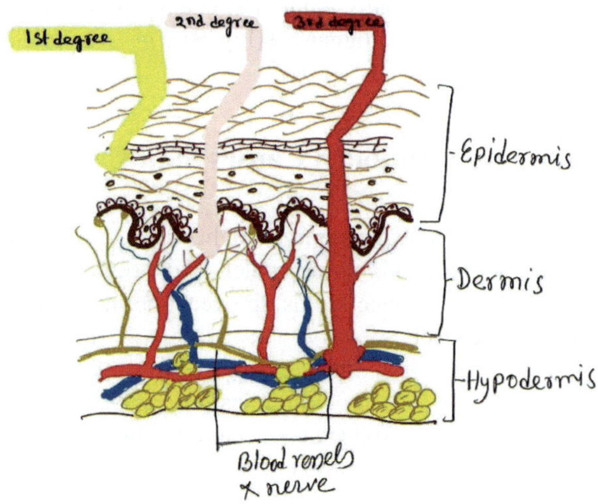

Fig. 31.5 Degree of burn

31.7 How Melanin Protects the Skin from Cancer! [6]

There are two main types of melanin, eumelanin and pheomelanin. UV rays cause damage to nucleotides of DNA by generating reactive oxygen species (ROS). Eumelanin absorbed UV rays and blocked deeper penetration and DNA damage. However, pheomelanin promotes carcinogenesis by producing ROS when irradiated by UV rays. Dark skin complex contains more eumelanin and protects from UV rays; fair skin contains more pheomelanin and is more susceptible to skin cancer.

31.8 How Arsenic Causes Skin Cancer! [7]

Chronic arsenic exposure to the skin (direct skin contact or consumption with drinking water) leads to oxidative stress, chromosomal abnormalities, and altered growth factors, which lead to carcinogenesis. Hyperkeratosis and hyperpigmentation of the skin are hallmark signs of chronic arsenic exposure. Bowen's disease is the most common arsenic-induced skin cancer, which may transform into squamous cell carcinoma (SCC) and basal cell carcinoma (BCC).

[Arsenic exposure → G2/M cell cycle arrest → DNA aneuploidy → p53 dysfunction → leads to cell cycle deregulation → leads to skin cancer].

31.9 Characteristics of Arsenic-Induced Skin Cancers

(a) Occur mainly in sun-protected body parts. (Because in a sun-exposed area, UVB rays inhibit mutant p53 and ki-67 expression, which leads to apoptosis of cells, and leads to the inhibitory effect of proliferation) [7].
(b) Recurrent and multiple lesions. (Because chronic arsenic exposure leads to decreased peripheral CD4+ counts, a decreased number of Langerhans cells, which leads to immune dysfunction, causing recurrent and multiple lesions [7].

31.10 Brief about Different Types of Skin Malignancy

31.10.1 Squamous Cell Carcinoma (SCC)

Arise from mutated keratinocytes. Often appear wart-like or as scaly, flaky, reddish patches that often bleed. It may metastasize.

31.10.2 Basal Cell Carcinoma (BCC)

Arise from the basal layer of the epidermis. Most commonly occur in sun-exposed parts of the body. Appear Pinkish White papule with telangiectasia. They easily ulcerate. They are less likely to metastasize.

31.10.3 Melanoma

Arise from melanocytes. They can be found anywhere on the skin. Lesions can be irregularly pigmented or amelanotic. They have the highest metastatic potential, and it depends on the depth of the lesion.

31.10.4 Langerhans' Cell Histiocytosis

In this carcinoma, Langerhans' cells accumulate and form granuloma, it's appearing as skin blisters, skin rashes, or erythematous papules. It may present as pancytopenia due to overcrowding of Langerhans' cells. It may be associated with pituitary gland dysfunction.

31.10.5 Markel Cell Carcinoma

It is a neuroendocrine small cell carcinoma of Merkel cells. It is a very rare tumor but very aggressive in nature. It often spreads to lymph nodes and organs.

31.10.6 Kaposi Sarcoma

It occurs in the lining cells of lymphatic or blood vessels. Mostly occurs in people who have weak immune systems with human herpes virus 8 carriers (HHV-8). HIV-positive people have weak immune systems and are commonly associated with Kaposi sarcoma.

31.10.7 Dermatofibrosarcoma Protuberance

It occurs from the dermis and is a rare type. Very slow-growing and rarely spreads. It may reappear after surgery.

31.11 Genetic Syndrome Associated with Various Skin Cancers [8]

31.11.1 Basal Cell Carcinoma (BCC)

1. *Basal cell nevus syndrome or Gorlin syndrome or Gorlin-Goltz Syndrome or nevoid BCC syndrome*: It is an autosomal dominant disorder. It is present as BCC before 20 years of age or an excessive number of BCC, odontogenic keratocyst of the jaw before age 20 years, palmar or plantar pitting, lamellar calcification of falx cerebri, medulloblastoma, macrocephaly, skeletal abnormality, rib abnormality, and cleft lip or palate.

31.11.2 Squamous Cell Carcinoma (SCC)

1. *Oculocutaneous albinism*—It is an autosomal recessive disease. Type 1 is associated with the long arm of Ch 11, and Type 2 is associated with the OCA2 gene.
2. *Epidermolysis bullosa*
3. *Fanconi anemia*—It is an autosomal recessive disease, rarely an X-linked recessive disease. It is associated with leukemia, skin, GIT, gynecological, and head and neck cancers.

31.11.3 Melanoma

1. *CDKN2A*—It is a germ-line tumor suppressor gene. Pathogenic variant associated with increased melanoma risk.
2. *Xeroderma pigmentosum*—It is an autosomal recessive disorder. It occurs due to a defective nucleotide excision repair mechanism. It increases the risk of melanoma, SCC, and BCC.

31.11.4 Pre-Management Workup

- Proper history and examination (ask for recent changes in color, shape, and size of existing mole, freckles, or other skin spots). Examine skin, including scalp, palms, feet, around genitalia, and buttocks. Any suspicious lesion found, note size, shape, color, texture, and any bleeding or not. Examine under the microscope or magnifying glass if feasible. Examine the regional lymph node.

- Biopsy from lesion- excisional biopsy that removes the entire growth is often sufficient to treat the skin cancer. Shave biopsy, Punch biopsy, and incisional biopsy are other options.
- If there is a palpable regional lymph node, take a biopsy from the lymph node.
- After confirmation, further tests to be done as per requirement (imaging, sentinel lymph node biopsy, etc.)
- BCC is mostly local and does not metastasize, but Merkel cell carcinoma and melanoma are more prone to spread and need imaging (X-rays, CT scan, MRI, PET scan).
- *AJCC staging is most commonly used for skin cancers.*
- *Brigham and Women's Hospital staging system for skin SCC is also used* [9].

Stage	Descriptions
T1	No high-risk factors
T2a	1 high-risk factor
T2b	2–3 high-risk factors
T3	≥4 high-risk factors

[a]High risk factors include tumor diameter >2 cm, poorly differentiated histology, perineural invasion of nerve >0.1 mm, or tumor invasion beyond subcutaneous fat

References

1. Lopez-Ojeda W, Pandey A, Alhajj M, Oakley AM. Anatomy, skin (integument). In: StatPearls. Treasure Island: StatPearls Publishing; 2024. Available from: http://www.ncbi.nlm.nih.gov/books/NBK441980/.
2. Brown TM, Krishnamurthy K. Histology, dermis. In: StatPearls. Treasure Island: StatPearls Publishing; 2024. Available from: http://www.ncbi.nlm.nih.gov/books/NBK535346/.
3. Kobayashi N, Muramatsu T, Yamashina Y, Shirai T, Ohnishi T, Mori T. Melanin reduces ultraviolet-induced DNA damage formation and killing rate in cultured human melanoma cells. J Invest Dermatol. 1993;101(5):685–9.
4. D'Orazio J, Jarrett S, Amaro-Ortiz A, Scott T. UV radiation and the skin. Int J Mol Sci. 2013;14(6):12222–48.
5. Maresca V, Flori E, Briganti S, et al. UVA-induced modification of catalase charge properties in the epidermis is correlated with the skin phototype. J Invest Dermatol. 2006;126(1):182–90.
6. Kollias N, Sayre RM, Zeise L, Chedekel MR. Photoprotection by melanin. J Photochem Photobiol B. 1991;9(2):135–60.
7. Yu HS, Liao WT, Chai CY. Arsenic carcinogenesis in the skin. J Biomed Sci. 2006;13(5):657–66.
8. PDQ Cancer Genetics Editorial Board. Genetics of skin cancer (PDQ®): health professional version. In: PDQ cancer information summaries. Bethesda: National Cancer Institute (US); 2002. Available from: http://www.ncbi.nlm.nih.gov/books/NBK65895.
9. Jambusaria-Pahlajani A, Kanetsky PA, Karia PS, et al. Evaluation of AJCC tumor staging for cutaneous squamous cell carcinoma and a proposed alternative tumor staging system. J Clin Oncol. 2013;31(18):2312–9. https://doi.org/10.1200/JCO.2012.48.5320.

Chapter 32
Miscellaneous Pediatric Solid Tumors

Kanika Sood Sharma and Amita Prakash Ambasta

32.1 Introduction

Pediatric solid tumors comprise of <1% of all cancers and differ from adult cancers in their biology, clinical presentation, and response to treatment. Pediatric cancers, though less common than adult malignancies, present a unique set of challenges that require specialized approaches in diagnosis, treatment, and care. These cancers can affect children of all ages, from infants to adolescents, each presenting distinct biological and clinical characteristics. The journey through pediatric cancer care demands not only advanced medical interventions but also a compassionate, family-centric approach that addresses the emotional and psychological needs of both the young patients and their families.

Although pediatric tumors vary widely in demography, they are generally curable with optimal treatment. As research continues to unravel new insights and therapies, the goal remains steadfast: to increase survival rates while ensuring the best possible quality of life for the children and their caregivers.

Neuroblastoma, Wilms tumor, bone sarcomas, rhabdomyosarcoma, and hepatic tumors comprise 7%, 5%, 4%,3%, and <1% of all malignancies in the 0–14-year age group [1]. This chapter aims to provide an overview of a few pediatric solid tumors. Through a comprehensive pathological evaluation, including detailed histopathological examination, immunohistochemical staining, and genetic analysis, clinicians can accurately diagnose pediatric cancers, assess prognosis, and tailor treatment strategies to optimize outcomes for young patients.

K. S. Sharma (✉) · A. P. Ambasta
Department of Radiation Oncology, Dharamshila Narayana Superspeciality Hospital, New Delhi, India

S. Pradhan et al. (eds.), *Evidence Based Handbook on Diagnosis and Staging in Oncology*, https://doi.org/10.1007/978-981-95-9701-7_32

32.2 Neuroblastoma

Neuroblastoma is an embryonal neuroendocrine tumor that arises from immature nerve cells (neural crest progenitor cells) of the sympathetic nervous system. [2] It can be found anywhere along the tract, with the most common site being adrenals (30%–40%), abdomen and pelvis (25%) followed by thorax (15%) and head and neck (5%). It typically affects infants and young children. It is the most common extracranial solid tumor found in children that accounts for approximately 15% of pediatric cancer deaths [3]. 90% of neuroblastoma is seen in <10 years of age, and the median age is 18 months. In some cases, it may regress or mature to form a benign ganglioneuroma.

1. *Clinical presentation*

In many cases, neuroblastoma remains silent due to spontaneous regression. However, the signs and symptoms vary depending on the location and extent of the tumor:

1. *Pain*: Pain is the most common symptom and may result from local visceral invasion or metastasis to bone.
2. *Palpable mass*: Often detected by parents or physicians during a routine examination, it generally presents as a non-tender, bluish mass in the abdomen, chest, or neck.
3. *Constitutional symptoms*: These include fever, weight loss, anorexia, and malaise.
4. *Skin metastasis*: This may appear as multiple ecchymotic patches, also known as the "blueberry muffin" sign.
5. *Spinal cord compression*: A dumbbell-shaped tumor extending through the neural foramina can cause loss of power in the lower extremities.
6. *Hypertension*: This can occur due to renal artery compression or catecholamine secretion by the tumor.
7. *Paraneoplastic syndromes*:

    - *Opsoclonus-myoclonus syndrome*: Characterized by rapid, multidirectional eye movements and muscle jerks.
    - *Secretory diarrhea*: Caused by the secretion of vasoactive intestinal peptide.

2. *Differential diagnosis*

Wilms Tumor A kidney tumor most commonly found in children, often presenting as an abdominal mass. It can cause symptoms such as abdominal pain, swelling, and sometimes blood in the urine. Early detection and treatment are crucial for a favorable outcome.

Rhabdomyosarcoma A malignant cancer that originates in the soft tissues, such as muscles, connective tissues, or bone. It primarily affects children and adolescents and can manifest in various parts of the body, including the head, neck, and genitourinary tract.

Ewing Sarcoma A highly aggressive cancer that occurs in the bones or soft tissues surrounding the bones. It predominantly affects teenagers and young adults, commonly presenting with pain and swelling in the affected area, often mistaken for sports injuries or infections.

Hepatoblastoma A rare liver cancer that primarily affects children under the age of three. It may present with abdominal swelling, pain, or a palpable mass, and can sometimes be associated with elevated alpha-fetoprotein levels in the blood.

Lymphoma A type of cancer that begins in the lymphatic system, which is part of the body's immune system. In children, lymphoma can present with symptoms such as swollen lymph nodes, fever, weight loss, and night sweats. It is categorized into Hodgkin and non-Hodgkin lymphoma, each with distinct characteristics and treatment protocols.

Other Abdominal Masses A differential diagnosis should also consider benign conditions, such as cysts, which can present as abdominal masses. These non-cancerous growths might still require medical intervention to prevent complications or alleviate symptoms.

3. *Clinical evaluation*

- History and physical examination:
- Detailed medical history, including symptoms and family history of cancer.
- Thorough physical exam focusing on the abdomen and possible metastasis sites.
- Laboratory tests:
  - Urine catecholamines: Elevated levels of VMA and HVA are diagnostic. It is elevated in >90% of patients with stage IV disease. A ratio of VMA to HVA of >1.5 is associated with a favorable prognosis in patients with metastatic neuroblastoma. Urinary assay of VMA can be used to screen infants for neuroblastoma.
  - Blood tests: CBC, liver function tests, LDH, and ferritin should be assayed. Anemia may be due to bone marrow invasion.

4. *Radiological evaluation*

Radiological imaging plays a critical role in the diagnosis, staging, and treatment planning of pediatric cancers. Various imaging modalities provide detailed insights into the nature and extent of the disease, guiding effective management strategies.

X-Ray Often the initial imaging modality, X-rays can reveal characteristic features of certain tumors. In the case of neuroblastoma, X-rays may show speckled calcification in approximately 85% of cases, which is indicative of the tumor's presence and can aid in initial diagnosis.

Contrast-Enhanced Computed Tomography (CT) CT scans, particularly with contrast enhancement, offer detailed cross-sectional images that help in assessing the extent of the disease. They provide vital information about lymph node involvement, hepatic metastasis, and the resectability of the tumor. This modality is crucial for planning surgical interventions and determining the feasibility of tumor removal.

Magnetic Resonance Imaging (MRI) MRI is superior to CT in providing detailed images of soft tissues. It is especially valuable for evaluating tumors with complex anatomy or involvement of critical structures. MRI is the preferred modality for assessing blood vessel encasement, intraspinal extension (as seen in dumbbell tumors), diffuse hepatic replacement, and bone marrow involvement. Its superior contrast resolution allows for a clearer differentiation of tumor margins and involvement of adjacent structures.

Meta-Iodo Benzyl Guanidine (MIBG) Scan The MIBG scan is highly specific for imaging neuroblastoma. MIBG, a molecule taken up by neurosecretory granules in both normal and neoplastic tissues of neural crest origin, enables visualization of primary and metastatic sites of neuroblastoma. This scan boasts a sensitivity of 85–90% and a specificity of 95% in detecting metastatic neuroblastoma, making it an invaluable tool in the diagnostic and staging process.

Positron Emission Tomography (PET) Scan PET scans are used selectively for staging and evaluating the response to treatment in pediatric cancers. This modality provides metabolic information about the tumor, which can complement the anatomical details obtained from other imaging techniques. PET scans are particularly useful in assessing the activity of the disease and monitoring its progression or regression in response to therapy.

Each of these imaging modalities contributes unique and complementary information, enabling a comprehensive evaluation of pediatric cancers and guiding the multidisciplinary approach to treatment planning.

5. *Pathological evaluation*

Pathological evaluation is essential for the definitive diagnosis, classification, and management of pediatric cancers. This process involves a combination of biopsy techniques, histopathological analysis, immunohistochemistry, and genetic and molecular studies.

Biopsy Techniques

- *Needle biopsy*: This minimally invasive procedure involves using a fine needle to extract a small sample of tissue from the suspected tumor site. Needle biopsies are often used for initial diagnosis as they are less invasive and can be performed quickly with minimal discomfort to the patient.
- *Open biopsy*: In cases where more extensive tissue analysis is needed, an open biopsy is performed. This involves a surgical procedure to remove a larger section of the tumor. The increased tissue sample allows for more comprehensive histopathological examination and provides sufficient material for multiple diagnostic tests.

Histopathological Features

- *Neuroblastoma*: Under microscopic examination, neuroblastoma is characterized by small, round, blue tumor cells arranged in dense nests of hyperchromatic cells. A hallmark feature is the presence of Homer-Wright rosettes, which are circular groupings of tumor cells with a central fibrillary core. Additionally, areas of necrosis, hemorrhage, and calcification are often observed within the tumor. These histopathological features help in confirming the diagnosis and differentiating neuroblastoma from other pediatric malignancies.

Immunohistochemistry

- Immunohistochemistry utilizes antibodies to detect specific proteins within the tumor cells, aiding in accurate diagnosis. In neuroblastoma, immunohistochemical staining is positive for neuron-specific enolase (NSE), synaptophysin, and chromogranin A, which are markers indicative of neural origin. Conversely, neuroblastoma cells typically test negative for muscle-specific markers and leukocyte common antigen, which helps distinguish it from other childhood cancers such as rhabdomyosarcoma and lymphomas.

Genetic and Molecular Markers

- *MYCN amplification*: The amplification of the MYCN gene is a significant prognostic marker in neuroblastoma [4]. It is associated with aggressive disease and poor prognosis, categorizing the patient as high-risk and often influencing the intensity and approach of treatment.
- *ALK mutations*: Mutations in the ALK (anaplastic lymphoma kinase) gene can be present in some cases of neuroblastoma [5]. Identifying these mutations is crucial as they can influence treatment decisions, including the use of targeted therapies designed to inhibit ALK activity.
- *Chromosomal abnormalities*: Specific chromosomal abnormalities are frequently observed in neuroblastoma. These include the gain of chromosome 17q and the loss of chromosome 1p, among others [6]. These genetic changes can provide insights into the tumor's biology, potential behavior, and response to therapy.

32.3 Retinoblastoma

Retinoblastoma is a relatively rare disease but stands as the most common intraocular malignancy in childhood, accounting for approximately 2% of childhood cancers [7]. It is typically diagnosed at an average age of 2 years. Although it profoundly affects vision, prompt diagnosis and treatment can achieve a cure rate of around 95%, with vision restoration in most cases. The disease arises from the exponential growth of retinoblasts. Metastatic spread can occur to regional lymph nodes, liver, lungs, bones, and brain.

1. *Clinical presentation*

   Retinoblastoma generally presents within the first year of life in cases of bilateral disease and within 3 years in cases of unilateral disease. Bilateral cases are usually hereditary.

   - *Leukocoria*
     - This is the most common presenting sign, characterized by a whitish pupillary reflex described as a "cat's eye" reflex.
   - *Strabismus*
     - This is the second most common presentation. All patients with strabismus should be examined for retinoblastoma.
   - *Other Signs*
     - Red or inflamed eye.
     - Poor vision or visual disturbances.
     - Pain in the eye (less common).

2. *Differential diagnosis*

   Several other conditions can mimic the presentation of retinoblastoma, including the following:

   - *Coats disease*: A condition characterized by abnormal development of blood vessels behind the retina, leading to retinal detachment.
   - *Persistent fetal vasculature (PFV)*: A condition where the fetal vasculature fails to regress normally.
   - *Retinal detachment*: Separation of the retina from its underlying layer, which can also present with visual disturbances.
   - *Ocular enlargement*: Conditions causing enlargement of the eye, which may present with similar symptoms.
   - *Calcification of the globe*: Calcifications within the eye that can be mistaken for tumors.

3. *Clinical evaluation*

   - *Direct ophthalmoscopy*
     - This is a simple, non-invasive procedure that can be performed in a clinical setting to detect the characteristic white reflex, or leukocoria.
   - *Examination under anesthesia*
     - This is conducted to thoroughly evaluate the corneal diameter, anterior chamber, and intraocular pressure, which can provide critical information about the extent of the disease.

4. *Radiological evaluation*
   1. *Ultrasound (USG)*
      (a) Ultrasound helps differentiate retinoblastoma from Coats disease and assess the size and location of the tumor.
   2. *Magnetic resonance imaging (MRI)*
      (a) MRI is crucial for assessing the involvement of the optic nerve and extra-ocular structures, which are important for staging the disease and planning treatment.

   5. *Pathological evaluation*

- *Gross pathology*
  - Retinoblastoma typically appears as a creamy white, chalky area with calcification and necrosis.
- *Microscopic pathology*
  - Microscopically, retinoblastoma is composed of small, round, blue cells with hyperchromatic nuclei and scant cytoplasm. The presence of Flexner-Winter Steiner rosettes, a characteristic but not always present feature, can aid in diagnosis.
- *Genetic marker*
  - The RB1 gene is a crucial genetic marker for retinoblastoma [8]. Identification of RB1 mutations helps assess the risk in siblings and offspring, guiding surveillance and early detection strategies.

32.4 Hepatoblastoma

Hepatoblastoma is a tumor of embryonic origin and the most common primary malignant liver tumor in children [9], occurring almost exclusively in infants. Isolated instances in older children and young adolescents have been documented. The tumor is more frequently found in males.

1. *Clinical presentation*
   Hepatoblastoma can present with a variety of symptoms, including the following:
   - *Abdominal distension*: The most common presentation, where the abdomen appears swollen due to the growing liver mass.
   - *Anorexia*: Loss of appetite, which may contribute to weight loss and poor nutrition.

- *Vomiting*: Frequent episodes that can result from the pressure exerted by the tumor on surrounding organs.
- *Anemia*: Low red blood cell count, which can cause fatigue and pallor.
- *Fever*: Often indicative of an inflammatory or systemic response to the tumor.
- *Jaundice*: Yellowing of the skin and eyes due to liver dysfunction.
- *Isosexual precocity*: Premature development of secondary sexual characteristics due to human chorionic gonadotropin (HCG) secretion or testosterone production by the tumor.

2. *Differential diagnosis*

   Several conditions need to be considered when diagnosing hepatoblastoma:

- *Hepatocellular carcinoma (HCC)*: Another primary liver cancer, more common in adults but possible in children.
- *Focal nodular hyperplasia*: A benign liver condition that can mimic malignant tumors.
- *Hepatic adenoma*: A benign liver tumor, typically hormone-related.
- *Lymphoma*: A type of blood cancer that can affect the liver.
- *Metastases*: Secondary cancers that have spread to the liver from other primary sites.

3. *Clinical evaluation*

   A comprehensive clinical evaluation is crucial for diagnosis and management:

- *Complete history and physical examination*: Essential to assess overall health and detect any signs indicative of hepatoblastoma.
- *Blood tests for serum alpha-fetoprotein (AFP)*: Elevated AFP levels are found in 84%–90% of patients with hepatoblastoma and are a key diagnostic marker [10]. Other tumor markers include HCG and cystathionase.

4. *Radiological evaluation*

   Imaging studies are vital for evaluating the extent of the disease:

- *Abdominal ultrasonography*: Used to evaluate liver masses and detect satellite lesions.
- *Multiphase computed tomography (CT)*: Hypervascular lesions in the liver with delayed contrast excretion are highly suggestive of a malignant liver tumor.
- *Magnetic resonance imaging (MRI)*: Superior to CT in defining tumor margins, vessel involvement, and adenopathy, providing detailed images of the tumor and its relationship to surrounding structures.

5. *Pathological evaluation*

   While biopsy is a critical tool for definitive diagnosis, it may not always be necessary or safe for very young children (6 months to 3 years) with significantly elevated AFP levels due to risks of hemorrhage, tumor seeding, and dissemination. However, biopsy remains highly recommended for a definitive diagnosis unless there are urgent life-threatening circumstances such as tumor invasion of the right atrium or tumor rupture.

- *Gross pathology*: Hepatoblastomas typically appear as large, well-circumscribed liver masses, usually single.
- *Histology*: The tumor can be classified as epithelial, mesenchymal, or mixed based on microscopic examination.
- *Genetic associations*: Hepatoblastoma is linked to several genetic conditions, including Beckwith-Wiedemann syndrome, familial adenomatous polyposis, congenital anomalies like hemihypertrophy and cleft palate, Wilms tumor, and glycogen storage diseases [11].

32.5 Langerhans Cell Histiocytosis

Langerhans cell histiocytosis (LCH) arises from early myeloid cells in the bone marrow. It is a rare dendritic cell disorder, affecting fewer than 1 in 200,000 children [12]. Also known as histiocytosis X, eosinophilic granuloma, Letterer-Siwe disease, and Hand-Schüller-Christian disease, LCH is characterized by the presence of Langerin-positive granulomatous infiltrates throughout the body, potentially impacting organs such as the skin, gastrointestinal (GI) tract, and central nervous system (CNS) [13].

1. *Clinical presentation*

   LCH typically presents in children aged 2–3 years but can occur at any age. Clinical manifestations vary widely depending on the organs involved:

- *Rashes*: The most common presentation, these skin lesions can be mistaken for seborrheic or atopic dermatitis. LCH rashes range from single lesions to widespread involvement, presenting as scaly papules and nodules, and are often associated with petechiae and bloody crusting.
- *Multisystemic disease*: This can include hepatosplenomegaly (enlargement of the liver and spleen) and pancytopenia (a reduction in the number of red and white blood cells, as well as platelets).
- *Bony involvement*: Patients may experience pain due to the infiltration of LCH cells into the bones, often leading to lytic bone lesions.

2. *Differential diagnosis*

   Several conditions can mimic the clinical presentation of LCH:

- *Osteomyelitis*: An infection in the bone that can present with similar symptoms.
- *Seborrheic dermatitis*: A common skin condition that causes a red, scaly, itchy rash.
- *Lymphoma*: A type of cancer that can involve the lymph nodes and other organs.
- *Leukemia*: A cancer of blood-forming tissues, including the bone marrow, which can present with similar systemic symptoms.

3. *Clinical evaluation*

   A thorough clinical evaluation is essential for diagnosing LCH:

   - *Complete history*: A detailed history should be taken, focusing on the nature and duration of symptoms.
   - *Complete blood assay*: This can provide insights into the involvement of multiple systems and help in identifying complications such as pancytopenia.

4. *Radiological evaluation*

   Imaging studies play a critical role in the evaluation of LCH:

   - *Chest radiograph*: Useful for detecting lung involvement.
   - *Skeletal radiograph*: Important for identifying lytic bone lesions, which are characteristic of LCH.

5. *Pathological evaluation*

   The pathogenesis of LCH is not fully understood, but it involves complex immunological and molecular mechanisms:

   - *Excessive production of cytokines and enzymes*: Affected bone tissue shows increased production of interleukin-1 (IL-1), interleukin-17a (IL-17a), prostaglandins, and metalloproteases (MMP9 and MMP12). Prostaglandin E2 is also elevated.
   - *Osteoclastic activation*: These molecular changes lead to the activation of osteoclasts, the cells responsible for bone resorption, contributing to the lytic lesions seen in LCH.

32.6 Carotid Body Tumor

Carotid body tumors (CBTs) are extra-adrenal paragangliomas that arise from the chemoreceptive cells of the carotid body situated near the bifurcation of the common carotid artery [14]. They are rare and are typically benign and hyper vascular. They. They grow slowly and have the potential to turn malignant [15]. Due to their location and potential local invasion, they can cause significant morbidity and mortality. Gender preponderance has not been definitely established, but many reports suggest increased incidence among females [16].

The pathogenesis is not clearly understood, but it arises due to chronic hypoxia as seen in individuals living at high altitudes [17]. In children, it is found in association with hereditary syndromes, such as Multiple Endocrine Neoplasia (MEN) type 2, von Hippel-Lindau disease, and familial paraganglioma syndromes.

1. *Clinical presentation*

   (a) They are slow-growing, painless masses that can present as.
       A palpable, firm, non-tender mass in the lateral neck.
       Pulsatile mass with possible bruit on auscultation
   (b) Horner's syndrome (ptosis, miosis, anhidrosis) if the sympathetic chain is involved.
   (c) Cranial nerve palsies (IX, X, XI, XII) if the tumor is extensive.
   (d) Dysphagia, hoarseness, or cough due to local compression.

2. *Differential diagnosis*

   (a) Branchial cleft cysts
   (b) Thyroid nodules or goiter
   (c) Lymphadenopathy (reactive or malignant)
   (d) Metastatic lymph nodes (from primary head and neck cancers)
   (e) Schwannomas and neurofibromas
   (f) Other paragangliomas (e.g., glomus vagale)

3. *Clinical evaluation*

   On clinical examination, CBT can be palpated as a firm, pulsatile mass that can be moved side-to-side but not vertically (Fontaine's sign). Auscultation may reveal a bruit due to the tumor's hyper vascular nature.

4. *Radiological evaluation*

   (a) *Ultrasound*: It identifies the location, size, and vascularity of the mass.
   (b) *Computed tomography (CT) and magnetic resonance imaging (MRI)*: These modalities provide detailed information on the tumor's size, extent, and relationship to surrounding structures. MRI, with its superior soft-tissue contrast, is particularly useful for planning surgery.
   (c) *Angiography*: Digital subtraction angiography (DSA) can delineate the tumor's vascular supply and is often used preoperatively for embolization to reduce intraoperative blood loss.
   (d) *Positron emission tomography (PET)*: PET scans with fluorodeoxyglucose (FDG) can be used to assess metabolic activity and detect metastases or multifocal disease, especially in malignant cases.

5. *Pathological evaluation*

   Grossly, they are well circumscribed with a pseudo capsule. They have a rubbery texture with areas of hemorrhage in the cut section.

   They have a characteristic growth pattern called "zellballen," which is a well-developed nested or organoid growth pattern of the tumor cells with an intervening stromal component of delicate fibrovascular tissue and supporting cells.

   Biochemical tests to measure catecholamine levels (e.g., metanephrines and normetanephrines in plasma and urine) are essential, as some CBTs secrete these hormones, causing systemic symptoms like hypertension and tachycardia.

   In hereditary cases, the SDH mutation is evaluated.

32.7 Esthesioneuroblastoma

Esthesioneuroblastoma is a rare neuroectodermal tumor that arises from the olfactory nerve in the upper nasal cavity. Intracranial extension is commonly seen at the time of diagnosis. Also called olfactory neuroblastoma. Although it majorly presents in the fifth to the sixth decade, some incidences have been found in teenagers too [18]. It is very rare in the pediatric population.

1. *Clinical presentation*

   (a) Unilateral nasal obstruction—may present as stuffiness
   (b) Epistaxis—painless nasal bleed
   (c) Decreased perception of smell
   (d) Exophthalmos—orbital infiltration may present as exophthalmos
   (e) Nasopharyngeal mass

2. *Differential diagnosis*

   (a) Sinonasal undifferentiated carcinoma
   (b) Squamous cell carcinoma of the maxillary antrum

3. *Clinical evaluation*

   A thorough clinical examination of the nose and neck is mandatory. Clinical evaluation may reveal a nasal mass or cervical lymphadenopathy. In extensive disease, signs of cranial nerve involvement may be elucidated.

4. *Radiological evaluation*

   (a) CT scan—It gives information about bony erosion and the extent of disease. The tumor may be seen as a soft tissue mass in the nasal cavity, often associated with erosion of the cribriform plate, fovea ethmoidalis, or other adjacent bony structures.
   (b) MRI—It gives details about the extent of nerve and soft tissue involvement. Intracranial extension is better identified in an MRI scan.
   (c) PETCT—It is used to identify regional and distant metastasis.

5. *Pathological evaluation*

   Homer-Wright rosettes (tumor cells arranged around a central fibrillary space) are a characteristic but not pathognomonic feature. Tumor cells are round to oval shaped with scanty cytoplasm. They stain positive for S100 and neuron-specific enolase stains but negatively for epithelial markers.

32.8 Take-Home Message

Early detection and multidisciplinary care are crucial in managing pediatric tumors. Awareness of symptoms, timely diagnosis, and access to specialized treatment can significantly improve outcomes. Collaborative efforts between healthcare providers, families, and support networks play a vital role in ensuring comprehensive care and enhancing the quality of life for young patients.

References

1. LaQuaglia MP, Gerstle JT. Advances in the treatment of pediatric solid tumors: a 50 year perspective. J Surg Oncol. 2022;126:933–42.
2. Matthay KK, Maris JM, Schleiermacher G, Nakagawara A, Mackall CL, Diller L, Weiss WA. Neuroblastoma. Nat Rev Dis Primers. 2016;2:16078.
3. Maris JM. Recent advances in neuroblastoma. N Engl J Med. 2010;362:2202–11.
4. Campbell K, Gastier-Foster JM, Mann M, Naranjo AH, Van Ryn C, Bagatell R, Matthay KK, London WB, Irwin MS, Shimada H, et al. Association of MYCN copy number with clinical features, tumor biology, and outcomes in neuroblastoma: a report from the Children's Oncology Group. Cancer. 2017;123:4224–35. https://doi.org/10.1002/cncr.30873.
5. Ogawa S, Takita J, Sanada M, Hayashi Y. Oncogenic mutations of ALK in neuroblastoma. Cancer Sci. 2011;102:302–8.
6. Bown N. Neuroblastoma tumour genetics: clinical and biological aspects. J Clin Pathol. 2001;54:897–910. https://doi.org/10.1136/jcp.54.12.897.
7. American Cancer Society. Cancer facts & figures 2020. Atlanta: American Cancer Society; 2020.
8. Zahn J, Chan MP, Wang G, Patel RM, Andea AA, Bresler SC, Harms PW. Altered Rb, p16, and p53 expression is specific for porocarcinoma relative to poroma. J Cutan Pathol. 2019;46(9):659–64.
9. Hiyama E. Pediatric hepatoblastoma: diagnosis and treatment. Transl Pediatr. 2014;3:293. https://doi.org/10.3978/j.issn.2224-4336.2014.09.01.
10. Czauderna P, López-Terrada D, Hiyama E, Häberle B, Malogolowkin MH, Meyers RL. Hepatoblastoma state of the art: pathology, gentics, risk stratification, and chemotherapy. Curr Opin Pediatr. 2014;26:19–28. https://doi.org/10.1097/MOP.0000000000000046.
11. Cohen MM Jr. Beckwith-Wiedemann syndrome: historical, clinicopathological, and etiopathogenetic perspectives. Pediatr Dev Pathol. 2005;8:287–304.
12. Arceci RJ. The histiocytoses: the fall of the Tower of Babel. Eur J Cancer. 1999;35:747–67; discussion 767–49.
13. Rodriguez-Galindo C, Allen CE. Langerhans cell histiocytosis. Blood. 2020;135(16):1319–31.
14. Fan D, Luster S, Eid IG, Saied CA. A multidisciplinary approach to carotid body tumors surgical management. J Surg Case Rep. 2020;2020:rjaa030.
15. Robertson V, Poli F, Hobson B, Saratzis A, Naylor AR. A systematic review and meta-analysis of the presentation and surgical management of patients with carotid body tumours. Eur J Vasc Endovasc Surg. 2019;57:477–86.
16. Ikeda A, Shiga K, Katagiri K, Saito D, Miyaguchi J, Oikawa SI, Tsuchida K, Asakage T, Ozawa H, Nibu KI. Multi-institutional survey of carotid body tumors in Japan. Oncol Lett. 2018;15:5318–24.
17. Knight TT Jr, Gonzalez JA, Rary JM, Rush DS. Current concepts for the surgical management of carotid body tumor. Am J Surg. 2006;191:104–10.
18. Dumon B. Esthesioneuroblastoma in children, adolescents and young adults. Bull Cancer. 2020;107:934–45.

GPSR Compliance

The European Union's (EU) General Product Safety Regulation (GPSR) is a set of rules that requires consumer products to be safe and our obligations to ensure this.

If you have any concerns about our products, you can contact us on ProductSafety@springernature.com

In case Publisher is established outside the EU, the EU authorized representative is:

Springer Nature Customer Service Center GmbH
Europaplatz 3
69115 Heidelberg, Germany

Batch number: 10726133

Printed by Printforce, the Netherlands